HOME HEALTH NURSING

Assessment and Care Planning

Fourth Edition

Karen McGough Monks, RN, MSN
Unit Based Educator
Yuma Regional Medical Center Home Care
Yuma, Arizona

T0372047

An Affiliate of Elsevier

Mosby
An Affiliate of Elsevier

11830 Westline Industrial Drive
St. Louis, Missouri 63146

Home Health Nursing: Assessment and Care Planning, ed 4

Notice

Nursing is an ever-changing field. Standard safety precautions must be followed, but as new research and clinical experience broaden our knowledge, changes in treatment and drug therapy may become necessary or appropriate. Readers are advised to check the most current product information provided by the manufacturer of each drug to be administered to verify the recommended dose, the method and duration of administration, and contraindications. It is the responsibility of the licensed health care provider, relying on experience and knowledge of the patient, to determine dosages and the best treatment for each individual patient. Neither the Publisher nor the editor assumes any liability for any injury and/or damage to persons or property arising from this publication.

Previous editions copyrighted 1988, 1993, and 1997

Library of Congress Cataloging-in-Publication Data

Monks, Karen McGough.
  Home health nursing: assessment and care planning—4th ed. / Karen McGough Monks. p. ; cm.
  Rev. ed. of: Home health nursing / Marie S. Jaffe, Linda Skidmore-Roth. c1997.
  Includes bibliographical references and index.
  ISBN-13: 978-0-323-01865-4   ISBN-10: 0-323-01865-3 (alk. paper)
  1. Home nursing—Planning. 2. Nursing assessment. 3. Nursing care plans.
I. Jaffe, Marie S. Home health nursing. II. Title.
  [DNLM: 1. Home Care Services—Handbooks. 2. Nursing Assessment—Handbooks. 3. Patient Care Planning—Handbooks. WY 49 M745h 2003]
RT120.H65 J34 2003
362.1′4—dc21

                                                                2002029591

Vice President and Publishing Director, Nursing: Sally Schrefer
Senior Editor: Loren Wilson
Sr. Developmental Editor: Nancy L. O'Brien
Project Manager: Catherine Jackson
Design Manager: Kathi Gosche

KI/RDC

Printed and bound by CPI Group (UK) Ltd, Croydon, CR0 4YY

Transferred to digital print 2013

REVIEWERS

CHRISTINE ROVINSKI-WAGNER, MSN, ARNP
Division Clinical Manager, Northeast Division
Tender Loving Care Staff Builders Home Care
Fort Pierce, Florida

JEANIE STOKER, BSN, RN, BC, MPA
Director of Home Care Services
AnMed Home Care Services
Anderson, South Carolina

To my family:
Patrick, my husband
Laura, my daughter
Joseph and Victoria, my son and daughter-in-law
For your support and encouragement

PREFACE

The fourth edition of *Home Health Nursing: Assessment and Care Planning* assists those providing home nursing services with a guide to appropriate interdisciplinary approaches for all aspects of care necessary to achieve an overall goal of optimal health and function of the homebound client. It continues to recognize and reflect agency and insurance requirements related to providing nursing care in the home setting.

This book uses the nursing process format to supply guidelines for the nurse to provide treatment of diseases and associated conditions, including comprehensive assessments and instructions to promote self-care, health promotion, and disease prevention. These guidelines provide for the organization and consistency of care that is even more crucial with the implementation of the Medicare prospective payment system (PPS). Home and community health nurses and administrators, clinical nurses, and nursing students will benefit from this small, compact, easily carried reference with its comprehensive home care–specific content and nursing process format.

In addition to maintaining features of the third edition, this edition includes the following:

- OASIS data items (recognized by M0 prefixes) identified throughout the Assessments section. OASIS items are intended to be answered as written. Each answer should be based on the client's status most of the time during the day of the assessment. It is best to observe the client when assessing functional status rather than relying totally on what the client verbalizes. Input from therapists involved in the case is also necessary to provide accurate assessments.
- Commonly used primary diagnoses and their corresponding International Classification of Diseases, Ninth Revision, Clinical Modification (ICD-9-CM) codes. The accuracy of the primary diagnosis and ICD code is crucial for proper identification of the home health resource group (HHRG) used to determine episode reimbursement under PPS. Correct diagnoses and detailed ICD codes will lead to that accuracy by identifying the main purpose for skilled services. Detailed codes contain as many digits as

needed to accurately describe the diagnoses. It is recommended that at least four digits (000.0) be used. When searching for the correct diagnosis and code in the ICD code book, go from generalized to specific terms. For example, when looking for the ICD code for Pressure Ulcer, first look up Ulcer. For Myocardial Infarction, look up Infarction.

· The most recent version of the North American Nursing Diagnosis Association (NANDA)-approved Nursing Diagnoses are used, including Wandering, Suicide, Powerlessness, and Risk for Falls.

· Increased inclusion of suggested therapy referrals, including physical therapy, occupational therapy, speech-language pathology, and medical social work. Many nurses do not understand all of the potential skills of the therapists, especially those of the occupational therapist and the medical social worker. The physical therapist is skilled in rehabilitation relating to mobility. The occupational therapist is skilled in rehabilitation relating to activities of daily living, upper extremity mobility, energy conservation, and home management. The speech-language pathologist is skilled in rehabilitation relating to dysphasia and dysphagia. The medical social worker is skilled in assisting the client in seeking community resources and providing counseling services to improve social and emotional functioning.

The conditions selected for inclusion in this book are identified by medical diagnoses and have been chosen based on their relevance to the population of clients served in the home setting. It is important to note that conditions that may be cared for in the home vary in different regions of the country. Some conditions included in this book, such as hypertension, are not ones expected to be a primary diagnosis for the home care client, but are still present in these clients and may require attention by the nurse.

Appropriate care planning and documentation are required by government and third-party payors to determine reimbursement for care given in the home and the future care needs of clients. It is hoped that this fourth edition will benefit those giving home care to clients and ultimately will allow clients to continue to receive care in a familiar and less threatening environment.

ACKNOWLEDGMENTS

I want to express my appreciation to the following individuals for sharing their nursing and home health expertise:

Janis Burger, MSN, RN, Northern Arizona Homecare
Esther Howe, MS, RN, Yuma Regional Medical Center Homecare
Pamela Miller, BS, RN, Yuma Regional Medical Center Homecare
Leone Neegan, MLS, Yuma Regional Medical Center Medical Library

Karen McGough Monks

GUIDELINES FOR USING THIS BOOK

The following outline presents an overview of the book's contents, with an explanation of each section and suggestions for use.

1. *Assessments* provides guides for a comprehensive client assessment and resources for collection of data that will be analyzed to determine appropriate problem identification in the nursing process. Offered are assessment guides that are related to body systems, body functions, psychosocial concerns, family concerns, and environmental considerations. The related OASIS items, identified with the M0 prefix, are included with the appropriate data. The guides are referred to in most care plans and are to be used as comprehensive tools with which the nurse may view the client by using those items pertinent to a particular problem or condition.

2. *Care Plans* are grouped under major body systems in alphabetical order and reflect general practice rather than specialty practice in home nursing care. The organization and content of each plan follow a logical progression and include the following:

   a. An introductory paragraph defining and describing the condition, the primary concern of home care, and client goals. This paragraph concludes with suggested primary diagnoses and corresponding ICD codes commonly used for clients with the condition.

   b. Nursing diagnoses related to the condition, which are taken from NANDA's 2001-2002 approved list. The suggested diagnoses that relate to an individual client may be used, and additional diagnoses may be added as needed from the comprehensive list offered in the appendix.

   c. Related (or risk) factors follow each nursing diagnosis. One or more may be given that may or may not be used, but the possibility of using other relationships based on specific client problems should not be precluded.

   d. Defining characteristics are signs and symptoms or possible observations that are related to a particular nursing diagnostic stem and its related factors. The nursing diagnosis, related factors, and defining characteristics provide a valuable background for each problem in the care plan.

e. Outcomes include short-term and long-term goals that are expected to be achieved to solve a specific problem identified by the nursing diagnosis. These are offered as an aid for the nurse to develop goals with the client and include the behaviors and physical evidence that one would expect to suggest goal achievement. As with the nursing diagnosis material, the outcomes may be used as they are or may be supplemented by client-specific and mutually developed goals and their associated observations. Each short-term or long-term goal includes a time frame for outcomes, which at best is an estimate, and may be longer or shorter as a client's individual condition warrants. The time frames serve only as a guide for the nurse to determine what is realistic and workable for a client.

f. Interventions/instructions are divided into nurse and client/caregiver actions for each nursing diagnosis. This organization assists in determining who is responsible for what actions to implement the plan of care and is home care user–friendly to include any caregiver in the home. The nursing interventions are primarily oriented toward assessments, tasks, and instruction/information to be performed by the nurse; the client/caregiver interventions are the actions to be performed after the nurse performs the instruction/information component of the care plan. Other interventions for the nurse or client may be added as needed. Each nursing intervention includes visit time frames for implementation, which are intended to be suggestions; they are flexible enough to accommodate changes appropriate to individual client needs and agency policy. (The nurse needs to remember that the visit frequencies and duration should reflect the client's needs, not the number of visits the payor is willing to reimburse.) Referrals to other disciplines that may be appropriate to achieve client goals are included, whether these are available in or outside the agency.

3. *Appendixes* contain material that may be used to supplement the care plans. They include a listing of NANDA-approved nursing diagnoses; indications for therapy/social service referrals; standard precautions; medication administration; insurance payment guidelines; tips on documentation; guidelines for

client self-determination; a selection of common laboratory values; and a listing of selected home care resources, along with their web site addresses.

It is intended for the user of the care plans to modify and/or supplement any material that has been offered in this book to better suit the identified needs of a specific client or family/caregiver.

CONTENTS

ASSESSMENTS, 1

✿ *Assessments* ✿

❋ *Health History and Review of Systems*

IDENTIFYING INFORMATION

Name (M0040), identification number (M0020), social security number (M0064), residence (M0300), state (M0050), zip code (M0060), telephone number, age or date of birth (M0066), sex (M0069), race/ethnicity (M0140), religion, marital status or significant person/contact person name, language, education, occupation, Medicare number (M0063), Medicaid number (M0065), financial/insurance information (M0150/160), source of information, advance directive (see Appendix).

PAST HISTORY

- Statement about general health
- Other medical conditions and dates of onset or occurrence (M0190/M0210/M0220); health status in past year; medical/treatment changes (M0200)
- Surgeries and injuries and dates; known or suspected allergies (food, drugs, environmental allergens)
- Hospitalizations for injuries, surgery, or medical problems (condition, date, duration) (M0175/M0180)
- Admittance to long-term care facility (reason, date, duration)
- Immunizations and dates
- Military history, travel and dates
- Childhood diseases and ages of occurrence
- Psychiatric illness and treatment
- Usual health care patterns and kind of practitioner used
- Use of rehabilitative and support personnel; past home care services
- Lifestyle patterns and personal habits in sleep, nutrition, fluid intake, urinary and bowel elimination, activity, sexual pattern, personal hygiene, others

PRESENT HISTORY

- Start-of-care date (M0030); primary physician (M0072)
- Chief complaint or health concern (in client's words if possible)
- Onset and development of problem, where it took place, what was done
- Primary diagnosis (M0230), other current diagnoses (M0240)
- Signs and symptoms, location, severity, duration, frequency, changes and effect on client, meaning of illness to client, prognosis (M0260), rehabilitative prognosis (M0270)
- Factors that alleviate or aggravate symptoms
- Client's knowledge of disease, procedures, and planned therapy
- Client's adaptation to chronic disorder; life expectancy (M0280)
- Laboratory and diagnostic tests and procedures performed and results
- Medications and treatments ordered since discharge (M0250/M0825)
- Homebound status

FAMILY HISTORY

- Spouse, children, parents, siblings, including health status, ages, occupations, deaths and causes; pets in the home
- Roles and responsibilities of family members; relationship with family members; activities; response to stress or crisis
- Support systems within family, marital relationship
- History of abuse by family members or relatives
- Adaptation of family members to care of client in the home; assisting persons (M0350/M0360); type and frequency of assistance (M0370/M0380)

PSYCHOSOCIAL HISTORY

- General appearance
- Health goals and practices
- Alcohol, caffeine, and tobacco consumption (M0290) (type, amount, frequency)
- Living arrangement (alone or with others and relations with them) (M0300/M0340); structural barriers (M0310); safety hazards (M0320); sanitation (M0330)
- Occupation and income; ability to pay for health care; insurance plan (Medicare, Medicaid, Civilian Health and Medical Program

of Uniformed Services [CHAMPUS], private insurance, workers' compensation)
- Education; degrees, profession if applicable
- Recreation and interests; social and other activities; hobbies; travel; retirement if applicable
- Friends; community involvement; clubs; organizations; church activities
- Use of community agencies (Meals on Wheels, hospital or clinic, day care, transportation, home cleaning services, shopping services)
- English as a second language or no English spoken
- Review of a usual day's activities
- Emergency contact and telephone number

MEDICATIONS AND TREATMENTS

- Prescribed and over-the-counter drugs (name, type, dose, frequency, route, length of use, side effects, desired effect, conditions being treated, drug form and how administered, contraindications, risk for toxicity)
- Herbs
- Oxygen and other inhalation medications or treatments
- Wound care products (i.e., duoderm)
- General compliance with medication regimen
- Management of medications (oral [M0780], inhalant [M0790], injection [M0800])
- Management of equipment for treatments (M0810/M0820)
- Street or recreational drugs
- Aids to ensure safe, correct self-administration of medications
- Effect of client's age on absorption and excretion
- Treatment for adverse effects, allergies

REVIEW OF SYSTEMS

- Height, weight, vital signs, and temperature

▌*Pulmonary System*

- Upper or lower respiratory disease or infections (acute or chronic)
- Dyspnea (at rest or exertional); pain in sinus, nose, throat, or chest; congestion or discharge from nose (rhinorrhea, epistaxis, snoring); hemoptysis; cough (productive or nonproductive, with sputum characteristics); hoarseness; olfactory perception; wheezing; abnormal breath sounds

▌*Cardiovascular System*
- Heart disease (chronic, acute, congenital); vascular disease (hypertension, arterial or venous circulatory disorders)
- Chest, arm, throat, or jaw pain; leg pain or claudication; paresthesias; edema; cyanosis; varicosities or ulcer; dyspnea (exertion, nocturnal); palpitations; orthopnea; murmur; abnormal heart sounds

▌*Neurologic System*
- Neuromuscular or neurosensory conditions; head or spinal trauma; seizure activity; vertigo or syncope; headache; tremors or spasms; paralysis; paresis; paresthesias; mentation changes (memory, orientation, level of consciousness); motor changes (gait, coordination); sensory perception changes (touch, taste, smell, vision, hearing); presbycusis; presbyopia; tinnitus; eye or ear pain or drainage; pruritus; photophobia; blurring; diplopia; floaters; use of glasses, contact lenses, hearing aid; sleep and rest pattern (rested, fatigue, muscle cramps); speech pattern (aphasia, slurred, alternate speech method)

▌*Gastrointestinal System*
- Gastrointestinal (GI), hepatic, biliary disorders; abdominal pain; nausea; vomiting; diarrhea; constipation; indigestion; heartburn; rectal bleeding; hematemesis; flatus; eructation (belching); jaundice; dysphagia (swallowing difficulty); chewing difficulty; anorexia; changes in appetite; presence and fit of dentures; caries; oral pain, bleeding, or lesions; halitosis; changes in gustatory perception; recent weight loss or gain; food intolerances, dislikes, and habits; special diet; 24-hour dietary intake review; bowel pattern review

▌*Endocrine System*
- Glandular dysfunction (thyroid, pancreas, adrenal, pituitary); polyuria; polydipsia; changes in metabolic function, skin color and texture, hair, tolerance to heat and cold; Cushing's response to corticosteroid therapy

▌*Hematologic System*
- Anemia, type and cause; weakness; pallor; night sweats; lymph node enlargement; skin hemorrhages; bruising; petechiae; bleeding from any site; previous transfusions (blood or blood products)

▌*Musculoskeletal System*

· Bone or joint disease; fracture; pain or stiffness in joints and muscles; redness, swelling, or heat at joint sites; deformity; limited range of motion (ROM) and movement; fatigue; weakness; energy and endurance; ability to perform activities of daily living (ADL) (total, assisted); deficits and use of assistive devices; limb prosthesis; exercise or activity pattern review; rehabilitation services; reaction to disability; Katz index of ADL independence

▌*Renal/Urinary System*

· Upper or lower renal tract disorders; urinary pattern review; difficulty in urination (dysuria, dribbling, urgency, frequency, oliguria, nocturia, retention, incontinence); hematuria; calculi; dialysis; urinary tract infection; presence of catheter; 24-hour fluid intake and output (I&O)

▌*Integumentary System*

· Skin color, eruptions, elasticity, turgor, texture, scarring, dryness or moisture; pruritus; alopecia; hair and nails characteristics and changes; corns; calluses; infection; pattern of daily skin-, hair-, nail-care review

▌*Reproductive System*

· Breasts and male or female genital or organ disorders; sexually transmitted diseases; infection; lesions; discharges; bleeding; pain (testicular, pelvic, dyspareunia); infertility; impotence; pattern of sexual activity and changes; menstrual information (menarche, last period, abnormal bleeding or irregularities, menopause); pregnancies (live births, abortions, complications); penile implant

▌*Psychosocial/Psychiatric/Mental*

· General appearance; depression; sadness; chronic anxiety or worry; dementia; delirium; mood swings; stressors; self-concept and self-esteem; delusions; combativeness; cognitive impairment (memory, attention span, orientation, judgment); intellectual function; disengagement or reclusiveness; thoughts of suicide; Mini-Mental State Examination; Short Portable Mental Status Questionnaire; Beck Depression Inventory; Yesavage Geriatric

Depression Scale; Older Adults Resources and Services Social Resource Scale (OARS); Family Adaptation, Partnership, Growth, Affection, and Resolve (APGAR)

✳ *Pulmonary System Assessment*

PAST HISTORY

▌*Lung and Airway Disorders*
- Chronic bronchitis (chronic obstructive pulmonary disease [COPD])
- Asthma
- Emphysema (COPD)
- Tuberculosis (TB)
- Pneumonia
- Pleurisy, pleural effusion
- Lung, larynx malignancy
- Influenza, colds, sinusitis, pharyngitis (frequency)
- Chest surgery (tracheostomy, lobectomy, pneumonectomy) or trauma (rib fracture, pneumothorax)

▌*Signs and Symptoms of Respiratory Disorders*
- Dyspnea with or without exertion; breathlessness
- Coughing and sneezing (amount, frequency)
- Sputum (amount, consistency, color)
- Chest, throat pain
- Wheezing; prostration

▌*Family History*
- Respiratory disorders, acute and chronic
- Allergies; eczema

▌*Allergies*
- Plants
- Animals
- Foods

- Drugs
- Environmental, occupational pollutants

■*Immunizations*
- Pneumonia
- Influenza

■*Activities of Daily Living*
- Position during sleep for optimal breathing
- Amount of exercise (tolerance, effect on breathing)
- Abilities for personal ADL self-care

■*Psychosocial History*
- Tobacco, alcohol, and caffeine consumption (type, amount, frequency)
- Anxiety and adaptation associated with acute illness or chronic pulmonary disease
- Home environment and exposure to irritants (odors, smoke, sprays, allergens, air conditioning and heating system, humidity, ventilation)

■*Past Treatments and Diagnostic Procedures (M0500)*
- Past or recent hospitalizations
- Desensitization therapy
- Pulmonary rehabilitation
- Medications taken for respiratory condition (oral, inhalant, injection)
- Diagnostic procedures and results

PRESENT HISTORY
- Chief complaint, including onset and length of time present

■*Signs and Symptoms*
- Respiratory rate: ease, depth, rhythm, use of accessory muscles; factors precipitating increases or other changes
- Dyspnea (M0490); orthopnea; tachypnea; bradypnea; cyanosis; pallor
- Chest, throat, sinus pain
- Fatigue; activity intolerance
- Productive or nonproductive cough and characteristics (amount, consistency, color)

▮*Present Treatment and Diagnostic Procedures*

- Assisted ventilation
- Oxygen
- Medications (bronchodilators, corticosteroids, decongestants, antitussives, expectorants, antihistamines, antimicrobials, antituberculars, oxygen, others)
- Breathing treatments (nebulizer, physiotherapy, breathing exercises)
- Lung biopsy; thoracentesis; bronchoscopy; radiography; nuclear study; pulmonary function; sputum culture; measurement of arterial blood gases

▮*Knowledge of Disease and Planned Home Therapy*

PHYSICAL EXAMINATION

▮*Inspection*

- Chest for symmetry (shape, expansion, movement, anteroposterior diameter ratio)
- Lips, ears, nails, nasal and throat mucosa for color
- Breathing pattern for use of mouth, diaphragm, chest, abdomen, accessory muscles, chest expansion
- Capillary refill; fingers for clubbing
- Nares for symmetry, discharge, patency; septum for alignment; pharynx for color, lesions, discharge; tonsils for presence, color, size, exudate
- Restlessness; confusion; fatigue; diaphoresis

▮*Palpation*

- Chest wall and intercostal muscles for skin smoothness, warmth, firmness, tenderness, bulging or masses, retraction, crepitus, symmetry of movement and chest expansion
- Trachea for midline alignment
- Tactile and vocal fremitus and location of increases or decreases

▮*Percussion*

- Posterior, anterior, lateral chest wall resonance for hyperresonance, dullness, flatness, tympany (pitch, intensity, duration with bilateral comparison)

▌*Auscultation*

- Posterior, anterior, lateral chest wall for vesicular breath sounds (posterior), bronchovesicular breath sounds (upper right posterior), bronchial breath sounds (over trachea) and whether diminished or absent and location
- Breath sounds heard in areas where not expected
- Voice sounds for intensity at airways and periphery by egophony or bronchophony (clarity, muffled sounds)
- Adventitious sounds, such as crackles, rhonchi, wheezes, friction rub

ANATOMIC AND FUNCTIONAL CHANGES ASSOCIATED WITH THE AGING CLIENT

- Weaker chest muscles, affecting bronchopulmonary movement, and increased use of accessory muscles and diaphragm for breathing
- Increased stiffness of rib cage and anteroposterior chest diameter in relation to lateral diameter, which reduces chest expansion
- Reduced reflex activity; ciliary movement; drying and atrophy of mucous membranes, affecting ability to cough and efficiency of bronchoelimination
- Shallow and more rapid respiratory rate, increasing with anxiety or exertion; pattern in rate and depth becoming uncoordinated with exertion or chronic respiratory disease
- Loss of lung elasticity; reduced compliance with air retained in lung bases, causing lower vital capacity and higher residual air and affecting breathing pattern
- Elastin and collagen property and distribution changes that result in loss of lung and blood vessel elasticity; change in volume pressure of the lungs; and decreased lung recoil, causing collapse of smaller bronchioles
- Progressive hyperventilation as lung elasticity is lost, causing slight hyperresonance on percussion and decreased or slightly quieter breath sounds on auscultation
- Fewer numbers of and increased size of alveoli; loss of lung capillaries; decrease in respiratory rate, oxygen saturation, and expired carbon dioxide, which results in reduction in gas exchange

- Reduced rate of gas movement across alveolocapillary membrane; increased use of oxygen during stress, which affects perfusion and diffusion, resulting in a greater risk for impaired gas exchange

✳ *Cardiovascular System Assessment*

PAST HISTORY

▪Cardiac and Vascular Disorders
- Hypertension
- Congestive heart failure
- Myocardial infarction
- Stroke
- Arterial insufficiency disorders (atherosclerosis, claudication, Buerger's disease)
- Venous insufficiency disorders (thrombophlebitis, varicose veins, leg ulcer)
- Surgery: heart (bypass, valvular, pacemaker), vascular (endarterectomy, venous ligation)

▪Signs and Symptoms of Cardiovascular Disorders
- Chest, arm, throat, jaw, or extremity pain; leg pain at rest or during activity
- Heart palpitations; dizziness; weakness
- Dyspnea; orthopnea
- Neck vein distension
- Dependent edema
- Extremity coldness, numbness, tingling
- Extremity discoloration

▪Family History
- Heart or vascular condition, acute or chronic
- Hypertension; stroke
- Diabetes mellitus

- Asthma
- Obesity

▌*Allergies*
- Medications
- Foods

▌*Activities of Daily Living*
- Sleeping in semi-Fowler's or high Fowler's position
- Abilities for personal self-care and/or ADL
- Exercising and effect on pulse and respirations
- Homebound status

▌*Psychosocial History*
- Tobacco, caffeine, and alcohol consumption (type, amount, frequency)
- Personality traits
- Occupation and work-related stress
- Adaptation to chronic illness or condition

▌*Past Treatments and Diagnostic Procedures*
- Past or recent hospitalizations
- Holter monitor
- Cardiac rehabilitation
- Special diet: low cholesterol and fat, low calorie, low sodium
- Medications taken for cardiac or vascular conditions (oral, sublingual)
- Diagnostic procedures and results

PRESENT HISTORY
- Chief complaint, including onset and length of time present

▌*Signs and Symptoms*
- Blood pressure; pulse rate (beats/minute) and regularity; apical pulse; apical radial pulse; factors that cause changes in baselines; changes with position or posture (sitting, standing, lying)
- Onset; duration; precipitating factors if any; alleviating factors if relevant to symptoms
- Pain in chest, arm, throat, jaw; aching in legs; pain, redness, and swelling in leg calf; lesions slow to heal

- Dyspnea; orthopnea; palpitations; changes in pulse regularity (slow or rapid)
- Edema; weight gain
- Changes in mentation; headache; insomnia; restlessness; fatigue
- Changes in skin color (pallor, redness, cyanosis)

Present Treatments and Diagnostic Procedures

- Oxygen
- Medications (antianginals, antiarrhythmics, anticoagulants, antihypertensives, β-adrenergic blockers, calcium channel blockers, diuretics, inotropics, lipid-lowering agents, thrombolytics, vasopressors, others)
- Electrocardiogram (ECG); cardiac angiography; echocardiography; cardiac nuclear scan; cardiac enzymes; lipid panel; electrolytes; prothrombin or thromboplastin time

Knowledge of Disease and Planned Home Therapy

PHYSICAL EXAMINATION

Inspection

- Chest, legs, and arms for symmetry
- Anterior chest wall for contour or retractions
- Skin of arms, hands, legs, and feet for color and texture (pink, warm, smooth, dry); color change in extremities when dangling or elevated (return to normal in 10 seconds)
- Legs and arms for hair distribution; fingers for clubbing
- Extremities for rashes, scars, ulcers and exudate, and discoloration (brownish color, eschar, irregular shape of ulcer, chronic venous stasis)
- Veins flush with skin surface or venous enlargement
- Pulsations in the aortic, pulmonary, right ventricular, apical, or left ventricular areas
- Nail beds for capillary refill in fewer than 3 seconds

Palpation

- Skin of extremities smooth, dry, warm to touch
- Chest and extremities for masses, pain, or tenderness
- Extremity veins smooth and full or dilated and tortuous
- Legs for edema, dependent or pitting
- Calf for tenderness, tension, redness, warmth, presence or absence of Homans' sign

- Cardiac thrills (pulsations of the heart that feel like the throat of a purring cat) or heaves
- Brachial artery of arms for rate, rhythm, amplitude, symmetry of blood pressure measurement
- Femoral, popliteal, carotid, temporal, and dorsalis pedis pulse for rate, regularity, amplitude, contour, and symmetry (60 to 90 beats/minute)
- Radial pulse for rate (tachycardia, bradycardia), regularity (trigeminal, bigeminal, pulsus differens), amplitude (pulsus alternans, pulsus biferiens, bounding pulse, pulsus paradoxus)

▌*Auscultation*

- Brachial blood pressure in both arms with client in lying position (same or no more than 5- to 10-mm Hg variance) and in standing position (decrease of 10 to 15 mm Hg systolic and 5 mm Hg diastolic); pulse pressure calculation
- Apical pulse, point of maximum impulse for rate, regularity, intensity
- Apical-radial pulse for rate, regularity, pulse deficit
- Carotid artery for bruits
- Chest for areas of aortic valve (right sternal border at second interspace), tricuspid valve (midclavicular line at left fifth intercostal), pulmonic valve (left sternal border at second interspace), second pulmonic valve (left sternal border at third interspace) for heart sounds (S_1 and S_2 heard in all areas) and extra heart sounds (S_3 and S_4, which should be absent)
- Heart murmurs for location, timing, duration, pitch, intensity, quality, sound distribution or pattern
- Pericardial friction rub; clicks, snaps for timing, intensity, pitch

ANATOMIC AND FUNCTIONAL CHANGES ASSOCIATED WITH THE AGING CLIENT

- Reduced heart size as a result of cardiac chronic illness and immobility; possible heart displacement from abnormal curvature of the spine
- Thickening and sclerosing of endocardium; thickening and rigidity of valves, which causes resistance to blood flow
- Reduced work of left ventricle and blood pumped by the heart at rest that decreases cardiac output and diminishes cardiac reserve; less capable of responding to increased demands when needed

- Loss of muscle fibers in heart from increased collagen and reduced elastin, causing reduced contractility and filling capacity and stiffness and enlargement of intramuscular vessels
- Increased arterial wall changes (atherosclerosis), reducing lumen size; occlusion of coronary arteries, causing decrease in blood flow
- Decrease in ability of heart to use oxygen, resulting in oxygen-activity imbalance and ischemia
- Reduced transport of nutrients and oxygen and removal of waste products from tissues, resulting from decreased capillary permeability and circulation
- Loss of elasticity in arterial walls; increased lability of vasopressor control that causes a decrease in the ability of vessels to stretch or expand, affecting blood pressure
- Increases in peripheral resistance from arteriole constriction, causing an increase in blood pressure and work of the heart; systolic increases faster than diastolic, causing a wider pulse pressure; both systolic and diastolic increase until humans are approximately 70 years of age
- Exercise-induced increases in blood pressure take longer to return to baseline; the baroreceptors in the aorta and carotid arteries have reduced sensitivity to pressure changes, causing slow response to postural changes
- Reduced effectiveness of venous valves and reduced muscle tone, causing decreased return of blood to the heart and distended superficial veins associated with inactivity
- Cellular changes; fibrosis of conduction system, neurogenic effect that impairs vasomotor response of vessels causing changes in ECG; prolonged intervals of QRS complex, PR segment, and QT prolongation; possible decreased voltage of all waves

❋ *Neurologic System Assessment*

PAST HISTORY

▌*Neurologic Motor and Sensory Disorders*
- Multiple sclerosis
- Cerebrovascular accident
- Transient ischemic attacks
- Muscular dystrophy
- Seizure disorder
- Head or spinal cord injury
- Brain or spinal cord tumor
- Motor or sensory aberrations
- Parkinson's disease
- Auditory, visual, speech, tactile impairments
- Surgery: brain (craniotomy), spinal column (laminectomy), eye (cataract, corneal transplant)

▌*Signs and Symptoms of Neurologic Disorders*
- Headache; dizziness
- Mentation changes; mental retardation
- Tremors; seizure activity
- Paralysis; muscle weakness; gait disturbances
- Speech changes; aphasia
- Behavioral changes (confusion, disorientation, mood, affect)

▌*Family History*
- Neurologic disorders, acute or chronic
- Hypertension
- Stroke
- Epilepsy
- Alzheimer's disease; dementia
- Huntington's chorea
- Diabetes mellitus

▌*Allergies*
- Medications

▌*Activities of Daily Living*
- Abilities for personal self-care and/or ADL
- Amount of independence or dependence
- Use of assistive aids (glasses, contact lenses, hearing aid)
- Rest/sleep/nap patterns (hours per 24 hours, frequency, times, length, use and effect of prescribed or over-the-counter sleeping aids, factors that promote or prevent sleep)
- Homebound status

▌*Psychosocial History*
- Tobacco and alcohol consumption (daily and over period of years)
- Occupational exposure to toxic agents that affect mental function
- Personality traits
- Adaptation to chronic illness or condition

▌*Past Treatments and Diagnostic Procedures*
- Past or recent hospitalizations
- Cervical or pelvic traction
- Medications taken for neurologic conditions
- Diagnostic procedures and results

PRESENT HISTORY
- Chief complaint, including onset and length of time present

▌*Signs and Symptoms*
- Anxiety
- Insomnia
- Headaches; back or neck pain (M0420)
- Syncope; vertigo
- Fatigue; mood and communication problems; aphasia (M0410)
- Memory deficits; changes in level of consciousness and behavior
- Sensory problems (paresthesias, visual, auditory)
- Motor problems (balance, paralysis, rigidity, tic, coordination)
- Quadriplegia; paraplegia

▌*Present Treatments and Diagnostic Procedures*
- Medications (sedatives, hypnotics, analgesics, anticonvulsants, antidepressants, antiglaucoma agents, antiparkinson agents,

antipsychotics, central nervous system stimulants, skeletal muscle relaxants)
- Lumbar puncture; cerebral angiography; electroencephalography; skull or spinal radiography; myography; electromyography; magnetic resonance imaging; nuclear and computed tomographic scans; visual and auditory tests; cerebrospinal fluid analysis

▌*Knowledge of Disease and Planned Home Therapy*

PHYSICAL EXAMINATION

▌*Inspection*
- Vital signs and temperature
- General appearance (posture, personal hygiene, facial expression)
- Muscles for symmetry of size, loss of mass, ROM in all joints
- Motor function (gait, coordination, balance, tremors during rest or intentional, ataxia, speech difficulty, dysphagia, muscle tone for spasticity or flaccidity, muscle strength in upper and lower extremities, involuntary muscle movements, deep reflexes)
- Sensory function (tactile, pain, proprioception, visual, auditory, discriminatory sensation, temperature)
- Mental function (level of consciousness; orientation to time, place, person, and event; memory; attention span; ability to make judgments and solve problems; ability to communicate; anger; agitation; euphoria; lability; depression)

▌*Spinal Nerve Innervation*
- Cervical 4 through 8 (C4 to C8): Motor function from neck downward to include ability to raise arms, flex and extend elbow, dorsiflex wrist, flex finger
- Thoracic 1 through 12 (T1 to T12): Ability to abduct finger, move thoracic and abdominal musculature
- Lumbar 1 through 5 (L1 to L5): Ability to flex hip, extend knee and large toe, dorsiflex ankle
- Sacral 1 through 5 (S1 to S5): Ability to plantar flex ankle, move perianal muscle

▌*Cranial Nerve Innervation*
1. Olfactory (sensory—smell): Odor identification
2. Optic (sensory—vision): Visual acuity; periphery and confrontation tests

3. Oculomotor (motor—pupil constriction; eyelid and extraocular movements): Response to penlight; size and shape of pupil; ptosis; accommodation to finger moving toward nose

4. Trochlear (motor—eye movement inward and downward): Convergence of eyes inward when finger moves toward nose

5. Trigeminal (motor—temporal, masseter muscles and lateral jaw movement; sensory-maxillary, mandibular facial, and ophthalmic sensitivity): Jaw and mastication muscle movement and ability to open and close jaws; sensitivity to sharp (pinprick) and dull (blunt pin end) object to extremity with eyes closed and to cornea with application of cotton wisp

6. Abducens (motor—eye abduction): Eye muscle movement for disconjugate gaze, eyes not moving together

7. Facial (motor—facial expressions; sensory—taste): Face and scalp muscle movement; grimacing; closing eyes tightly; discriminating salty and sweet tastes

8. Acoustic (sensory—hearing with cochlear division and balance with vestibular division): Weber's and Rinne tests for acuity; balance test

9. Glossopharyngeal (motor—pharynx; sensory—taste and pharyngeal sensation): Swallowing ability and gag reflex; rise of uvula when saying "ah"; taste sensation at posterior tongue; hoarseness

10. Vagus (motor—pharynx, larynx, palate; sensory—pharynx, larynx): Ability to speak, phonation, swallowing, and gag reflex with cranial nerve IX

11. Accessory (motor—sternocleidomastoid and trapezius muscle movements): Shoulder shrugging and turning head against resistance

12. Hypoglossal (motor—tongue): Tongue protrusion, deviation, and strength

Palpation

- Head and muscles for symmetry, shape, masses, depression
- Carotid and temporal pulses, comparing strength and quality bilaterally
- Muscles for tone, shape, size, and atrophy

Skeletal Muscle Reflexes

- Biceps; brachioradial; triceps; patellar; Achilles tendon (ankle); Babinski's (plantar)

▌*Auscultation*
· Bruits over eyes, temples, mastoid processes

ANATOMIC AND FUNCTIONAL CHANGES ASSOCIATED WITH THE AGING CLIENT

· Reduced size and weight of brain; atrophy of convolutions; widening sulci and gyri; increased dilation of ventricles; appearance of lesions and senile plaques
· Reduced number of neurons, which decreases transmission from brain to body areas, affecting arousal of organ or system
· Reduced dendrites in nerve; synapses; lesions on axons, which decrease peripheral nerve conduction and cause a slowing of reaction time
· Cerebral circulation changes affecting mental acuity, movement, sensory perception and interpretation, and ability to cope with multiple events
· Metabolic changes affecting synapses that cause neurotransmitter effects of brain that influence sleep, temperature control, and mood
· Slowing of reflexes but deep reflexes unchanged
· Electroencephalography readings are one cycle lower than for younger adults
· Sleep stages I and II last longer, stage III remains the same, and stage IV is reduced or omitted; changes in sleep stages can result in irritability, lethargy, fatigue, anxiety, tension, difficulty in falling asleep, frequently interrupted sleep with easier awakening as intensity of sleep is decreased
· Deterioration of tactile, olfactory, gustatory (reduced number of taste buds) perceptions that affect pain threshold, sensation of pressure and hot or cold, and anorexia or loss of interest in food

✳ *Gastrointestinal System Assessment*

PAST HISTORY

▌*Gastrointestinal Disorders*
- Peptic ulcer; gastritis
- Inflammatory bowel disease
- Enteritis; irritable bowel
- Diverticular disease
- Esophageal reflux, varices
- Hepatitis
- Cirrhosis
- Gallbladder disease
- Hernia
- Hemorrhoids; rectal disorders
- Surgery (partial or complete gastrectomy or colectomy, cholecystectomy, liver transplant, herniorrhaphy, hemorrhoidectomy, oral surgery)

▌*Signs and Symptoms of Gastrointestinal Disorders*
- Nausea; vomiting
- Diarrhea; constipation
- Dysphagia
- Indigestion; heartburn
- Anorexia
- Weight changes
- Malnutrition
- Blood in vomitus, feces
- Abdominal pain, distension
- Rectal pain, itching

▌*Family History*
- GI disorders, acute and chronic
- Ulcers
- Hemorrhoids
- Colorectal malignancy
- Hepatitis
- Obesity

▮*Allergies*
- Foods
- Medications

▮*Patterns of Bowel Elimination and Nutritional Intake*
- Food likes and dislikes; appetite; cultural influences; eating pattern (meal frequency and time)
- Ability to chew and swallow; dentures and fit
- Caloric intake for 24 hours; special diet: high or low calories, high fiber, bland or low residue
- Bowel elimination pattern, characteristics, amount, color, frequency; flatus; incontinence (M0540)
- Use of laxatives or enema, type and frequency

▮*Activities of Daily Living*
- Abilities for self-care (feeding and toileting) (M0710/M0680)
- Use of assistive aids for meals and elimination
- Homebound status

▮*Psychosocial History*
- Tobacco, alcohol, and caffeine consumption (daily and over period of years)
- Personality traits
- Stress, anxiety, chronic illness and effect on elimination and nutrition
- Adaptation to chronic illness or condition

▮*Past Treatments and Diagnostic Procedures*
- Past or recent hospitalizations
- Presence of bowel diversion (type, care, response), ostomy (M0550)
- Medications taken for GI conditions (oral, rectal)
- Diagnostic procedures and results

PRESENT HISTORY
- Chief complaint, including onset and length of time present

▮*Signs and Symptoms*
- Pain and characteristics
- Anorexia; nausea; vomiting
- Heartburn; flatulence; eructation

- Constipation; diarrhea; impaction; incontinence (M0540)
- Weight changes
- Jaundice; pruritus
- Blood in vomitus (coffee ground), feces (black, tarry)

■ *Present Treatments and Diagnostic Procedures*

- Medications (antacids, antiemetics, antidiarrheals, H_2-receptor antagonists, laxatives, stool softeners, suppositories, vitamins, anticholinergics, antidiabetics, antimicrobials, lipid-lowering agents)
- Proctoscopy; gastroscopy; colonoscopy; esophagoscopy; gastric and bowel radiography; gallbladder radiography; GI and hepato-biliary nuclear and computed tomography scans; paracentesis; tissue biopsy; ultrasonography; gastric acid tests; motility tests; feces for culture, occult blood, ova, parasites, toxins; liver function tests; enzymes; complete blood count (CBC); electrolytes
- Enemas; bowel irrigation
- Nasogastric, gastrostomy feedings; total parenteral nutrition
- Gastric decompression, suctioning

■ *Knowledge of Disease and Planned Home Therapy*

PHYSICAL EXAMINATION

■ *Inspection*

- Weight: actual and ideal for age, size, sex, and frame; height in relation to weight
- Contour of abdomen for shape, size, and protrusion of umbilicus
- Abdominal skin for smoothness, rash, scars, ascites
- Oral cavity for pain, color, texture, caries, mucositis, lesions, bleeding, odor, irritation by dentures
- Teeth for number, color, surface
- Tongue for color, texture, coating, lesions; hard and soft palate for color, shape, movement
- Anus for pain, itching, inflammation, bleeding, drainage
- Jaundice of skin, sclera, mucous membranes
- Feces and vomitus for abnormal constituents or consistency
- Drainage from nasogastric tube or ostomy, condition of stoma

■ *Auscultation*

- Presence of bowel sounds in four quadrants, including frequency, pitch, loudness, rushing, swishing, gurgling

· Absence of bowel sounds for 1 minute in each quadrant

❚*Percussion*

· Four quadrants for dull (bladder distension), tympanic (stomach and intestinal distension or gas), or wavelike sounds
· Liver and spleen for dullness

❚*Palpation*

· Abdomen for tone, masses, pain, distension, tautness, warmth or coldness in four quadrants
· Liver and kidneys for smoothness, firmness, and palpability
· Inguinal nodes for contour, mobility, tenderness, and palpability
· Rectal sphincter for tightness, smooth rectal walls

ANATOMIC AND FUNCTIONAL CHANGES ASSOCIATED WITH THE AGING CLIENT

· Thinning of teeth and wearing down of grinding surfaces with erosion of roots and crowns, which affects biting and chewing; saliva pH becomes alkaline, causing tendency for tooth decay; denture fit affected as oral structures change and bone loss occurs
· Thinning and drying of oral epithelium as volume of saliva decreases; reduced salivary enzyme that affects the beginning digestion of starches; taste buds reduced in number, affecting taste and appetite
· Decreased metabolic rate with gradual weight reduction; change in fat distribution with increased body fat and decreased lean body mass and subcutaneous tissue
· Weaker abdominal and pelvic musculature, affecting defecation
· Reduced size of liver; pancreatic atrophy occurs
· Reduced stomach, hepatic, pancreatic enzymes and thinning and atrophy of tract mucosa, slowing digestion and absorption, drug metabolism and detoxification
· Decreased gag reflex, affecting swallowing, which can result in aspiration
· Reduced peristalsis and motility, affecting delayed emptying and esophageal reflux, gastrocolic reflex, and contraction of sphincter muscles, which contribute to constipation

✳ *Endocrine System Assessment*

PAST HISTORY

▌*Endocrine Gland Disorders*
- Diabetes mellitus
- Diabetes insipidus
- Addison's disease
- Hyperthyroidism or hypothyroidism
- Hyperparathyroidism or hypoparathyroidism
- Thyroid malignancy
- Pituitary tumor
- Surgery (thyroidectomy)

▌*Signs and Symptoms of Endocrine Disorders*
- Weight; appetite; hydration changes
- Vital sign changes; presence of dyspnea, palpitations
- Mentation, visual disturbances
- Weakness; fatigue; muscle activity changes
- Elimination pattern changes (bowel and urinary)
- Frequent infections

▌*Family History*
- Endocrine disorders, acute or chronic
- Diabetes mellitus
- Thyroid disease
- Hypertension
- Obesity

▌*Allergies*
- Foods
- Medications
- Iodine

▌*Activities of Daily Living*
- Abilities for self-care and/or ADL
- Ability to follow regimen for diabetes mellitus

- Exercise requirements
- Homebound status

▌*Psychosocial History*
- Tobacco and alcohol consumption (daily and over periods of years)
- Personality traits
- Stress from occupation or chronic condition
- Cultural preferences in diet; special diet: diabetic, low calorie, low fat
- Adaptation to chronic illness

▌*Past Treatments and Diagnostic Procedures*
- Past or recent hospitalizations
- Exposure to or treatment with radiation
- Medications taken for endocrine conditions (oral, subcutaneous)
- Diagnostic procedures and results

PRESENT HISTORY
- Chief complaint, including onset and length of time present

▌*Signs and Symptoms*
- Weakness; fatigue; muscle weakness, twitching, spasms, numbness, tingling, cramping, tremors, wasting; reduced strength
- Bone pain, aching
- Polyuria; polydipsia; polyphagia
- Heat/cold intolerance
- Anorexia; nausea; vomiting
- Headache; malaise
- Nervousness; irritability; drowsiness; confusion; insomnia
- Anxiety; depression; apathy; syncope
- Pruritus; thick, leathery skin; brittle nails; coarse hair
- Libido changes; impotence; amenorrhea

▌*Present Treatments and Diagnostic Procedures*
- Medications (hormones, antidiabetics, antithyroid agents, β-adrenergic–blocking agents, glucocorticoids)
- Radiography; nuclear scans; biopsy; CBC; electrolytes; glucose studies; ketones; thyroid function studies; growth hormone studies; cortisol; aldosterone; urinalysis

∎*Knowledge of Disease and Planned Home Therapy*

PHYSICAL EXAMINATION

∎*Inspection*
- Vital signs, height, and weight
- Extremities for symmetry; edema (location, type, grade)
- Skin for color, turgor, dryness, oiliness, texture, edema, distribution of fat
- Nail texture; hair amount, texture, and distribution
- Moon face; protruding eyeballs; tongue for thickening; hoarseness; breath for odor
- Neck for symmetry, masses visible on swallowing

∎*Palpation*
- Decreased or absence of deep reflexes
- Thyroid for size, shape, hardness, nodules; nodes for size, fixation

ANATOMIC AND FUNCTIONAL CHANGES ASSOCIATED WITH THE AGING CLIENT
- Reduced weight of pituitary gland with increased connective tissue and decrease in vascularity; some atrophy of the parathyroid gland; follicular distension and fibrosis of thyroid gland
- Decreased production of triiodothyronine hormone by the thyroid; follicle-stimulating hormone by the pituitary; parathyroid hormone by the parathyroid; cortisol hormone by the adrenals; anabolic steroids by the gonads; progesterone by the ovaries, testes, and adrenals; and testosterone in males; cessation of estrogen in females
- Changes in metabolic rate; atrophy of uterus, vagina, and ovaries; menopause; muscle loss; decreased sexual drive resulting from reduced production and secretion of hormones
- Pancreatic alveolar degeneration and duct obstruction; reduced number of insulin receptors on cells, decreased insulin release with carbohydrate intake, reduced glucose tolerance and amount of insulin secreted, placing one at risk for type 2 diabetes

✳ *Hematologic System Assessment*

PAST HISTORY

▌*Blood and Blood-forming Organ Disorders*
· Anemias
· Leukemias; lymphomas
· Hemophilia
· Immune disorders
· Other blood dyscrasias
· Surgery (splenectomy)

▌*Signs and Symptoms of Hematologic Diseases*
· Weight loss
· Fatigue; weakness; pallor; shortness of breath
· Pain in bones or joints
· Bleeding from any site; bruising on body parts
· Enlarged nodes

▌*Family History*
· Hematologic disorders, acute and chronic
· Anemias
· Hemophilia
· Sickle cell trait
· Malignancies

▌*Allergies*
· Foods
· Medications
· Chemicals

▌*Activities of Daily Living*
· Abilities for self-care and/or ADL
· Amount of dependence or independence
· Homebound status

▌*Psychosocial History*
· Tobacco, caffeine, and alcohol consumption (amount, type, frequency)

- Personality traits and lifestyle
- Occupation and exposure to chemicals, heavy metals, other toxic agents, or environmental pollutants
- Adaptation to chronic illness or condition

■ *Past Treatments and Diagnostic Procedures*
- Past or recent hospitalizations
- Bone marrow transplant
- Transfusions of blood or blood products and response
- Medications taken for hematologic conditions (oral, parenteral)
- Special diet: high iron, folate
- Diagnostic procedures and results

PRESENT HISTORY
- Chief complaint, including onset and length of time present

■ *Signs and Symptoms*
- Change in behavior, level of consciousness, orientation
- Fatigue; weakness; dizziness; headache; pallor; dyspnea
- Pain in bones or joints, mouth or tongue
- Anorexia; nausea; emaciation
- Night sweats
- Infections
- Skin hemorrhages; bleeding from any site (prolonged or excessive)

■ *Present Treatments and Diagnostic Procedures*
- Medications (antimicrobials, antianemics, antineoplastics, glucocorticoids, immunosuppressants, analgesics, antianxiety agents)
- Bone marrow analysis; node biopsy; nuclear scan; CBC; platelet and reticulocyte counts; prothrombin and thromboplastin time; iron studies

■ *Knowledge of Disease and Planned Home Therapy*

PHYSICAL EXAMINATION

■ *Inspection*
- Vital signs, height, and weight
- General appearance for dehydration, cachexia
- Ecchymoses or petechiae

- Skin color, texture; pruritus; nail bed color
- Oral cavity for redness, edema, bleeding, ulceration

▌*Palpation*
- Liver and spleen size
- Joint swelling
- Lymph node enlargement: tenderness; mobility; consistency in neck, axilla, and inguinal areas

ANATOMIC AND FUNCTIONAL CHANGES ASSOCIATED WITH THE AGING CLIENT

- Lymphoid tissue changes affecting immunity; decreased immunocompetence reducing chances for survival from illness
- Degeneration of thymus gland, affecting secretion of thymic hormone and production and efficiency of T-lymphocytes, which reduces ability to respond to antigen stimuli and to prevent tumor formation
- Reduced ability of bone marrow to produce leukocytes and erythrocytes, which affects response to infection and anemia
- Decreased antibodies, which affects response to antigens, and increased autoantibodies, affecting susceptibility to autoimmune disease

✳ *Musculoskeletal System Assessment*

PAST HISTORY

▌*Muscle, Bone, and Joint Disorders*
- Arthritis and type
- Bursitis
- Fractures
- Low back syndrome
- Osteoporosis
- Paget's disease
- Ruptured disk
- Bone malignancy

- Bone infections
- Deformities
- Neuromuscular disease
- Musculoskeletal surgery or trauma (amputation, laminectomy, hip or knee replacement)

Signs and Symptoms of Musculoskeletal Disorders
- Pain, swelling in joints
- Muscle weakness, twitching, or deterioration
- Coordination or balance in walking and other movements
- ROM, activity and mobility
- Paralysis
- Burning, numbness, tingling in extremities
- Contractures; abnormal body alignment
- Pathologic fractures

Family History
- Joint or bone disorders, acute and chronic
- Neurologic motor deficits
- Neuromuscular disease
- Musculoskeletal disease

Allergies
- Foods
- Medications
- Chemicals

Activities of Daily Living
- Ability for self-care and/or ADL
- Ability to use hands and fingers to grasp, hold objects
- Ability to walk/transfer; energy and endurance and effect on joints (M0700/M0690)
- Use of aids for eating, toileting, dressing, personal hygiene, and grooming
- Homebound status

Psychosocial History
- Tobacco, alcohol, caffeine, and chemical consumption (daily and over period of years)
- Personality traits

- Occupation and need for mobility and dexterity; proneness to accidents
- Adaptation to disability or chronic illness

▌*Past Treatments and Diagnostic Procedures*

- Past or recent hospitalizations
- Cast, splint, or traction for bone or joint disorder or surgery
- Physical and occupational therapy and rehabilitation
- Transcutaneous electrical nerve stimulation; cold or heat applications
- Medications taken for musculoskeletal conditions (oral, injections)
- Diagnostic procedures and results

PRESENT HISTORY

- Chief complaint, including onset and length of time present

▌*Signs and Symptoms*

- Pain in affected area
- Redness, swelling, warmth in affected area
- Weakness; fatigue
- Loss of mobility, coordination or balance, or weight-bearing ability
- Limited ROM
- Loss of sensation in extremity
- Muscle spasms; reduced muscle strength and mass
- Diminished peripheral pulse in extremities; delayed capillary refill

▌*Present Treatments and Diagnostic Procedures*

- Medications (anticholinergics, antimicrobials, antigout agents, antiparkinson agents, analgesics, nonsteroidal analgesics, glucocorticoids, immunosuppressants, skeletal muscle relaxants, antianxiety agents, minerals)
- Radiography; nuclear and computed tomography scans; myelography; electromyography; biopsy; electrolytes; uric acid; rheumatoid factor; CBC; sedimentation rate; alkaline phosphatase
- Special diet: high calcium, low calorie
- Use of trapeze, cast, brace, traction, aids for ADL
- Bed rest; amount of activity allowed and tolerated
- Limb prosthesis

█*Knowledge of Disease and Planned Home Therapy*

PHYSICAL EXAMINATION

█*Inspection*
- Legs, arms, shoulders, clavicles, scapulas, musculature (hypertrophy or atrophy) for symmetry
- All joints for full ROM, degree of motion, and symmetry
- Ability to sit, lie, get up, stand, walk (M0700), transfer (M0690) and posture in all positions
- Deformities or contractures; deviations; changes in contour
- Presence of scoliosis; kyphosis; lordosis; hammer toe
- Gait; coordination; balance; endurance
- Body alignment in supine, prone, side-lying positions
- Amputation (arm or leg and site of amputation)
- Enforced immobilization
- Casted extremity or body part for circulatory and neurologic function

█*Palpation*
- Joint(s) or injury for warmth, swelling, tenderness
- Crepitus from joint motion
- Muscles for strength, mass, tone, spasticity, flaccidity, rigidity
- Presence of reflexes
- Tenderness on pressure or movement
- Thickening, bony enlargement around joints

ANATOMIC AND FUNCTIONAL CHANGES ASSOCIATED WITH THE AGING CLIENT

- Loss of muscle fiber, muscle mass, bone minerals, and bone mass, causing muscle wasting and reduction in weight, strength, endurance, and agility and brittle bones because bone resorption is faster than new bone formation, resulting in an increased risk for fractures
- Shortened vertebral column, hip and knee flexion, and curvature of spine, reducing height and effecting postural change that causes change in body balance and risk for falls
- Reduced motor coordination and manual skills, affecting reaction time; change in extrapyramidal system, causing muscle stiffness, slowness, and tremors at rest
- Decreased storage of muscle glycogen and change in enzyme function, causing loss of energy and muscle fatigue

- Joint changes from increased synovial membrane and synovial fluid thickness
- Muscle cramping and paresthesias of legs, resulting in pain and loss of sleep
- Mechanical and dermatologic changes in feet caused by long-term stress of weight bearing on feet

✳ *Renal/Urinary System Assessment*

PAST HISTORY

▌*Kidney and Bladder Disorders*
- Renal failure
- Urinary tract infection (M0510) (cystitis, pyelonephritis)
- Glomerulonephritis
- Calculi
- Neurogenic bladder
- Prostatic hypertrophy
- Hypertension
- Malignancy
- Surgery: kidney (nephrectomy, nephrostomy, transplant), bladder (urinary diversion, cystectomy, prostatectomy)

▌*Signs and Symptoms of Renal/Urinary Disorders*
- Pain in kidney or bladder area
- Urinary incontinence (M0520/M0530); bladder distension
- Retention; hesitancy; dribbling; urgency; frequency; burning; nocturia; dysuria
- Polyuria; oliguria; anuria
- Urine amount, color, odor, sedimentation, hematuria, pus, mucus, clarity
- Type of fluid I&O for 24 hours
- Weight gain
- Edema; fever; bruising; restlessness; insomnia
- Dryness, itching, poor turgor of skin; dryness of lip and mucous membranes
- Mentation changes

■ *Family History*
- Renal or bladder disorders, acute or chronic
- Congenital or familial renal or urinary conditions
- Hypertension
- Connective tissue disorder
- Diabetes mellitus

■ *Allergies*
- Foods
- Medications

■ *Activities of Daily Living*
- Abilities for personal self-care (toileting) (M0680)
- Use of assistive aids for elimination
- Homebound status

■ *Psychosocial History*
- Tobacco, alcohol and caffeine consumption (type, amount, frequency)
- Personality traits
- Sexually transmitted diseases
- Exposure to environmental or occupational nephrotoxic substances (heavy metals, carbon tetrachloride, phenols, pesticides)
- Adaptation to chronic illness or condition

■ *Past Treatments and Diagnostic Procedures*
- Past or recent hospitalizations
- Presence of urinary diversion (type, care, response)
- Medications taken for renal or urinary conditions (oral, injections)
- Diagnostics and results

PRESENT HISTORY

- Chief complaint, including onset and length of time present

■ *Signs and Symptoms*
- Pain
- Weight gain; edema
- Changes in urinary pattern; incontinence (M0520/M0530)
- Changes in urinary characteristics; urinary tract infection (M0510)

- Anorexia; nausea; vomiting
- Thirst; dry skin; poor skin turgor
- Weakness; muscle cramping
- Pruritus; visual changes
- Fluid imbalance
- Electrolyte imbalance

∎ *Present Treatments and Diagnostic Procedures*

- Medications (analgesics, diuretics, antimicrobials, anticoagulants, cholinergics, electrolytes, immunosuppressants, glucocorticoids)
- Intravenous pyelography; cystography; radiography; nuclear scan; ultrasonography; kidney biopsy; blood urea nitrogen (BUN); creatinine and creatinine clearance; urinalysis; urine culture
- Urinary drainage devices or catheterization
- Fluid inclusions or restrictions
- Hemodialysis or peritoneal dialysis
- Special diet: low salt, potassium, calcium, or protein

∎ *Knowledge of Disease and Planned Home Therapy*

PHYSICAL EXAMINATION

∎ *Inspection*

- Blood pressure for elevation
- Skin for color, pruritus, petechiae, ecchymoses, dryness, urate crystals
- Hands, feet, sacral region, legs for edema; abdomen and neck vein for distension
- Urinary output and characteristics with or without an indwelling catheter
- Behavior changes (alertness, confusion, cognitive ability, level of consciousness)
- Breath for fruity or urine odor; urine for foul odor
- Condition of urinary diversion site, dialysis shunt or abdominal site, urinary catheter site

∎ *Palpation*

- Kidneys for size and movement
- Kidney, bladder area for pain
- Bladder or abdominal distension

▌*Percussion*
· Dullness over bladder if distended

ANATOMIC AND FUNCTIONAL CHANGES ASSOCIATED WITH THE AGING CLIENT

· Reduced renal tissue growth and number of nephrons, decreasing kidney size and affecting renal function efficiency
· Sclerosis of glomeruli and atrophy of afferent arterioles, which results in degeneration of glomeruli and glomerular filtration rate (GFR)
· Reduced cell mass and water content of adipose tissue, causing decreased intracellular body water and total body water, with extracellular body water remaining unchanged
· Reduced blood flow, GFR, and tubular function, affecting ability to concentrate urine and drug clearance
· Reduced resorption of glucose and sodium, reduced creatinine production and clearance, and increased BUN, causing prolonged time for acid-base abnormalities to return to normal and necessitating age adjustments in evaluating laboratory values
· Bladder becomes funnel-shaped, and capacity and smooth muscle tone are decreased, causing urinary frequency and nocturia
· Enlarged prostate in men, resulting in urgency, frequency, and dribbling
· Increased weakness of bladder and perineal muscles in women, causing retention and stress incontinence
· Bladder emptying incomplete, resulting in urinary stasis and risk for urinary tract infection
· Reduced inhibitory neural impulses to the bladder, affecting bladder contractions and voluntary control over bladder function, which causes incontinence

✳ *Integumentary System Assessment*

PAST HISTORY

▌*Integumentary Disorders*
- Dermatitis
- Eczema
- Infestations; scabies; pediculosis
- Infections of skin, nails, scalp
- Skin malignancy
- Surgery (graft, cosmetic)

▌*Signs and Symptoms of Integumentary Disorders*
- Alopecia
- Dandruff
- Itching; breaks in skin
- Brittleness, ridging, redness, edema of nails and cuticles
- Tendency to skin infections, herpes simplex
- Sensitivity to sun, soaps, deodorants, perfumes, others
- Dryness; oiliness; excessive moisture; body odor
- Skin color changes
- Lumps or growth on the skin
- Bruising; delayed healing
- Ulcer on extremity (M0468-M0476)

▌*Family History*
- Integumentary disorders, acute and chronic
- Allergies; eczema

▌*Allergies*
- Foods
- Medications
- Cosmetics
- Environmental contacts

▌*Activities of Daily Living*
- Abilities for personal self-care (bathing, grooming, dressing) (M0670/M0640/M0650-M0660)

- Pattern of bathing, frequency and time; soap, toothpaste, shaving cream, powder, lotions used; razor or electric shaver; use of assistive aids for personal hygiene
- Pattern of hair and nail care; shampoo, rinse, nail polish, hair tint used; trimming of toenails and fingernails, use of assistive aids or professionally done
- Homebound status

Psychosocial History
- Home environment exposure to allergens or irritants
- Personality traits; anxiety
- Occupational exposure to irritants such as dyes, sprays, perfumes, allergens
- Effect on body image if dermatitis or scarring present
- Adaptation to chronic skin condition

Past Treatments and Diagnostic Procedures
- Past or recent hospitalizations
- Medications used for integumentary conditions (topical, oral)
- Diagnostic procedures and results

PRESENT HISTORY
- Chief complaint, including onset and length of time present

Signs and Symptoms
- Changes in skin color, eruptions, breaks, and precipitating factors
- Hair loss and precipitating factors
- Nail changes and precipitating factors
- Injury from burns, with extent and degree of damage to skin and pain

Present Treatments and Diagnostic Procedures
- Medications (antipruritics, antianxiety agents, antimicrobials, glucocorticoids, antihistamines, sedatives, analgesics)
- Skin biopsy; skin culture; CBC
- Desensitization therapy
- Braden scale for pressure ulcer prediction

▌*Knowledge of Disease and Planned Home Therapy*

PHYSICAL EXAMINATION

▌*Inspection*

- Skin for cyanosis, redness, jaundice, pallor, pigmentation, bleeding, bruising
- Skin for striae, rashes, urticaria, bites, wrinkling
- Skin for dryness, moisture, oiliness, sweating, peeling, scaling, crusting
- Pruritus; odor; exudate; cleanliness
- Edema; pain; breaks; incisions and scars; sagging parts
- Blisters; cellulitis; calluses; corns; superficial infection
- Lesions (M0440), lipomas, keloids, warts, nevi, with measurements, location and distribution; pressure ulcer (M0445/M0450/M0460/M0464); stasis ulcer (M0468/M0470/M0474/M0476); surgical wound (M0482/M0484/M0486/M0488)
- Senile lentigines, senile ectasias, seborrheic keratosis, sebaceous hyperplasia in the aging client
- Nails for cleanliness, texture, thickness, angle, infection, ingrown nails or hangnails
- Hair for cleanliness, quantity, texture, distribution, color, odors, brittleness, oiliness or dryness, baldness
- Scalp for infestation, lesions, dandruff

▌*Palpation*

- Skin temperature (warm, hot, cold), texture (rough, bumpy, smooth, thin, thick)
- Skin turgor, elasticity, moisture, mobility, elevated lesions with measurement
- Tumors, cysts, or any lumps on skin or scalp
- Bony prominences and response to pressure
- Capillary return in nails and movement of nail plate when pressure applied

ANATOMIC AND FUNCTIONAL CHANGES ASSOCIATED WITH THE AGING CLIENT

- Change in distribution of body fat with loss of subcutaneous fat, especially over the arms and legs, which causes loss of body insulation and support for vessels

- Reduced formation of collagen with loss of elasticity of skin, causing sagging, wrinkles, lines in face and neck, ptosis of eyelids, and elongation of ear lobes
- Reduced cell replacement in dermis and epidermis, affecting wound healing and risk for decubitus ulcers
- Atrophy of skin layers and reduced vascularity and elasticity, which causes loss of water content and storage in skin layers, reduced skin turgor, stiffness, and loss of pliability
- Reduced water content of skin and function of eccrine and sebaceous glands, causing rough, scaly texture and pruritus from dryness; risk for pressure ulcers; trauma; and reduced ability of body to cool itself
- Decreased circulation to skin and appendages, affecting blood supply of oxygen and nutrients to skin
- Neurosensory changes in skin, affecting tactile perception of pain associated with lesions or tumors
- Excessive skin pigmentation on exposed areas, causing aging spots, and overgrowth epidermal tissue, causing senile telangiectasia and hyperkeratotic warts
- Nail ridges; thickness, brittleness, and splitting of nails increased, causing reduced growth and strength, increased risk for fungal infections with lifting of nail plate
- Density of hair follicles reduced; loss of axillary, pubic, and head hair and melanin production, causing graying, increased hair growth in ears, nares, eyebrows

❋ *Reproductive System Assessment: Female*

PAST HISTORY

▮*Reproductive Disorders*
- Sexually transmitted diseases
- Pelvic inflammatory disease
- Endometriosis
- Tubal pregnancy
- Abortions

- Infertility
- Menstrual disorders
- Breast, uterine, ovarian, vaginal malignancy
- Surgery: breast (simple or radical mastectomy), uterus (hysterectomy), pelvic reproductive organs (salpingectomy, oophorectomy, tubal sterilization), vaginal (cystocele or rectocele repair)

Signs and Symptoms of Reproductive Organ Disorders
- Breast tenderness, discharge, lump or mass; change in nipple
- Dyspareunia
- Dysmenorrhea; amenorrhea; other menstrual irregularities
- Rashes or irritations of genitalia with pruritus
- Discharge from meatus, vagina
- Dysuria; urinary frequency; retention; incontinence

Family History
- Breast or reproductive organ malignancy
- Reproductive organ disorders, acute or chronic

Allergies
- Scented feminine powders, pads, tampons

Activities of Daily Living
- Ability for personal self-care and/or ADL (toileting [M0680], menstrual hygiene)
- Amount of independence or dependence
- Presence of indwelling catheter and ability for care (M0520)
- Breast self-examination and frequency
- Birth control use and effectiveness
- Homebound status

Psychosocial History
- Age at menarche; menstrual frequency, amount, duration, regularity, and pain; last menstrual period
- Number of pregnancies, children
- Date or age of menopause; hot flashes; discharge; pain
- Intercourse frequency if active; satisfaction level
- Sexual orientation; multiple partners if appropriate
- Ability to carry out role function to satisfaction
- Adaptation to infertility or other chronic condition

▌*Past Treatments and Diagnostic Procedures*
- Past or recent hospitalizations
- Intrauterine device; birth control implant
- Medications taken for gynecologic conditions (oral, vaginal)
- Diagnostic procedures and results

PRESENT HISTORY
- Chief complaint, including onset and length of time present

▌*Signs and Symptoms*
- Abdominal pain; menstrual dysfunction
- Vaginal discharge and characteristics
- Genital irritation, pruritus
- Dyspareunia; dysuria

▌*Present Treatments and Diagnostic Procedures*
- Medications (hormones, antimicrobial, analgesics, fertility agents, antineoplastic agents, birth control agents)
- Breast self-examination and frequency
- Ultrasonography; mammography; laparoscopy; amniocentesis; breast, endometrial, or cervical biopsy; CBC; typing and Rh factor; pregnancy test; pap smear
- Presence of urinary catheter (M0520), birth control device

▌*Knowledge of Disease and Planned Home Therapy*

PHYSICAL EXAMINATION

▌*Inspection*
- Breast(s) for size, symmetry, contour, dimpling, texture, rash, moles, venous pattern
- Nipples for size, shape, color, discharge, induration; areolae for size, shape, surface
- External genitalia (urethra, clitoris, introitus, perineum) for color, inflammation, swelling, ulcerations or lesions, discharge, episiotomy
- Pediculosis pubis
- Vaginal wall for bulging, mucous membrane color, inflammation, masses, and lesions
- Cervical color, position, ulceration, bleeding, discharge

▌*Palpation*
- Breast elasticity, fullness, tenderness, nodes; nipple elasticity and discharge with pressure

- Breast mass size, shape, location, consistency, tenderness, mobility
- Axillary nodes present or absent
- Perineum for bulging; glands or duct openings for smoothness, discharge
- Vaginal wall smoothness, muscle tone, tenderness, nodules
- Cervical size, shape, position, mobility, patency
- Uterine size, position, shape, consistency, mobility, tenderness, mass

ANATOMIC AND FUNCTIONAL CHANGES ASSOCIATED WITH THE AGING CLIENT

- Sparser pubic hair
- Reduced size of uterus, cervix, and ovaries; reduced size and firmness of breast tissue
- Reduced subcutaneous tissue, which causes sagging breasts and flattening and folding of labia
- Shorter and narrower vaginal canal with increased thinning and loss of elasticity of the lining, which causes atrophic vaginitis and dyspareunia
- Vaginal secretions alkaline and reduced in amount, causing a need for more lubricant before intercourse
- Pelvic muscle tone weakness, which increases risk for uterine prolapse and stress incontinence
- Decreased estrogen secretion, which results in hot flashes; follicular maturation, which affects the stimulation to the uterine lining; and Bartholin's gland secretion, which results in reduced lubrication of the vagina

✳ *Reproductive System Assessment: Male*

PAST HISTORY

▌*Reproductive Disorders*

- Sexually transmitted diseases
- Prostatitis; prostatic hypertrophy
- Epididymitis

- Hydrocele
- Hernia
- Malignancy (prostate, testis)
- Surgery (prostatectomy, orchiectomy, penile implant, vasectomy, herniorrhaphy)

Signs and Symptoms of Reproductive Organ Disorders
- Pain in scrotum, testes
- Discharge from penis
- Lesions on penis
- Impotency; libido or sexual dysfunction
- Urinary difficulty with urgency, frequency, weak stream, difficulty in starting or stopping, incontinence (M0530), inability to empty bladder

Family History
- Reproductive disorders, acute or chronic

Activities of Daily Living
- Ability for self-care and/or ADL (toileting, genital hygiene)
- Presence of indwelling catheter and ability for care (M0520)
- Use of incontinence pads or undergarments
- Homebound status

Psychosocial History
- Personality traits
- Intercourse frequency if active; satisfaction level
- Sexual orientation; multiple partners if appropriate
- Ability to carry out role functions to satisfaction
- Effect of sexual dysfunction on self-concept
- Adaptation to illness, impotence, or other chronic condition

Past Treatments and Diagnostic Procedures
- Past or recent hospitalizations
- Penile implant or device
- Scrotal self-examination and frequency
- Medications taken for reproductive conditions (oral)
- Diagnostic procedures and results

PRESENT HISTORY
- Chief complaint, including onset and length of time present

▌*Signs and Symptoms*
- Pain
- Urinary dysfunction
- Bleeding or discharge from penis
- Genital irritation, pruritus
- Penile lesions, ulcers, soreness

▌*Present Treatments and Diagnostic Procedures*
- Medications (hormones, analgesics, antimicrobials, antispasmodics, antineoplastics)
- Cystoscopy; nuclear scan; prostate biopsy; CBC; urinalysis; urine culture; anal and meatal smear
- Use of aids or device for impotence
- Presence of urinary catheter (M0520)

▌*Knowledge of Disease and Planned Home Therapy*

PHYSICAL EXAMINATION

▌*Inspection*
- Breasts and nipples for symmetry, lesions, drainage, induration
- Pediculosis pubis; pubic hair distribution
- Penis, urethral meatus, scrotum for ulceration, scars, rashes, discharge, swelling, tenderness
- Circumcision and cleanliness
- Size and shape of penis for age, contour of scrotal sac with testes in place, position of urethral meatus

▌*Palpation*
- Breasts and nipples for masses, tenderness, discharge on pressure
- Penile shaft for masses, tenderness, induration
- Testes for size, shape, consistency, tenderness, symmetry, irregularities
- Hernia via inguinal ring and canal
- Prostate via rectal examination for softness, contour, enlargement, tenderness

ANATOMIC AND FUNCTIONAL CHANGES
ASSOCIATED WITH THE AGING CLIENT

· Increased size of prostate with urinary problems, and decreased size and firmness of testes, which causes reduced sperm production; scrotum sac hangs lower and more loosely
· Reduced volume and viscosity of seminal fluid, which decreases force of ejaculation
· Erection time increased with need for more stimulation, affecting orgasm and enhanced satisfaction
· Decreased testosterone secretion, causing reduced sexual energy

✳ *Eye, Ear, Nose, and Throat Assessment*

PAST HISTORY

▎*Eye, Ear, Nose, and Throat (EENT) Disorders*
· Infections (tonsillitis, conjunctivitis, otitis, pharyngitis)
· Glaucoma
· Cataracts
· Retinal detachment
· Deviated septum; nasal polyps
· Allergic rhinitis
· Macular degeneration
· Dry eye
· Presbyopia; presbycusis
· Surgery: eye (cataract, keratoplasty, corneal transplant, enucleation), ear (tympanoplasty, stapedectomy), nose (polypectomy, submucous resection), throat (tonsillectomy)

▎*Signs and Symptoms of EENT Disorders*
· Pain; headaches
· Discharge from eye, ear, nose
· Multiple colds
· Halitosis

- Buzzing or roaring in ears
- Vertigo; loss of equilibrium
- Nystagmus
- Hoarseness
- Runny or stuffy nose; epistaxis
- Changes in visual (M0390), auditory acuity (M0400)

Family History
- EENT disorders, acute and chronic
- Allergies

Allergies
- Foods
- Medications
- Animals
- Chemicals
- Environmental pollutants

Activities of Daily Living
- Ability for self-care and/or ADL
- Effects of visual or auditory impairment on independence or dependence
- Use of glasses, contact lenses, eye prosthesis, hearing aid, lip reading, signing
- Ability to care for assistive visual and auditory aids and instill eyedrops, eardrops, or nose drops
- Response to noise levels, mouthwash or rinses, hair sprays, ear cleansing with cotton swabs
- Homebound status

Psychosocial History
- Effect of impairment on self-concept and occupation
- Effects of age and emotions on impairments or disease
- Personality traits, anxiety, or depression
- Home environment exposure to allergens and irritants
- Adaptation to impairment or illness

Past Treatments and Diagnostic Procedures
- Past or recent hospitalizations
- Last hearing or vision test
- Desensitization therapy

- Medications taken for EENT conditions (oral, inhalant, topical)
- Diagnostic procedures and results

PRESENT HISTORY

- Chief complaint, including onset and length of time present

▌*Signs and Symptoms*
- Pain or soreness in affected area
- Onset, duration, precipitating factors
- Dysphagia; hoarseness; loss of voice
- Discharge from eye, ear, nose, throat
- Redness, swelling of eye, throat, nasal mucosa
- Epistaxis
- Temperature elevation
- Changes in visual (M0390) or auditory perception and acuity (M0400)

▌*Present Treatments and Diagnostic Procedures*
- Medications (antimicrobials, glucocorticoids, antihistamines, analgesics, antiglaucoma agents, antipyretics)
- Radiography; computed tomography; CBC; culture of throat, nasal, ear, eye secretions
- Eye, ear, throat irrigations
- Nasal packing; eye covering and dressing

▌*Knowledge of Disease and Planned Home Therapy*

PHYSICAL EXAMINATION

▌*Inspection*
- Ophthalmoscopic and otoscopic examination
- Visual acuity, visual fields, extraocular muscle intactness and movement tests
- Eyelids for symmetry, position, blinking, color, edema, lesions; eyebrows for movement, quantity and distribution, symmetry
- Conjunctiva and sclera for color, edema, lesions, opacities; iris for marking, color, and shape
- Cornea surface, transparency, sensitivity
- Pupil for size, shape, equality, reaction to light and accommodation

- Lacrimal glands for roundness, intactness; eyes for moisture or dryness
- External ears and auricles for lesions, deformities, color, size, and symmetry of position
- Ear canals for redness, edema, swelling
- Nose for deformities, shape, symmetry, color, edema, drainage, bleeding, and septal alignment
- Lips for color, dryness, cracking, edema, ulcers
- Throat for color, swelling, bleeding, inflammation, lesions
- Tonsils (if present) for redness, swelling, pus, or other exudate

▌*Palpation*
- Pinnae for firmness, masses, elasticity, pain
- Nose for structure
- Frontal or maxillary sinuses and lacrimal glands for tenderness

ANATOMIC AND FUNCTIONAL CHANGES ASSOCIATED WITH THE AGING CLIENT

- Reduced size of pupils, affecting night vision or a slow adaptation to the dark
- Reduced sensitivity of cones in retina, which causes decreased discrimination and blending of colors
- Sclera becomes yellow with pigmented deposits and cornea with white-yellow deposits around iris (arcus senilis), which becomes more translucent; inner canthus develops yellow plaques (xanthelasma)
- Loss of elasticity and increased opacity of lens, affecting focus and accommodation, night vision, color vision, reduced peripheral vision and tolerance to glare, and high risk for development of cataracts
- Reduced secretion by lacrimal glands, which causes dry conjunctiva and eye irritation; resorption of intraocular fluid; and a shallower anterior chamber, which can all increase risk for glaucoma
- Thinner and more wrinkled lids, loss of supporting tissue, which causes a sunken appearance of the eye into the socket
- Atrophy or sclerosis of tympanic membrane and increased rigidity of middle ear bones, which affect the transmission of nerve impulses from the ear to the brain, causing difficulty in hearing high-frequency sounds, which later progresses to include low-frequency sounds, hearing if noise is present, sound distortion,

and phonetic regression; keratin in cerumen is increased, hardens, and accumulates, affecting hearing

---

✳ *Psychosocial Assessment*

MENTAL/COGNITIVE/LEARNING

▌*Past History*
- Educational level and achievements
- Attitude toward learning; motivation
- Difficulty in achieving educational or vocational goals
- Learning disabilities
- Interest in and willingness to learn about care and procedures
- Ability to listen to and comprehend information given
- Ability to read and follow written instructions
- Vocabulary level and attention span
- Memory and ability to recall events, past and present
- Hearing, visual impairments
- English spoken or English as a second language

▌*Present History*
- Knowledge and understanding of illness and prognosis
- Cerebral function (M0560), including orientation (M0570), memory, recall, attention and concentration, comprehension, judgment, dementia, level of consciousness, communication pattern (articulation)
- Thought processes with ability to think rationally and logically and to solve problems
- Sensory function, including vision, hearing
- Physical ability; strength for self-care
- Ability to express needs and maintain record of care and procedures
- Administration of Short Portable Mental Status Questionnaire or Mini-Mental State Examination

PSYCHIATRIC

▌*Past History*
- Psychiatric conditions, treatments, therapist
- Institution, including length of stay and discharge date

- Attitude toward treatments
- Medications taken (prescribed, over-the-counter, recreational, street)
- Alcohol intake, amounts and length of time
- Hypochondriasis
- Suicide potential and precipitating factors
- Family history of mental disorders
- Relationships with family members and feelings about family

▌*Present History*

- Personal appearance, including hygiene, clothing, physical characteristics, posture, mannerisms, facial expression, gestures
- Communications, including tone, quality, flow, speed, use of associative looseness, flight of ideas, blocking, mutism, circumstantiality, word salad, echolalia, eye contact
- Mood; affect; stressors present
- Behaviors (M0600)
- Orientation to time, place, person, and event
- Delusions; hallucinations; illusions; paranoia (M0610/M0620)
- Coping ability and skills; use of defense mechanisms
- Presence of chronic anxiety (M0580), worry, depression (M0590), insomnia
- Lives alone or with others; isolates self; support of significant others
- Participation in social interactions and activities
- Administration of Beck Depression Inventory, Yesavage Geriatric Depression Scale
- Receiving Psychiatric Nursing Services (M0630)

ADVANCE DIRECTIVES

- Patient Self-Determination Act and its requirements and need for written information about advance directives (see Appendix)
- Presence of an advance directive or form for health care and location of the document(s) or a copy available
  - Living will
  - Durable power of attorney for health care
  - Do not resuscitate order
- Family understanding of and conflicts about client's directives
- Knowledge of rights of autonomy and consent to or refusal of care in the home, initiation of 911 call for client in home

SPIRITUAL

- Religious beliefs and practices; identified spiritual leader
- Feelings about a supreme being and how this view affects illness
- Feelings about what will happen during illness
- Specific people helpful in religious life
- Religious symbols of importance (Bible, prayer, rosary, literature)
- Rituals of importance (communion, Sacrament of the Sick, lighting Sabbath candles, quiet time)
- Religious restrictions (dietary laws, fasting, blood transfusion, medical treatment, birth control, abortion, autopsy)
- Need for church attendance; priest, minister, or rabbi visits

OCCUPATIONAL/RECREATIONAL

Past History

- Type of and feelings about past employment
- Effects on health
- Reasons for leaving or changing vocation, profession
- Presence of occupational hazards
- Hobbies and avocational activities

PRESENT HISTORY

- Type of present employment or retirement; loss of employment
- Feelings about work or retirement
- Activity involved in work; telephone use (M0770)
- Effect of work environment on health (stress, chemicals, allergens)
- Plans for returning to work
- Housekeeping tasks: laundry (M0740), housekeeping (M0750), shopping (M0760) (amount, kind, participation)
- Need for more education or wish for vocational retraining
- Type, frequency, and degree of participation in play, recreational activities
- Effect of illness on recreational interests or hobbies
- Alternative interests and activity options during illness
- Need to change recreational activities permanently
- Adaptation to retirement and role changes

FUNCTIONAL CHANGES ASSOCIATED WITH THE AGING CLIENT

- Intelligence remains basically the same but can be affected by sensory deficits
- Learning capacity can be slowed initially but can keep pace with other learners; there is a tendency to continue with familiar solutions for problems rather than develop new attitudes and methods
- Retention ability more limited and easily affected by external distractions
- More difficult to perform more than one task at a time
- Slowing of memory if information not continued to be used
- Personality traits remain the same but can become more psychologically diverse

Functional Assessment

GENERAL

- Homebound status; complete bed rest; activity restrictions
- Independence or dependence in self-care and ADL and desire and willingness to perform and adapt to limitations
- Degree of disability or handicap or deficit
- Presence of artificial limb, eye, dentures
- Rehabilitation therapy by physical and/or occupational therapist (M0825)
- General review of activities of a typical day to include personal care, social, and leisure routines
- Katz index of ADL for actual functional status

BATHING/GROOMING

- Ability to wash body (shower, tub bath, sponge bath) (M0670)
- Use of aids to bathe (long handles for sponge, mitt on hand, bars, skid proof mat, stool in bath or shower stall, soap on rope hanging around neck)
- Ability to brush teeth, cleanse dentures, comb or brush hair (M0640)

- Use of aids to brush teeth (long and built-up handles, extension handles, cup for soaking teeth, mounted dryer or brush with suction cup, squeeze bottles for shampoo and toothpaste)
- Ability to shave or apply makeup (electric or safety razor, make-up kit)
- Use of aids to shave and apply makeup (shaving cream, built-up handles, mirror mounted with suction cups or hanging around neck)

DRESSING/UNDRESSING

- Type of clothing that is easy to put on and remove (loose fitting, elastic at waist, closures with zipper or Velcro, wide openings to slip over head or slip on with front opening, shoes that slip on or have Velcro closures)
- Ability to dress and undress (buttons, zipper, tie laces, putting on shoes and socks/nylons), dress upper body (M0650), dress lower body (M0660)
- Use of aids for dressing (hooks, zippers, long handles for shoes)

TOILETING

- Ability to use bathroom, commode, bedpan, urinal (M0680)
- Use of aids for toileting (grab bars, mounted toilet seat with side arms, tongs or mounts for toilet tissue)

FEEDING

- Ability to feed self (M0710), partial or total assistance; ability to prepare meal (M0720)
- Use of aids for eating (china and flatware with suction cups, flatware with swivel, extension handles on flatware, bumper guard on plate, bib for droppings, cuff to hold utensils)
- Use of aids for drinking (grippers on cup or glass, large handles, long and bending straws, suction cups for cup or glass)

MOBILITY

- Ability to walk (M0700), sit, stand, or lie down; transferring (M0690), amount of assistance needed
- Use of aids for mobility and movement (wheelchair, walker, crutches, cane, brace, elevated chair, adjustable seat or ejector chair, footstool, trapeze, holding rails, mechanical lift, electric or semielectric hospital bed)

GENERAL ACTIVITIES

- Book holder, tilted table, clipboard, pencil holder, card or pad holder, mounts on chair for radio and books, remote control for electric appliances
- Cars (M0730) with special modifications, use of vans or buses with wheelchair lift
- Magnifiers; large-print reading materials and telephone amplifier; special wiring for turning lights on or to alert deaf client
- Automatic dialer and speaker phone attachment
- Pets for visual and auditory assistance

✳ *Environmental Assessment*

HOME EXTERIOR

- Primary entrance
- Steps or ramp available if needed
- Homebound or able to leave home safely

HOME INTERIOR

- Condition and cleanliness; noise; waste disposal
- Space storage for extra equipment and supplies
- Counter space for preparation of supplies, cleaning of equipment
- Refrigeration for foods, medications, supplies
- Location of fuse or circuit breaker box
- Proper lighting; frayed or loose wiring or electrical connections; grounding of equipment
- Heating and air conditioning adequacy
- Wood stove or kerosene heater use and ability to fuel fire
- Ventilation; temperature control; drafts
- Laundry facilities for clothing, linens, supplies
- Doorways and if adequate to move through easily, to accommodate wheelchair and commode, and to allow for delivery of equipment

- Floors and pathways clear, dry, and not slippery; arrangement of furniture out of pathways but close enough to use for support when ambulating; small rugs and carpet edges out of pathways
- Stairway, number of stairs and height of stairs; room on first floor or need for client to be transported upstairs
- Safety bars and holding aids for movement in environment
- Hot and cold running water or means to heat water; indoor plumbing versus drawn water
- Bathroom, commode within easy access; raised commode; grab bars
- Presence of allergens, dust, animals, plants, sprays, odors

SAFETY FACTORS

- Client's feeling of safety in home
- Functioning smoke alarm
- Hospital bed; trapeze connection
- Side rails up or bed in low position if using hospital bed
- Call bell, water, tissues, wastebasket, telephone within reach
- Chair to assist to standing position
- Scales for weight in bathroom or near bed
- Proper body alignment and positioning if on bed rest
- Use of restraints
- Safe smoking precautions
- Isolation or protective isolation procedures needed
- Nonslip mats in bath or shower
- Night lights if out of bed at night to use bathroom or commode
- Safety aids for ADL to prevent falls, promote self care; amount of assistance needed; proper fitting nonskid foot covering
- Proper handwashing technique when required
- Proper administration of medications and use of aids to ensure accuracy
- Proper cleansing and disinfection of reusable supplies, removal and disposal of hazardous wastes
- Available emergency numbers to call

✳ *Family Assessment*

PHYSICAL HISTORY

- Chronic illness of family members
- Functional abilities or disabilities
- Energy levels of family members and how physical needs of its members are met
- Physical strength and ability to perform procedures
- Ability to manage equipment (M0820)
- Rigidity in functioning within family system
- Health practices
- Types of practitioners used
- Medications taken by family members

PSYCHOSOCIAL HISTORY

▌*Emotional Status/Mental Status*

- Changes in family life and roles caused by client needs
- Family unable to meet emotional needs of its members
- Ability of family members to express feelings
- Ability of family to accomplish developmental tasks
- Ability to communicate clear message, solve problems, and make decisions
- Family attitude; overconcern toward illness or disability; relationship of client and family members
- Family patterns in use of coping mechanisms (denial, rationalization, projections, defensiveness) and ability to adapt
- Family organization (arguments, separations, divorces)
- Willingness to perform procedures and care for client
- Support of client by member most likely to become caregiver
- Family APGAR for family function

PSYCHIATRIC DISORDERS

- General mental health of family
- Psychosomatic tendency
- Chronic anxiety in family members
- Depression in family members
- Behavior disorder of family member
- Presence of alcoholism, family violence, suicides, drug abuse

CULTURAL INFLUENCES

- General values and ethnic identity of family
- Spiritual beliefs; religious affiliation
- Language barriers; English as a second language
- Beliefs regarding health care and health professionals

✳ *Economic Assessment*

FINANCIAL RESOURCES

- Ability to perform financial responsibilities (M0160) and handle money; power of attorney to manage finances
- Ability to access preventive health care and screening
- Ability to purchase food, pay for rent and utilities
- Ability to purchase or rent equipment, supplies, and services used in the home
- Retirement income and/or effect of illness on limited or fixed income
  - Social security
  - Retirement program
  - Private pensions
  - Public assistance
- Occupation, effect of illness on work and ability to continue with the same occupation
- Programs available to assist
  - Social Security Supplement
  - Foundations
  - Churches
  - National associations
  - Voluntary agencies and support groups
  - Government grants
- Insurance for health, home, or hospital care
  - Medicare, Medicare Gap, or supplemental health insurance
  - Medicaid
  - Health maintenance organization

- Private health insurance
- Private home care insurance
- Private long-term care insurance
- Workers' compensation
- Veterans Administration
- CHAMPUS
- Catastrophic health insurance

RESOURCES FOR EQUIPMENT AND SUPPLIES

- Pharmacy and supply companies
- Home health agencies
- Home infusion and supply companies
- Durable equipment companies (purchase or rental)
- Medical supplies companies (disposable and reusable)
- Community organizations that offer medical supplies, financial assistance

❈ *Care Plans* ❈

PULMONARY SYSTEM

✳ Asthma

Asthma is an airway-reactive, obstructive pulmonary disease characterized by irritation and constriction of the bronchi and bronchioles, resulting in bronchospasms, excessive mucus production, dyspnea, and frequent wheezing, especially in acute episodes. The causes may be extrinsic (i.e., associated with allergic responses) or intrinsic (i.e., associated with stress, activity or exercise, or respiratory infection) or a combination of these.

Home care is primarily concerned with the teaching of medication regimens to prevent or control attacks, prevention of upper and lower pulmonary and sinus infections, and assistance in reducing stressors.

Primary Diagnoses:
Asthma—ICD code: 493.10
Asthma, Chronic Obstructive—ICD code: 493.20

NURSING DIAGNOSIS ANXIETY

▌**Related Factors:** Threat of death; threat to or change in health status

▌**Defining Characteristics:** Dyspnea; fear of suffocation; apprehension regarding recurrence of attacks; feelings of helplessness and tension; change in lifestyle needed to control breathing

OUTCOMES

▌**Short Term**
Reduction in anxiety, as evidenced by verbalization of anxiety and concern; relaxed posture; slower and quieter respirations; and statements that client feels better, is less anxious, is able to sleep better (expected in 2 to 7 days)

▌*Long Term*

Anxiety reduced to optimal coping capabilities, as evidenced by avoidance of physical and emotional stressors, compliance with treatment regimen with positive responses, and control of anxiety during dyspneic episodes (expected in 2 weeks and ongoing)

NURSING INTERVENTIONS/INSTRUCTIONS

1. Establish rapport and exhibit a caring, accepting attitude while client expresses anxiety and concerns about the condition, its symptomatology, its chronicity, and any perceived disability (each visit).
2. Assess mental and emotional status and effect of stressors on breathing (see Psychosocial Assessment, p.7, for guidelines) (first visit).
3. Assess client's inner personal resources and coping abilities; note reactions and responses to instructions and various treatment modalities (first visit).
4. Assist client in identification of stressors and realistic adaptation to avoiding them (first and second visits).
5. Instruct client in guided imagery and relaxation techniques and in music therapy (first and second visits).
6. Refer client to the medical social worker for counseling in coping strategies as indicated (each visit).
7. Instruct client in the importance of a measured, paced routine for all activities of daily living (ADL) and to avoid those that cause fear and uncertainty (first visit).
8. Provide continuing information about client's condition, tests, treatments, and progress; answer all questions honestly. Set up a telephone appointment to respond to these questions if information is not immediately available (each visit).
9. Initiate referral to self-help or support groups or to counseling if indicated (any visit).

CLIENT AND FAMILY/CAREGIVER INTERVENTIONS

1. Client attempts to prevent or discourage stressful situations and noxious stimuli.
2. Client practices guided imagery and visualization techniques during stressful and nonstressful episodes.
3. Client identifies present coping skills and refines or develops more effective skills to decrease anxiety.

4. Client has someone present during attack so that he or she is not alone; has telephone numbers for emergency assistance nearby and available.
5. Client asks questions about condition and reason for treatments if needed.
6. Client consults physician if unable to control anxiety and respirations are affected.
7. Client consults psychologic counselor to control breathing pattern and to reduce anxiety if necessary.

NURSING DIAGNOSIS: INEFFECTIVE AIRWAY CLEARANCE

■ *Related Factors:* Tracheobronchial secretions, obstruction

■ *Defining Characteristics:* Altered breath sounds (wheezing); changes in rate or depth of respirations; cough with or without sputum; excessive mucus; dyspnea

OUTCOMES

■ *Short Term*
Adequate oxygenation, as evidenced by respiratory rate, depth, and ease within baseline determinations; usual speech pattern; absence of dyspnea, cough, or wheezing; absence of complaints of chest tightness, pressure, or feelings of suffocation; pulse and blood pressure within preestablished baselines; airway clear of mucus, with chest clear and with normal breath sounds and air movement; skin pink, warm, and dry (expected in 1 to 2 days)

■ *Long Term*
Adequate respiratory functioning, as evidenced by breathing with optimal level of ease necessary to maintain desired or limited lifestyle (expected in 1 to 2 weeks)

NURSING INTERVENTIONS/INSTRUCTIONS

1. Assess respiratory status, rate, depth, and ease; wheezing that is more pronounced on expiration; dyspnea; difficulty in speaking; use of accessory muscles; hyperinflated appearance of chest; cough; tachycardia; diaphoresis; and factors that precipitate these signs and symptoms (see Pulmonary System Assessment, p. 8, for guidelines) (each visit).

2. Instruct client to take own respirations and pulse and record in log; allow for return demonstration (first visit).
3. Instruct client to control known allergens, noxious stimuli, emotional stressors, and environmental temperature changes (first visit).
4. Assess effect of activity on respiratory status and energy level; reinforce need to exercise moderately and regularly and to maintain activity tolerance. Instruct client to pace activities and rest if breathing is affected (first visit).
5. Instruct client in positioning during rest or sleep, generally semi-Fowler's (first visit). Evaluate effectiveness (second visit).
6. Instruct client in breathing exercises (first and second visits).
7. Instruct client to drink 2 to 3 L (2 to 3 qt or 10 to 12 glasses) of fluid daily unless restricted (first visit).
8. Administer oxygen by nasal cannula at 2 L/min as ordered, using compressed cylinder, concentrator, or liquid system; instruct client in self-administration, safety precautions, and care of equipment (each visit).
9. Instruct client in use of humidifier, incentive spirometer, nebulizer, and handheld inhaler (first visit).
10. Instruct client in use of prophylactic cromolyn bronchodilators (oral and inhalation), steroids, mucolytics, and expectorants; include dose, time, frequency, order of administration and reason, food and drug interactions, method of administration, and side effects. Instruct client to stop drug and call physician if side effects occur (first visit; reinstruct on second visit).
11. Initiate referral to respiratory therapist and durable medical equipment company as indicated (first visit).

CLIENT AND FAMILY/CAREGIVER INTERVENTIONS

1. Client and caregiver take and record rate and depth of respirations twice daily and log any changes in breathing pattern.
2. Client performs deep-breathing and physical exercise regimen daily.
3. Client uses humidifier and breathing apparatus as ordered.
4. Client and caregiver safely administer oxygen by cannula when needed.
5. Client maintains predetermined fluid intake over 24-hour period.

6. Client administers medications correctly by proper route. Client avoids taking any other drugs unless approved by physician; reports any adverse effects of medication to physician; carries bronchodilator inhaler at all times.
7. Client has laboratory tests for theophylline level when ordered.
8. Client avoids exposure to allergens and irritants, including house dust, dirty heating or air conditioning filters, pet hair, molds, pollens, and environmental pollutants; eliminates offending foods, odors, passive smoking, and other known irritants.
9. Client wears identification bracelet or carries card with information about condition, medications, and allergies.
10. Client is referred to American Lung Association and self-help groups for information and support.

NURSING DIAGNOSIS RISK FOR INFECTION

▌*Related Factors:* Inadequate primary defenses (decrease in ciliary action, stasis of body fluids); chronic disease; increased environmental exposure to infectious agents

▌*Defining Characteristics:* Inability to mobilize and remove secretions; change in sputum color and breathing pattern; temperature elevation; chest pain

OUTCOMES

▌*Short Term*

Prevention of respiratory infection, as evidenced by normal range of temperature; sputum clear, thin, and easily coughed up and removed (expected with daily assessment)

▌*Long Term*

Maintenance of a pulmonary system free of acute infection (acute bronchitis, pneumonia, influenza) (expected to be ongoing)

NURSING INTERVENTIONS/INSTRUCTIONS

1. Assess temperature for elevation; note amount and characteristics of sputum and compare with tenacious, yellowish or green or brown sputum of infectious process; auscultate lung fields for adventitious sounds (each visit).

2. Instruct client to avoid exposure to infection potential (first visit).
3. Instruct client in administration of antiinfective agents, including dose, frequency, method, route, food and drug interactions, and side effects (first visit).
4. Instruct client to examine sputum daily and in proper disposal of tissues (first visit).

CLIENT AND FAMILY/CAREGIVER INTERVENTIONS

1. Client takes temperature if feeling chilled or experiencing malaise or if sputum changes color, and reports to physician.
2. Client avoids exposure to persons with upper respiratory or pulmonary infections.
3. Client and caregiver maintain an environment that is free of irritants, is well ventilated, and is of optimal temperature and humidity.
4. Client covers mouth and nose when sneezing and coughing. Client disposes of tissues and contaminated articles in a waterproof bag; seals and disposes of properly.
5. Client washes hands as indicated to prevent transmission of infectious agents.
6. Client disinfects reusable equipment and supplies; air dries and stores in clean plastic bag.
7. Client administers prescribed antiinfective medications correctly; takes full course of medication and reports responses.

NURSING DIAGNOSIS	INEFFECTIVE THERAPEUTIC REGIMEN MANAGEMENT

▌**Related Factors:** Excessive demands made on individual; decisional conflicts

▌**Defining Characteristics:** Inappropriate choices of daily living for meeting the goals of a treatment or prevention program; verbalization that client did not take actions to include treatment regimens in daily routines or take actions to reduce risk factors for exacerbation of illness

OUTCOMES

▌Short Term

Performance of health behaviors consistent with therapeutic regimen, as evidenced by verbalization of specific behaviors needed for optimal health and prevention of complications or exacerbation of symptoms (expected in 1 week)

▌Long Term

Compliance with management of therapeutic regimen, as evidenced by active participation in therapy, demonstration of health behaviors consistent with goals of therapy, and dealing with social situations that oppose or present a conflict with regimen (expected in 1 month and ongoing)

NURSING INTERVENTIONS/INSTRUCTIONS

1. Provide client with detailed written instructions and a plan for specific behaviors, such as administering medication via oral and inhalation routes, controlling activity and environment, performing respiratory exercises, avoiding certain foods and other allergens, and taking other measures specific to client (first visit).
2. Advise client to use reminders or clues to perform or change a behavior (first visit).
3. Instruct client in monitoring behavior(s) regularly and recording for analysis and in the need for alternative behavior(s) or strengthening behavior(s) (first and second visits).
4. Instruct client in use of a structured method of performing aspects of therapeutic regimen, such as a checklist, calendar, or pill dispenser (first visit; reinforce second visit).
5. Encourage client to seek ongoing support groups for long-term opportunities to reinforce behavior(s) and to comply with regimen (any visit).

CLIENT AND FAMILY/CAREGIVER INTERVENTIONS

1. Client demonstrates accurate performance of specific health behavior(s) consistent with goals of therapeutic regimen.
2. Client engages in activities that assist in compliance with therapeutic regimen and strengthen coping ability.
3. Client uses alternative resources and support groups.
4. Client verbalizes plan to deal with situations that oppose therapeutic goals and exacerbate condition.

5. Client verbalizes, plans, performs, and records specific health-related activity, with analysis of behavior(s) to modify.

NURSING DIAGNOSIS DEFICIENT KNOWLEDGE

▌*Related Factors:* Lack of information about disease, preventive measures, relapse, or complications

▌*Defining Characteristics:* Expression of need for information about disease process, causes, risk for infection or other complications

OUTCOMES

▌*Short Term*
Beginning knowledge, as evidenced by statements of signs and symptoms of disease, causes of disease, complications of disease, and actions to take (expected in 3 to 7 days)

▌*Long Term*
Adequate knowledge, as evidenced by client's meeting requirements to achieve optimal level of health and functioning during progress to wellness (expected in 1 month)

NURSING INTERVENTIONS/INSTRUCTIONS

1. Assess lifestyle and ability to adapt, learning abilities and interests, and family participation and support (first visit).
2. Instruct client to avoid exposure to upper respiratory infections, smoking, and changes in environmental temperature (first visit).
3. Instruct client in signs, symptoms, and complications that may occur and to report them to physician (first visit).
4. Initiate referral to social services and support groups for educational materials (first visit).
5. Suggest influenza and pneumonia immunization if appropriate (last visit).

CLIENT AND FAMILY/CAREGIVER INTERVENTIONS

1. Client avoids allergens, respiratory irritants, persons with infections, and cigarette or cigar smoke.

2. Client complies with suggested physician visits for follow-up evaluation and reports any complaints.
3. Client contacts and participates in community support groups focusing on respiratory health.
4. If elderly, client secures influenza and pneumonia immunizations.

✳ *Chronic Obstructive Pulmonary Disease*

Chronic obstructive pulmonary disease (COPD) is a progressive disorder of the lungs and airways. It includes diseases such as emphysema and chronic bronchitis. The disorder is characterized by long-term destruction of the walls of the alveoli, which affects oxygen and carbon dioxide gas exchange, and by chronic inflammation and narrowing of the bronchioles, affecting air outflow. COPD is caused by smoking, air and chemical pollutants, α_1-antitrypsin deficiency, and the aging process. Changes in the respiratory system associated with the aging process, such as loss of elasticity, decreased vital capacity, and increased residual air, contribute to the prevalence and severity of the disorder.

Home care is primarily concerned with the teaching of medication regimens, which involve various routes, depending on the progression and severity of the disease; maintenance of daily well-being as the disease progresses to the end stage; and use of assistive mechanical ventilation. Emphasis is also placed on infection protection and control.

Primary Diagnoses:
Chronic Airway Obstruction—ICD code: 496.0
Obstructive Chronic Bronchitis—ICD code: 491.21
Emphysema—ICD code: 492.8

NURSING DIAGNOSIS ANXIETY

▌**Related Factors:** Threat of death; change in health status

▌**Defining Characteristics:** Apprehension; uncertainty about outcome; fear of suffocation; increased helplessness and tension

OUTCOMES

▌**Short Term**
Reduction in anxiety level, as evidenced by verbalization of anxiety and concerns and their causes; anxiety reduced and within manageable level during dyspneic episodes (expected in 2 days)

▌**Long Term**
Anxiety controlled, as evidenced by avoidance of anxiety-producing situations and by positive responses to therapy (expected in 1 month)

NURSING INTERVENTIONS/INSTRUCTIONS

1. Assess mental and emotional status and effect of stressors on breathing and lifestyle; inner personal resources and ability to cope and respond to treatment; environment for excessive stimuli (first visit).
2. Provide an accepting environment for expression of anxiety and concerns (each visit).
3. Identify coping mechanisms used by client and encourage client to use those that are effective (each visit).
4. Instruct client in relaxation techniques, music, guided imagery, and the use of autogenic technique during periods of dyspnea (first and second visits).
5. Refer client to medical social worker for counseling of coping strategies as indicated (each visit).
6. Instruct client to avoid stressful situations, excessive activity, and medications that are taken for anxiety that affect respiration (first visit).
7. Provide client with continuing information about status or condition, improvements, and treatments, and answer all questions (each visit).
8. Initiate referral to counseling or psychotherapy as indicated (any visit).

CLIENT AND FAMILY/CAREGIVER INTERVENTIONS

1. Caregiver maintains calm, caring attitude during episodes of dyspnea; stays with client.
2. Client attempts to prevent or discourage stressful situations.
3. Client develops and uses effective coping skills that decrease anxiety.
4. Client asks questions about medications, equipment, or the disease when information is needed.
5. Client adapts to chronic illness and long-term treatments.
6. Client seeks assistance from psychotherapist to manage anxiety.
7. Client consults physician if unable to control anxiety and respiration is affected.

NURSING DIAGNOSIS INEFFECTIVE BREATHING PATTERN

▋*Related Factors:* Anxiety; decreased energy; fatigue; decreased lung expansion; tracheobronchial obstruction

▋*Defining Characteristics:* Dyspnea; tachypnea; cough with or without sputum; changes in rate and depth of respiration; use of accessory muscles; altered chest excursion; crackles, rhonchi; assumption of three-point position; prolonged expiratory phase; increased anteroposterior diameter of chest; abnormal arterial blood gas levels

OUTCOMES

▋*Short Term*
Return to adequate breathing pattern and airway clearance, as evidenced by satisfactory respiratory rate, ease, and depth at baseline and by reduction in dyspneic episodes, hypoxia, stasis of secretions, and abnormal breath sounds (expected in 1 to 2 days)

▋*Long Term*
Maintenance of respiratory baselines, as evidenced by breathing at optimal level within disease parameters (expected in 1 month)

NURSING INTERVENTIONS/INSTRUCTIONS

1. Assess respiratory status, including rate, depth, and ease; presence of dyspnea; use of accessory muscles, with lengthened

expiratory phase; energy and fatigue level; ability to mobilize and remove secretions by coughing; breath sounds on auscultation for crackles or wheezes; hyperresonance on percussion; tactile fremitus (see Pulmonary System Assessment, p. 8, for guidelines) (each visit).

2. Provide postural drainage using gravity and percussion, avoiding any positions that may compromise the elderly client (first visit and as needed).

3. Instruct client to drink 2 to 3 L (2 to 3 qt or 10 to 12 glasses) of fluids per day, unless restricted, and to follow an activity regimen within tolerance level (first visit).

4. Demonstrate for client and instruct client in deep-breathing and coughing exercises, with pursed lip breathing and abdominal breathing (first visit).

5. Inform client of positions for sleeping that will allow for ease in breathing and chest expansion (first visit).

6. Instruct client in administration of oral bronchodilators, use of small-volume nebulizer and handheld measured-dose inhaler (carry at all times), and administration of corticosteroids orally and by handheld measured-dose inhaler (first visit).

7. Instruct client in oxygen administration via nasal cannula from compressed cylinder, concentrator, or liquid oxygen system (first and second visits).

8. Encourage client in continued participation in pulmonary rehabilitation program at home (first visit).

9. Initiate referral to respiratory therapist and durable medical equipment agency (first visit).

10. Instruct client to cease smoking and to enter program for support if necessary (first visit).

11. Draw blood sample, or advise client to visit laboratory, for theophylline-level check when ordered by physician (each visit).

12. Report to physician dyspnea not controlled by medication, inability to clear secretions from airway, confusion, or change in mentation (each visit).

13. Instruct client to wear identification bracelet or carry card in purse or wallet stating condition and medications (first visit).

14. Instruct client to contact American Lung Association for information and support services (first visit).

CLIENT AND FAMILY/CAREGIVER INTERVENTIONS

1. Client or caregiver assesses respiration for rate and ease twice daily.
2. Client performs deep-breathing exercises, four breaths four times per day.
3. Client performs isometric exercises to strengthen diaphragm and intercostal muscles and lifts 3-pound weights for upper body strengthening daily as part of a pulmonary rehabilitation regimen, which should also include swimming, walking, or bicycling.
4. Client maintains fluid intake of 10 to 12 glasses per day unless restricted.
5. Client uses positioning and formatter wedge or pillows for sleeping.
6. Client administers medications correctly; avoids over-the-counter drugs unless advised by physician; and reports adverse effects to physician.
7. Client or caregiver administers oxygen correctly at 2 to 3 L/min (portable and stationary) and takes safety precautions in the presence of oxygen.
8. Client avoids exposure to outside and home pollutants, such as sprays, fumes, smog or particulates in air; pet hair; or other allergens.
9. Client uses humidification in home and changes air conditioner and furnace filters monthly. (Humidification unit and filter should be cleaned weekly.)

NURSING DIAGNOSIS ACTIVITY INTOLERANCE

▌*Related Factors:* Generalized weakness; sedentary lifestyle; imbalance between oxygen supply and demand

▌*Defining Characteristics:* Tired, weak feeling; fatigue; exertional discomfort and dyspnea; awakening caused by dyspnea; hypoxia; increased pulse rate and blood pressure during activity

OUTCOMES

▌*Short Term*
Increased endurance and ability to perform ADL, as evidenced by maintenance of respiration, pulse, and blood pressure while

independently caring for self and performing routine tasks (expected in 1 week)

▌*Long Term*
Optimal activity level achieved and maintained within baseline respiratory and energy parameters (expected to be ongoing)

NURSING INTERVENTIONS/INSTRUCTIONS

1. Assess activity tolerance, pulse, and respirations before and after activity; assess for presence of dyspnea and increased work of breathing during activity; assess amount of sleep and rest (first visit).
2. Refer client to occupational therapist for assistance with energy-conservation upper body conditioning as indicated (first visit).
3. Instruct client to rest after each activity and to pace activities around rest periods and use of bronchodilator (first visit).
4. Instruct client to use oxygen during activities if appropriate (first visit).
5. Instruct client in use of energy-saving devices and aids (first and second visits).
6. Instruct client to build endurance by increasing activities every 2 to 3 days (each visit).
7. Arrange for home health aide (HHA) visits to assist with ADL (first visit).

CLIENT AND FAMILY/CAREGIVER INTERVENTIONS

1. Client exercises moderately and for short periods, as tolerated, and increases as energy and endurance increase.
2. Client takes pulse before and after activity; checks for increases of 10 or more beats/min.
3. Client rests every 3 hours and following activity such as bathing, walking, or using stairs.
4. Client uses stool to sit in shower, arm rests, aids for dressing, hand bars for support, aids for reaching and walking, and wheelchair if necessary.
5. Client uses inhaler before activity; performs activity when systemic bronchodilator is at optimal effect.
6. Client asks for assistance in ADL.
7. Client uses proper inspiration and expiration pattern when participating in an activity, such as lifting during expiration.
8. Client avoids continuing activity if dyspneic or fatigued.

NURSING DIAGNOSIS RISK FOR INFECTION

▌*Related Factors:* Inadequate primary defenses; chronic disease

▌*Defining Characteristics:* Stasis of secretions; inability to mobilize and remove secretions; loss of ciliary action; reduction of pulmonary macrophages

OUTCOMES

▌*Short Term*
Prevention of pulmonary infection, as evidenced by normal temperature and sputum that is clear and thin for easy removal (expected with daily assessment)

▌*Long Term*
Maintenance of pulmonary system free from acute infection (expected to be ongoing)

NURSING INTERVENTIONS/INSTRUCTIONS

1. Assess for temperature elevation, chest pain, change in color of sputum to yellow or green, and increased viscosity (each visit).
2. Instruct client in antibiotic administration (first visit).
3. Instruct client to examine sputum daily and to report changes in color and symptoms to physician (first visit).
4. Inform client of precautions to take to avoid exposure to potential infection (first visit).

CLIENT AND FAMILY/CAREGIVER INTERVENTIONS

1. Client takes temperature if feeling chilled and sputum changes color.
2. Client avoids smoking and exposure to groups or to persons with upper respiratory infections.
3. Client washes hands frequently, especially before treatments or eating and after using tissues for coughing and expectorating.
4. Client covers nose and mouth when coughing; disposes of tissues in bag that is waterproof; seals and discards daily.
5. Client and caregiver maintain environment that is humidified and well ventilated.
6. Client secures pneumonia and flu immunizations.

7. Client washes, rinses, and disinfects reusable equipment and supplies; air dries on clean towel or hangs over shower rail.
8. Client discards disposable supplies in sealed waterproof bag.
9. Client reports temperature elevation, chills, yellow or green sputum, or chest pain to physician.
10. Client takes prescribed antibiotics at proper intervals around the clock until all are used.

NURSING DIAGNOSIS DEFICIENT KNOWLEDGE

■ **Related Factors:** Lack of information about disease or complications

■ **Defining Characteristics:** Expression of need for information about disease process, causes, risk for infection, or other complications

OUTCOMES

■ **Short Term**
Adequate knowledge, as evidenced by statements of signs and symptoms of disease, causes of disease, complications of disease, and actions to take (expected in 3 to 7 days)

■ **Long Term**
Optimal knowledge, as evidenced by client's meeting requirements to achieve optimal level of health and functioning during progress to wellness (expected in 1 month)

NURSING INTERVENTIONS/INSTRUCTIONS

1. Assess lifestyle and ability to adapt, learning abilities and interests, and family participation and support (first visit).
2. Instruct client to avoid exposure to upper respiratory infections, smoking, and changes in environmental temperature (first visit).
3. Instruct client in signs, symptoms, and complications that may occur and to report them to physician (first visit).
4. Initiate referral to social services and support groups for educational materials and smoking cessation assistance (first visit).
5. Suggest influenza and pneumonia immunization if appropriate (last visit).

CLIENT AND FAMILY/CAREGIVER INTERVENTIONS

1. Client avoids respiratory irritants, persons with infections, and cigarette or cigar smoke.
2. Client complies with suggested physician visits for follow-up evaluation and reports any complaints.
3. Client contacts and participates in community support groups focusing on respiratory health.
4. If elderly, client secures influenza and pneumonia immunizations.

✳ *Pneumonia*

Pneumonia is an inflammation of the lungs caused by bacteria, viruses, fungi, or protozoa. It may also be caused by aspiration of food, water, or gastric contents into the alveolar system. It is usually the result of an upper respiratory infection and may involve segments of, a lobe of, or an entire lung. The disease progresses from an initial filling of the alveoli and bronchioles with exudate, to consolidation of the lung area as leukocytes attempt to destroy the organisms. The disease is especially life threatening in the elderly or chronically ill.

Home care is primarily concerned with the teaching of medication regimens (antiinfective agents based on identified causative pathogen) and prevention of complications.

> Primary Diagnoses:
> Pneumonia—ICD code: 486.0
> Aspiration Pneumonia—ICD code: 507.0

NURSING DIAGNOSIS | INEFFECTIVE BREATHING PATTERN

■ *Related Factors:* Chest pain; hypoventilation; decreased energy; fatigue; inflammatory process; tracheobronchial obstruction

■ *Defining Characteristics:* Dyspnea; tachypnea; respiratory depth changes; altered chest excursion; diminished breath sounds; cough with tenacious, purulent sputum; abnormal arterial blood gas values

OUTCOMES

▌*Short Term*
Adequate oxygenation, as evidenced by respiratory rate, depth, and ease within normal baseline determinations; absence of dyspnea; cough less frequent; chest clear with normal breath sounds and air movement (expected in 7 to 10 days)

▌*Long Term*
Adequate respiratory functioning, as evidenced by breathing with optimal level of ease to maintain usual lifestyle (expected in 1 month)

NURSING INTERVENTIONS/INSTRUCTIONS

1. Assess physical status of respiratory system (see Pulmonary System Assessment, p. 8 for guidelines); note lifestyle, history, and trends (e.g., frequent upper respiratory infections, chronic respiratory disease, chronic illness, smoking, alcoholism, immunosuppressive therapy) to identify predisposing factors and to determine their implications for care and future teaching (first visit).

2. Monitor respirations for ease, rate, and depth; auscultate and percuss chest for diminished breath sounds and dullness (each visit). Instruct client to take respirations and record in log (first visit).

3. Assess skin color, constitutional symptoms, chills and fever, and pleuritic chest pain, and note sputum and its viscosity, amount, and change in color (each visit).

4. Assess fluid maintenance needs based on age, weight and height, sex, general health, and insensible fluid losses. Instruct client to double fluid maintenance unless his or her status would be compromised (as with an elderly client or a client who has a cardiac or renal disorder) (first visit).

5. Note allergies to medications and instruct client in antiinfective and bronchodilation therapy, including dose, frequency, food or drug interactions, and side effects (first visit).

6. Instruct client in chest physiotherapy, splinting, deep-breathing and coughing exercises, and how to expectorate; allow for return demonstration (each visit).

7. Monitor sputum culture and x-ray results as available (each visit). Teach client to monitor own sputum (first visit).

8. Refer client to respiratory therapy as indicated (first visit).

9. Instruct client to avoid indiscriminate or trivial use of antibiotics (last visit).
10. Suggest visit to physician for influenza and pneumonia immunizations, especially if client is elderly (last visit).

CLIENT AND FAMILY/CAREGIVER INTERVENTIONS

1. Client takes respirations and records in log.
2. Client monitors sputum (not saliva) and reports to physician changes in color, amount, or consistency.
3. Client administers antiinfective, antitussive, and expectorant as ordered and takes complete course of antiinfective prescription.
4. Client drinks predetermined amount of liquid at specified intervals over 24-hour period.
5. Client and caregiver humidify environment and maintain optimal temperature and ventilation of environment.
6. Client performs deep-breathing and coughing exercises three to four times per day as tolerated.
7. Client disposes of used tissues properly and washes hands as appropriate.

NURSING DIAGNOSIS HYPERTHERMIA

❚ Related Factors: Illness

❚ Defining Characteristics: Increase in body temperature above normal range; increased respiratory rate

OUTCOMES

❚ Short Term
Absence of temperature elevation, as evidenced by normal temperature and absence of chills, shaking, or diaphoresis (expected in 3 to 4 days)

❚ Long Term
Afebrile; comfort at optimal level without recurrence of temperature elevation (expected in 1 week to 1 month)

NURSING INTERVENTIONS/INSTRUCTIONS

1. Monitor temperature for deviations from normal and instruct client to take own temperature and record in log and to return demonstration (first visit).

2. Assess for presence of chills and diaphoresis with temperature elevation (each visit).
3. Supervise administration of antiinfective medications (first visit; reinstruct on second visit).
4. Instruct client in administration of antipyretics based on temperature elevation (first visit).
5. Instruct client in use of sponge bath and appropriate clothing and room temperature for comfort (first visit).
6. As temperature decreases, monitor white blood cell count and sputum culture results if available (each visit).

CLIENT AND FAMILY/CAREGIVER INTERVENTIONS

1. Client takes temperature twice daily, when feeling chilled or as needed, and records in log.
2. Client takes antipyretics correctly.
3. Client maintains increased fluid intake unless restricted.
4. Client bathes by sponging or tub bath; maintains dry linens and room free of drafts at comfortable temperature and ventilation.

NURSING DIAGNOSIS ACUTE PAIN

Related Factors: Injuring agent of inflammatory process

Defining Characteristics: Verbal expression of pain descriptors; holding chest to guard or protect it; changes in respiratory pattern

OUTCOMES

Short Term
Control of pain, as evidenced by relaxed expression and posture, effortless respiration, and statements that pain has been relieved (expected in 2 to 7 days)

Long Term
Optimal comfort level, as evidenced by continued freedom from pain during respiration or ADL (expected in 1 week to 1 month)

NURSING INTERVENTIONS/INSTRUCTIONS

1. Assess pain location, frequency, severity, and characteristics and its relationship to condition and activity (each visit).

2. Instruct client in proper splinting (position, comfort, aids) before coughing and deep-breathing exercises (first visit).
3. Instruct client in administration of mild analgesic 30 minutes to 1 hour before pulmonary exercises and before pain becomes severe (first visit).
4. Encourage rest periods and pacing of activities (first visit).

CLIENT AND FAMILY/CAREGIVER INTERVENTIONS

1. Caregiver provides rest; assists with ADL.
2. Client administers analgesic correctly; avoids use if it affects respiration.
3. Client schedules activities around medication administration.
4. Client notifies physician if pain persists or symptoms escalate.
5. Client paces activities; rests when needed.

NURSING DIAGNOSIS   RISK FOR ACTIVITY INTOLERANCE

▮ *Related Factors:* Presence of respiratory disease; deconditioned status; work of breathing (weakness, fatigue)

▮ *Defining Characteristics:* Weakness; fatigue; inability to perform ADL

OUTCOMES

▮ *Short Term*
Minimal fatigue expressed and activity tolerance increased, as measured by increasing periods of wakefulness and progressive ability to perform ADL without fatigue (expected in 1 week)

▮ *Long Term*
Independence in return to self-care, as evidenced by optimal level of care achieved and return to wellness (expected in 1 month)

NURSING INTERVENTIONS/INSTRUCTIONS

1. Obtain history, including ADL, levels of independence and endurance, and family assistance and support (first visit).
2. Instruct client in performing personal hygiene and comfort measures; stress accessibility to personal items needed for care; and instruct to ask for assistance when needed (first visit).
3. Provide privacy, encourage rest, and instruct client to progressively increase activity at own pace (first and second visits).

4. Instruct client to exercise moderately for short periods as tolerated (first visit).
5. Refer client to occupational therapy for energy conservation as indicated (first visit).

CLIENT AND FAMILY/CAREGIVER INTERVENTIONS

1. Client performs daily personal care with assistance or independently as able, without rushing and at a tolerable pace.
2. Client schedules periods of activity and rest based on endurance and individual need.
3. Client uses services of the occupational therapist.

NURSING DIAGNOSIS DEFICIENT KNOWLEDGE

■ **Related Factors:** Lack of information about disease, preventive measures, relapse, or complications

■ **Defining Characteristics:** Expression of need for information about disease process, causes, risk for reinfection, or other complications

OUTCOMES

■ **Short Term**
Adequate knowledge, as evidenced by statements of signs and symptoms of disease, transmission and causes of disease, complications of disease, and actions to take (expected in 3 to 7 days)

■ **Long Term**
Adequate knowledge, as evidenced by client's meeting requirements to achieve optimal level of health and functioning during progress to wellness (expected in 1 month)

NURSING INTERVENTIONS/INSTRUCTIONS

1. Assess lifestyle and ability to adapt, learning abilities and interests, and family participation and support (first visit).
2. Instruct client to avoid exposure to upper respiratory infections, smoking, and changes in environmental temperature (first visit).
3. Instruct client in signs, symptoms, and complications that may occur (e.g., chest pain, dyspnea, persistent elevated temperature) and to report them to physician (first visit).

4. Initiate referral to social services and support groups for educational materials and smoking cessation assistance (first visit).
5. Suggest influenza and pneumonia immunization if appropriate (last visit).

CLIENT AND FAMILY/CAREGIVER INTERVENTIONS

1. Client avoids respiratory irritants, persons with infections, and cigarette or cigar smoke.
2. Client complies with suggested physician visits for follow-up evaluation and reports any complaints.
3. Client contacts and participates in community support groups focusing on respiratory health.
4. If elderly, client secures influenza and pneumonia immunizations.

✳ *Mechanical Ventilation/Tracheostomy*

Mechanical ventilation is a method of applying intermittent or continuous ventilation to support inflation of the lungs. It can provide temporary or permanent assistance to take over the action of the diaphragm and chest wall muscles. Clients with neuromuscular, skeletal, or hypoventilation conditions are candidates for part-time or continuous, 24-hour assisted ventilation, depending on the status or severity of the disease. Negative-pressure devices are applied to the outside of the chest wall to pull it out and to initiate inspiration to allow respiratory muscles to rest. Positive-pressure ventilators increase airway pressure above atmospheric pressure to inflate the lungs by pushing a volume of air into the lungs during inspiration, and they improve gas exchange by better distribution of gases in the lung. They can be invasive (e.g., artificial airway such as a tracheostomy tube) or noninvasive (e.g., facial or nasal mask). Positive-pressure ventilators are the most common type of ventilators used in the home and are small, portable, and easily moved in the environment. The type of ventilator selected depends on the medical diagnosis and is based on regulating the cycle (pressure, volume, and time cycled) before the client is discharged from the hospital; on daily requirements; on needed oxygen concentration; and on resources to acquire, maintain, and repair the equipment.

A tracheostomy is a surgically created opening in the skin of the neck and into the trachea (between the second and fourth tracheal cartilage rings) to allow for passage of air in and out of the airways. It is performed when upper airway obstruction is present (e.g., infections, edema, tumor, foreign body); in cases of underlying pulmonary disease; following lung, larynx, neck, or cardiac surgery; or in conditions that require long-term assisted ventilation. It can be temporary, or it can be permanent, depending on the underlying disease process. Tracheostomy tubes are made of plastic or metal (nondisposable) and consist of an inner and an outer cannula. The tubes can be cuffed or without a cuff and have a fenestration for those who are able to speak when off the ventilator.

Home care is primarily concerned with total management of the client who is ventilator dependent and the various levels of interventions needed to preserve respiratory status and to support the psychophysiologic adaptive capacities of the client and family. The assessment and instruction in the management of tracheostomy care with prevention of skin, tube, or infection complications (e.g., patent inner cannula, change of tube, stoma care, inflation of cuff); ventilator monitoring (e.g., settings, alarms, patency and cleanliness of circuitry, troubleshooting); and ADL and special needs (e.g., alternate feeding pattern, urinary catheter, ambulation, other activities) is essential. Of additional importance is the ability and capacity of the family to become trained and to participate in the total care of the client who is technology dependent.

> Primary Diagnoses:
> Vary According to Underlying Disease Process
> Mechanical Ventilation—ICD code: 96.7

NURSING DIAGNOSIS ANXIETY/FEAR (CLIENT AND FAMILY)

Related Factors: Change in health status; presence of ventilator and tracheostomy; threat of death; threatening situations (tube obstruction or accidental dislodgment, ventilator dysfunction)

Defining Characteristics: Difficulty breathing; fear of suffocation; apprehension; restlessness; facial tension; inability to speak; fear of responsibility of providing tracheostomy care

OUTCOMES

Short Term
Progressive reduction in anxiety and fear associated with care of tracheostomy, as evidenced by verbalizing increased ability to remain calm and by acquaintance with and competence in care measures as needed (expected in 2 to 4 weeks)

Long Term
Fear and anxiety at a manageable level, as evidenced by effective and ongoing support and performance of adequate care required for ventilator and tracheostomy (expected in 1 month and ongoing)

NURSING INTERVENTIONS/INSTRUCTIONS

1. Assess emotional and mental status of client and family members; their ability to adapt to the presence of assisted ventilation/tracheostomy; and their anxiety, fear, and concerns about care (see Psychosocial Assessment, p. 7, for guidelines) (first visit and any visit as needed).

2. Provide information about reasons for assisted ventilation, inform client and family of treatments and procedures involved in home management and how the client's safety and comfort will be facilitated; use easily understandable language (first and second visits).

3. Maintain a calm, quiet environment. Comfort client who is fearful when unable to produce sounds and inform that voice will return when the tube is removed, if temporary and if speech rehabilitation is provided, or when off ventilator, as appropriate (first visit).

4. Provide opportunity for family and/or caregiver to verbalize fears and concerns; encourage alternative modes of communication to replace lack of vocal sounds (each visit).

5. Suggest that caregiver stay with client during anxious times (first visit).

6. Assist caregiver to reduce feelings of apprehension, anxiety, and fear about the client's condition (each visit).

7. Provide link of communication between family and health professional referrals for information and problem solving (any visit as needed).

8. Initiate referral to a support group or community agency or to counseling as appropriate (any visit).
9. Refer to medical social worker for coping strategies, as indicated.

CLIENT AND FAMILY/CAREGIVER INTERVENTIONS

1. Client and family recognize anxiety associated with care of ventilator/tracheostomy and possibility of tube obstruction or other complications.
2. Client and family verbalize anxiety, frustration, fatigue, and stress related to management of total care.
3. Client and family maintain calm, supportive environment and control stimuli.
4. Client and family use relaxation techniques such as music, television watching, reading, and imaging.
5. Client and family use appropriate coping mechanisms and support resources if needed.

| NURSING DIAGNOSIS | INEFFECTIVE BREATHING PATTERN/AIRWAY CLEARANCE, IMPAIRED GAS EXCHANGE, RISK FOR ASPIRATION |

Related Factors: Decreased energy; fatigue; tracheobronchial obstruction (thick mucus); altered oxygen supply; loss of lung function; inflammatory/infectious process; decreased lung expansion; presence of tracheostomy tube; impaired swallowing

Defining Characteristics: Dyspnea; tachypnea; use of accessory muscles (retractions); nasal flaring; grunting; cyanosis ("dusky" skin color); tachycardia; irritability; diaphoresis; elevated temperature; restlessness; abnormal breath sounds (crackles, rhonchi); inability to clear increased thick secretions; hypoxia; hypercapnia; elevated peak inspiratory pressure on ventilator or ventilator asynchrony; inability or refusal to remove and clean tube

OUTCOMES

Short Term
Optimal ventilator function and airway patency with adequate ventilation (caregiver response to alarms) and oxygenation (deter-

mined by pulse oximetry) via tracheostomy, as established and evidenced by clearance or removal of loosened secretions by cough or suction; prevention of tube dislodgment; maintenance of skin and mucous membrane color based on racial baseline parameters with absence of hypoxia; breath sounds clear and equal bilaterally; and adequate rest, sleep, relaxation, and comfort (expected in 2 days and ongoing)

▌*Long Term*

Management of home respiratory care, as evidenced by respiratory baselines and gas exchange maintained with ventilator; absence of signs of respiratory distress with clear breath sounds; absence of injury associated with tracheostomy; complete and effective tracheostomy care demonstrated; progressive withdrawal of oxygen and/or ventilation support when and if appropriate (expected in 1 month and ongoing)

NURSING INTERVENTIONS/INSTRUCTIONS

1. Explain importance of and ensure that caregiver has been trained in cardiopulmonary resuscitation (CPR) before hospital discharge; collaborate with caregiver to develop a protocol to activate emergency medical service (first visit; reinforce on subsequent visits).

2. Assess caregiver knowledge and understanding of disease etiology of client's status and need for assisted ventilation, and of his or her ability to adapt and manage ventilator and care of tracheostomy (first visit; continue on second visit).

3. Provide information and instruction in pulmonary assessment and signs and symptoms to note and collaborate with caregiver to plan daily care based on respiratory status; use language that is easily understood or provide written instructions (first visit; reinstruct in plan changes as needed).

4. Assess and instruct caregiver to assess and monitor client's respiratory status for distress and chest expansion for symmetry, counting respiratory rate with ventilator cycle and client's respiratory efforts, including absence or presence of effort, depth, and normal rate and rhythm, to determine effectiveness of assisted ventilation and if settings need changing; include color of skin, oral mucous membranes, and nail beds for hypoxia; abnormal breath sounds on auscultation; and presence and characteristics of secretions in assessment (see Pulmonary System Assessment, p. 8, for guidelines) (every visit).

5. Assess client comfort on ventilator and follow orders for settings of rate, control or assist/control mode, tidal and sigh volume, fraction of inspired oxygen, peak flow, and pressure limits; note stability of these parameters (each visit).

6. Assess and instruct caregiver to assess all ventilator connections, settings, alarms, and function daily and to monitor for possible need of changes in ventilatory settings if infection or other stressors are present (first and every visit).

7. Instruct client in how to become synchronous with the ventilator; inform caregiver to stay with client and to provide emotional support when anxious (first visit; repeat on second visit).

8. Instruct caregiver in the daily cleaning and changing of the circuits, the machine, the suctioning equipment and supplies, and the resuscitation bag (first visit; reinstruct on second visit and as needed).

9. Administer and assist and instruct caregiver in providing supplemental humidified oxygen with ventilator via tracheostomy based on ordered pressure input and flow rate requirements of the ventilator and portability and availability of the oxygen system; advise caregiver to have a portable oxygen unit and resuscitation bag available (first and second visits).

10. Instruct client and caregiver in safety measures in use of oxygen (first visit).

11. Instruct caregiver to humidify inspired air by cascade, jet nebulizer, or humidifier to prevent drying of secretions and loss of body fluids and heat (first visit).

12. Instruct client and caregiver in medication administration ordered in conjunction with ventilation therapy (first visit; each visit as needed).

13. Instruct caregiver in tracheostomy tube care, including changing and cleaning of inner tracheostomy tube and ties, performing the procedure for tube removal, cleansing and disinfecting, and reinserting to remove mucus accumulation and to maintain airway patency (first visit; subsequent visits as needed).

14. Instruct caregiver in suctioning of secretions using clean technique if client is unable to remove by coughing. Instruction will emphasize the use of the correct amount of pressure, the correct number of thrusts for the appropriate amount of time for each thrust, and the use of resuscitation bag to preoxygenate and

oxygenate between each suctioning event (first visit; subsequent visits based on auscultation or sounds of gurgling).

15. Instruct client and caregiver to assess for possible tube dislodgment or decannulation and measures to take to secure tube by adjusting ties; assist in devising an emergency kit containing an extra tube, clean ties, suction tube, and scissors to keep on hand and nearby (first and second visits).

16. Instruct client and caregiver in deflation of cuff when off the ventilator and during food ingestion and in reinflation of cuff when on the ventilator (first and second visits).

17. Instruct caregiver to offer small amounts of easy-to-swallow food and to place client in upright position during meals to prevent aspiration or to perform nasogastric feedings as appropriate (first visit).

18. Demonstrate elevation of the head of the bed and positions of optimal comfort for sleeping and resting that will allow for diaphragmatic movement and chest expansion (first visit).

19. Provide information and instruction using language that is easily understood and provide written instructions and care plan (first visit; reinforce regularly).

20. Assess response to ventilatory assistance and tracheostomy status, and report to the physician untoward responses or any deviations from the established norm (each visit).

21. Suggest client wear loose, nonrestrictive clothing near neck (first visit).

22. Inform caregiver and family of availability of American Lung Association and local support groups for information and services (first visit).

CLIENT AND FAMILY/CAREGIVER INTERVENTIONS

1. Caregiver becomes CPR certified before client's discharge from hospital, obtains training in emergency procedures associated with ventilator, and places list of emergency activities and telephone numbers in strategic place for easy access.

2. Caregiver completes training or classes in all aspects of care before independent care of client receiving assisted ventilation.

3. Caregiver locates a resource and acquires special equipment and supplies (e.g., oxygen source and back-up tank with gauge, ventilator and accessories, suctioning equipment and supplies, extra tracheostomy tubes, ties, dressings); collaborates with social services to secure financial assistance if needed.

4. Caregiver develops trust in home care providers (nurse, respiratory therapist, nursing assistant) and confidence in own competence in managing total care.

5. Caregiver verbalizes understanding and rationale for physical care, airway management, treatments and procedures, and need for constant monitoring.

6. Caregiver assesses respirations for rate and effort compared with ventilator effectiveness, client's color during suctioning, and signs of respiratory distress or deterioration to report.

7. Caregiver demonstrates maintenance of ventilator function using ventilator checklist; complies with treatments, monitoring schedules, and equipment care and cleaning.

8. Caregiver correctly administers humidified oxygen (continuous or intermittent) and uses resuscitation bag when needed; provides adequate humidification to airway by increasing humidity to environment.

9. Caregiver follows safety precautions in oxygen use, including posting a sign stating oxygen in use, no sparks, no open flames, no oil or grease, no smoking.

10. Caregiver reviews potential nonmedical problem solving or troubleshooting of equipment malfunction, management of ventilator settings, and alarms outlined in the manufacturer's guidelines and corrective actions to take.

11. Caregiver provides tracheostomy tube care, removes ties and tube, cleanses with soapy water and pipe cleaners and rinses with water, reinserts, and secures in place with clean ties; inflates or deflates cuff as appropriate.

12. Caregiver suctions tracheostomy at correct pressure and length of time as frequently as needed using clean technique to remove thick mucus or mucus that is difficult to cough up or if respiratory status changes as a result of airway obstruction caused by mucus accumulation.

13. Caregiver cleanses reusable suction catheter and tracheostomy tube with soap and water and stores in clean plastic bags.

14. Caregiver ensures availability of portable suction apparatus by keeping on hand back-up batteries, portable oxygen tank, and resuscitation bag.

15. Caregiver positions client with formatter wedge or pillows to elevate head for sleep and rest; reports change in mentation or orientation following naps or changes in sleep patterns caused by hypercapnia.

16. Caregiver provides rest before frequent small high-calorie meals.
17. Client complies with ordered medication regimen.
18. Caregiver provides oral care for mouth dryness and comfort.
19. Caregiver and client make list of questions to ask for each home care visit.
20. Caregiver identifies any deterioration in respiratory status and reports to physician in a timely manner.
21. Caregiver notifies local power company and emergency services of client on ventilator.
22. Caregiver uses emergency services when life-threatening changes occur and cannot be resolved.

NURSING DIAGNOSIS RISK FOR INFECTION

▌Related Factors: Inadequate primary defenses (stasis of secretions); invasive procedure (tracheostomy); insufficient knowledge of caregiver to avoid exposure of client to pathogens

▌Defining Characteristics: Ineffective cough to remove secretions; change in odor and color of secretions from tracheostomy to yellow or green; increased secretions; temperature elevation; abnormal breath sounds

OUTCOMES

▌Short Term
Early detection of signs and symptoms of respiratory infection and use of clean technique to perform procedures, as evidenced by airway patency with colorless and odorless secretions removed and by afebrile status (expected with daily assessment)

▌Long Term
Adaptation to a lifestyle that promotes a clean, safe environment and preventive measures performed to minimize risk for pulmonary infections, as evidenced by patent, infection-free respiratory system (expected to be ongoing)

NURSING INTERVENTIONS/INSTRUCTIONS

1. Assess home and living hygienic conditions (see Environmental Assessment, p. 57, for guidelines) (first visit; follow-up for additional modifications on second visit).

2. Assess for changes in respiratory status, for diminished breath sounds on auscultation, and for changes in oxygen saturation (each visit).
3. Assess temperature for increases or decreases from baseline norm, increased viscosity, and change in color or odor of secretions from tracheostomy that indicate pulmonary infection (each visit).
4. Instruct caregiver in taking axillary temperature (first visit).
5. Instruct caregiver in washing hands and importance of washing hands before and after care (first visit).
6. Instruct caregiver in use of clean technique during tracheostomy suctioning procedure, cleansing tube, and changing dressing (first visit; review on subsequent visits).
7. Instruct caregiver in administration of ordered prophylactic or therapy and in responses to expect with oral antibiotic and antipyretic in proper form based on ability to swallow (first visit; reinforce on subsequent visits).
8. Instruct client and caregiver in precautions to prevent infection, such as washing hands and avoiding contact with those who have an upper respiratory infection, and in the importance of adequate nutritional intake and rest (first visit and ongoing).
9. Obtain sputum specimen, if possible, for culture if ordered (any visit).

CLIENT AND FAMILY/CAREGIVER INTERVENTIONS

1. Caregiver observes for yellow or green color, foul odor, or increased amount of sputum from tube, or any blood from the tube, and reports changes to the physician.
2. Caregiver suctions the tracheostomy using clean technique at correct suction pressure and length of time to prevent stasis if mucus is copious or thick.
3. Client or caregiver takes axillary temperature if sputum color or respirations change and reports elevations specified by physician.
4. Caregiver administers oral antibiotic therapy correctly until all medication is taken; notes and reports side effects.
5. Caregiver maintains personal hygiene, avoids use of contaminated articles when performing care, and avoids possible exposure of client to family members or others with suspected upper respiratory infections; wears face mask if appropriate.

6. Caregiver washes hands properly, especially before caring for client; uses clean technique during care and procedures; and washes and stores supplies appropriately.
7. Caregiver properly disposes of all articles and supplies according to standard precautions.

NURSING DIAGNOSIS RISK FOR IMPAIRED SKIN INTEGRITY

❚Related Factors: External factor of irritants (secretions); mechanical pressure of tracheostomy tube

❚Defining characteristics: Moisture caused by secretions; irritation, excoriation, or damage of peristomal skin or tissue around tube insertion site; redness and accumulation of crusting at site

OUTCOMES

❚Short Term
Skin at tracheostomy site dry and intact, as evidenced by absence of redness, irritation, bleeding, and pressure resulting from tube movement during care (expected in 1 to 2 days)

❚Long Term
Optimal skin integrity maintained, as evidenced by absence of any abnormal color, irritants, bleeding and breakdown at tracheostomy tube site, and stenosis or strictures at the stoma site (expected in 1 week and ongoing)

NURSING INTERVENTIONS/INSTRUCTIONS

1. Assess skin at tube site for signs indicating risk for breakdown, such as excessive moisture, irritation and redness, rash, or excoriation; lack of cleanliness and crusting; and that tube is not secured in proper position (see Integumentary System Assessment, p. 39, for guidelines) (first and every visit).
2. Demonstrate and instruct caregiver in assessing skin at least twice daily and in cleansing procedure around tube along with softening and removal of dried secretions twice daily, with careful attention to avoid manipulation of the tube; allow caregiver to return demonstration (first visit; reinstruct second visit if needed).

3. Instruct caregiver in application of antiseptic or antibiotic ointment at site if ordered (first visit).
4. Instruct and inform caregiver in changing tracheostomy ties and pad when needed and in rotating position of knots on ties to avoid pressure areas; allow to practice procedure under supervision (first and second visits).
5. Inform caregiver to increase environmental humidity to prevent dry skin and mucous membranes (first visit).
6. Instruct client to report to the physician any bleeding, rash, or excoriation at the tube site (first visit).

CLIENT AND FAMILY/CAREGIVER INTERVENTIONS

1. Caregiver assesses skin at tracheostomy site daily and reports changes or breakdown.
2. Caregiver maintains clean, dry, tracheostomy site with tube in secure position.
3. Caregiver avoids allowing secretions to accumulate or dry at tube site by cleansing, redressing, and changing ties and pad if wet, soiled, or loose.
4. Caregiver applies ointment or protective skin barrier at site as ordered.
5. Caregiver notes fit of tube and, if manipulation irritates site, consults with physician to replace tube if fit is too tight or loose.
6. Caregiver provides optimal humidity by cool room vaporizer to prevent drying or excess moisture of skin.

NURSING DIAGNOSIS IMPAIRED VERBAL COMMUNICATION

▌*Related Factors:* Tracheostomy

▌*Defining Characteristics:* Inability to speak with tube in place; unwilling to attempt other methods of communication

OUTCOMES

▌*Short Term*
Alternate modes of communication attempted, as evidenced by satisfactory nonverbal interactions among client, caregiver, and family members (expected in 3 to 4 days)

▌*Long Term*
Effective method of communication adopted (expected in 1 week and ongoing)

NURSING INTERVENTIONS/INSTRUCTIONS

1. Assess client's, caregiver's, and family's willingness to attempt different methods of communication with fenestrated tube in place; adaptation to possible alternative methods of communications; and coping skills and presence of frustration, anger, or depression (first and subsequent visits as needed).
2. Assist or suggest various modes of communications, such as slate, paper and pencil, flash cards, and letters of the alphabet, to aid in communication compatible with preference or lifestyle (first and second visits).
3. Initiate order for speech pathologist consultant (any visit).

CLIENT AND FAMILY/CAREGIVER INTERVENTIONS

1. Client maintains effective use of alternative modes of communication, such as computer, magic slate, paper and pencil, hand grasps, signs and signals, eye blinking or movements, mouth sounds, and picture cards.
2. Caregiver displays patience, encourages alternative modes of communication, and anticipates client's needs.
3. Client speaks using valve device available for use on tracheostomy tube or in-line while on ventilator, with fenestrated tube in place, in those able to be off the ventilator for a time and able to speak.

NURSING DIAGNOSIS IMPAIRED PHYSICAL MOBILITY

▌*Related Factors:* Decreased strength and endurance; intolerance to activity and limited movement with ventilator use; anxiety

▌*Defining Characteristics:* Inability to purposefully move in physical environment; imposed restriction of movement including mechanical apparatus; difficulty in performing ADL

OUTCOMES

▌*Short Term*
Progressive mobility independently or with assistance and with or without ventilator, as evidenced by position changes and use of assistive aids (expected in 1 week)

▌*Long Term*

Optimal independent movement and use of extremities within level of endurance while attached to ventilator, as evidenced by participation in self-care as able (expected in 3 weeks and ongoing)

NURSING INTERVENTIONS/INSTRUCTIONS

1. Assess energy level, physical restrictions while attached to ventilator, neuromuscular or musculoskeletal impairments, and ability to participate in movement and activities (first visit).
2. Assess availability of portable ventilator and wheelchair to support ventilator to enhance movement in environment; instruct client in use of devices to operate on chair (first and second visits).
3. Assess for response to activity, such as respiratory changes or distress (first and each visit).
4. Perform range-of-motion exercises and instruct caregiver to perform these daily (first visit; reinforce on subsequent visits).
5. Instruct client in different position changes as needed for use of extremities in performing self-care (first visit).
6. Obtain an order for physical and occupational therapy referral as appropriate, and reinforce teaching by therapist for exercises and mobility while client is receiving assisted ventilation.

CLIENT AND FAMILY/CAREGIVER INTERVENTIONS

1. Client schedules time for and assists or participates in daily activities as tolerated.
2. Client avoids extremes in activity while allowing for as much independence as possible.
3. Client discontinues activity if fatigue or respiratory distress results.
4. Client follows recommendations of therapists to maintain mobility, muscle tone, and range of motion.
5. Client uses resource to acquire wheelchair with a mount for ventilator if appropriate (any visit).

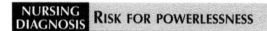

NURSING DIAGNOSIS **RISK FOR POWERLESSNESS**

▌*Related Factors:* Illness-related regimen

Defining Characteristics: Expressions of resentment, anger, guilt, passivity; dependence on others; expressions of having no control

OUTCOMES

Short Term
Improved perception of control over current situation as evidenced by relaxed facial expression and body posture (expected in 1 week)

Long Term
Optimal perception of ability to affect care outcome as evidenced by increased communication about desired care and by relaxed body posture (ongoing)

NURSING INTERVENTIONS/INSTRUCTIONS

1. Assess mental and emotional status; expressions of degree of control over situation; behavioral changes indicating resentment, anger, guilt, passivity, frustration; use of defense mechanisms and coping and problem-solving skills; ability to communicate (first visit).
2. Provide an accepting environment and a means to communicate to promote expressions of frustrations and concerns (all visits).
3. Encourage client to participate in administering and planning care within his or her capability. Provide choices in areas of client's control (all visits).
4. Initiate referral to social services, support groups, counseling, or psychotherapy as indicated (any visit).

CLIENT AND FAMILY/CAREGIVER INTERVENTIONS

1. Client expresses feelings about ability to control the situation.
2. Client participates in planning and administering care within his or her capability.
3. Client makes choices in areas of control.
4. Family/caregiver allows and encourages participation of client.
5. Client and caregiver use social services, support groups, and counseling as appropriate

NURSING DIAGNOSIS CAREGIVER ROLE STRAIN

Related Factors: Amount of caregiving tasks; duration of caregiving required; unpredictable illness course or instability in the care receiver's health; discharge of client with significant home care needs; inexperience with caregiving

■ *Defining Characteristics:* Worry about client's health, having enough time and energy to provide care needed; conflict in family about issues of providing 24-hour care and supervision of client; disturbed sleep; family disorganization and role changes; significant person's expression of inability to cope and feelings of fear, anxiety, guilt, and anger related to providing care; stress causing impatience with client's needs (ventilator/tracheostomy) and physical changes

OUTCOMES

■ Short Term
Identification of role strain, as evidenced by verbalization of stress, nervousness, or worry; interference with other important roles in life; loss of independence; and need for assistance and support; ability of family to plan and care for client (expected in 1 week)

■ Long Term
Resolution of role strain, as evidenced by provision of normal environment and continued, progressive, and safe care without compromise to caregiver's or family's physical and emotional needs (expected in 1 month and ongoing)

NURSING INTERVENTIONS/INSTRUCTIONS

1. Assess extent of client's care needs, and caregiver's ability and feelings of adequacy to perform role and care, feelings about the demands and complexity of care (e.g., exhaustion and resentment), and feeling of being alone and having no pride in caregiving activities (first visit).
2. Assess relationship between caregiver and family, stressors placed on the relationship caused by the receiver of care, breakdown in family relationships, and role confusion or competing demands of family and care responsibilities (first visit and ongoing).
3. Assist caregiver in monitoring his or her continued ability to perform care and treatments, day-to-day needs that need to be changed or learned, changes in strains or stressors, maintenance of routines, and need for additional resources or assistance (each visit).

4. Provide time for caregiver and family to discuss frustrations, anxiety, fear, and fatigue; praise attempts and accomplishments in coping and providing care (each visit).
5. Assist caregiver in locating respite care for client to give caregiver relief from constant attendance and care demands (any visit).
6. Encourage sharing of caregiver roles and responsibilities among family members, friends, and extended family to provide relief to immediate family (any visit).
7. Listen to family feelings, concerns, expectations, and preferences for caregiving; answer all questions (each visit).
8. Instruct caregiver in methods to develop appropriate coping skills and to meet family's medical and other needs (emotional, financial, food, respite, supplies, and equipment) by referral to social or counseling services (initiate on first visit and each visit as needed).

CLIENT AND FAMILY/CAREGIVER INTERVENTIONS

1. Caregiver prepares for emotional changes associated with caregiving during the discharge planning and teaching, develops trust in home care personnel, and collaborates in developing and modifying daily care.
2. Caregiver develops ability to cope with caregiver role; incorporates flexibility into day-to-day functioning.
3. Caregiver explores and uses community resources (e.g., United Way) to provide physical and psychologic assistance and relief from role strain (respite care).
4. Caregiver maintains own health and well-being in caregiver role and as much independence and privacy as possible; becomes involved in outside activities.
5. Caregiver develops new coping skills, and strategies for role changes by family members needed to support and participate in the care of the client.
6. Caregiver and family members preserve family relationships and minimize stressors by sharing feelings, fears, and concerns with one another.
7. Caregiver and family members progressively adapt to and accept client's need for ventilatory care.
8. Caregiver participates in outside support groups, refers to clergy or counseling as needed.

✳ *Tuberculosis*

Tuberculosis (TB) is an infectious disorder of the lungs, but it may also affect other organs or systems, such as bones and joints, the central nervous system, the genitourinary tract, and the adrenal glands. TB is caused by *Mycobacterium tuberculosis* and usually is contracted and transmitted by inhalation of air contaminated by droplets containing the organisms. This inflammatory pulmonary disorder causes the formation of tubercles, which leads to necrosis, caseation, fibrosis, and calcification in the affected areas of the lungs. The most susceptible groups include persons who are malnourished, persons who exhibit a low host resistance to the causative agent, and those who are immunosuppressed (e.g., individuals with acquired immunodeficiency syndrome [AIDS]).

Home care is primarily concerned with the teaching of daily personal hygiene, nutrition, rest, and medication regimens.

Primary Diagnosis:
Pulmonary Tuberculosis—ICD code: 011.0

NURSING DIAGNOSIS INEFFECTIVE BREATHING PATTERN

▊ *Related Factors:* Decreased energy; fatigue; inflammatory process

▊ *Defining Characteristics:* Shortness of breath; fremitus; respiratory depth changes; diminished breath sounds; altered chest expansion; productive or nonproductive cough; blood-tinged sputum

OUTCOMES

▊ Short Term

Adequate oxygenation, as evidenced by respiratory rate, depth, and ease within preestablished baselines and by reduced frequency of productive coughing (expected in 1 to 2 weeks)

▊ Long Term

Adequate respiratory functioning, as evidenced by client breathing with optimal level of ease to maintain desired or limited lifestyle, by x-ray studies showing arrested or inactive stage of the disease, and by sputum-culture conversion from positive to negative (expected in 2 to 5 months)

NURSING INTERVENTIONS/INSTRUCTIONS

1. Assess physical status of respiratory system (see Pulmonary System Assessment, p. 8, for guidelines) (first visit).
2. Monitor respirations for ease, rate, and depth; temperature for elevation; and cough and mucus production for frequency, type, and characteristics. Check for hemoptysis and dyspnea; also note dullness on percussion and crepitant crackles and rhonchi on auscultation. Instruct client in procedure for taking respirations and temperature and recording in a log (each visit).
3. Evaluate level of endurance when client is performing ADL; note onset of fatigue, cough, or pain. Instruct client in measures to minimize or reduce energy expended and in establishing a rest schedule (first visit; reinstruct monthly).
4. Instruct client in effective cough procedure that does not cause stress to the chest wall and in how to collect an early morning sputum specimen for laboratory analysis (first visit).
5. Suggest oral hygiene for frequent coughing and expectoration (first visit).
6. Monitor results of x-ray studies and sputum analysis as available, and incorporate information into clinical profile (each visit).
7. Refer client to self-help or support groups and local branches of organizations such as the American Lung Association and Smokenders (first visit).

CLIENT AND FAMILY/CAREGIVER INTERVENTIONS

1. Client takes and records temperature and respiratory rate and depth as needed.
2. Client adapts ADL to physical tolerance.
3. Client performs oral hygiene two to three times daily or as needed.
4. Client has laboratory tests performed on sputum (collect and transport sputum specimen to laboratory as ordered).
5. Client reports acute dyspnea or hemoptysis to physician.

NURSING DIAGNOSIS	IMBALANCED NUTRITION: LESS THAN BODY REQUIREMENTS

■ *Related Factors:* Inability to ingest nutrients because of biologic factors

■ *Defining Characteristics:* Anorexia; lack of interest in food; weakness; fatigue; weight loss; inadequate nutritional intake

OUTCOMES

■ *Short Term*
Adequate nutrition, as evidenced by stable weight, stable arm circumference, and adequate energy level to perform ADL (expected in 2 to 4 weeks)

■ *Long Term*
Optimal nutritional status maintained, as evidenced by normal weight for height and frame and compliance with prescribed diet, rest, and activity regimens (expected in 1 to 3 months)

NURSING INTERVENTIONS/INSTRUCTIONS

1. Assess nutritional status, food likes and dislikes, cultural and religious restrictions, caloric requirements, and economic resources (first visit).
2. Take height and weight and compare with standardized charts; instruct client in taking weight (first visit).
3. Take arm measurements for baseline and later comparisons (first visit).
4. Instruct client to maintain a food diary for 1 week, including type and amount of food consumed with times and method of preparation (first and second visits).
5. Instruct client in food selections for a high-protein, high-carbohydrate diet. Incorporate assessment data and food diary into menu planning (first and second visits).
6. Provide information for vitamin supplements (first visit).
7. Suggest oral hygiene before each meal (first visit).
8. Suggest eating more frequent meals in smaller amounts if appetite is poor (first visit).
9. Refer HHA to assist with ADL and meal preparation (first visit).
10. Refer to nutritionist as indicated (any visit).

CLIENT AND FAMILY/CAREGIVER INTERVENTIONS

1. Client weighs self weekly using same scale, at same time of day, and wearing same amount of clothing and records in a log.
2. Client maintains a 7-day food diary listing types, times, and amounts of all foods eaten.
3. Client performs oral hygiene with mouthwash before meals and brushes teeth after meals.
4. Client eats a high-protein, high-carbohydrate, high-calorie diet.
5. Client uses high-calorie supplements as needed.
6. Client takes vitamins daily.
7. Caregiver prepares foods that are preferred and related to cultural needs and that provide calorie requirements and social interaction.

NURSING DIAGNOSIS DEFICIENT KNOWLEDGE

Related Factors: Lack of information about measures to comply with medical regimen and about prevention of transmission of disease

Defining Characteristics: Expression of need for information about the disease, how it is transmitted, long-term medication regimen, and rest and activity requirements and limitations

OUTCOMES

Short Term
Adequate knowledge, as evidenced by client describing the causes, transmission, susceptibility, and progression of the disease; the signs and symptoms of complications; and the medication side effects; by skin testing of contacts; by compliance with medication regimen (expected in 1 to 2 weeks)

Long Term
Adequate knowledge, as evidenced by continued compliance with medication regimen and lifestyle adaptations and by x-ray films showing that the disease is in a dormant state; disease prophylaxis of contacts (expected in 2 to 5 months)

NURSING INTERVENTIONS/INSTRUCTIONS

1. Assess client's ability to perform ADL and his or her lifestyle, ability and willingness to adapt and learn, and family support system. Integrate information with disease staging and progression (see Functional Assessment, p. 55 and Psychosocial Assessment, p. 52, for guidelines) (first visit).

2. Assess respiratory, renal, hepatic, hematopoietic, neurologic, visual, and auditory changes; note known allergies; and ascertain pregnancy status (first visit and then monthly) (see respective assessments for guidelines).

3. Instruct client in causes, dormancy, and progression of disease and relate them to plan for care (first visit).

4. Instruct client contacts (in last 3 months) to obtain skin testing and, possibly, follow-up x-ray films at local health department (first visit; reinstruct each visit).

5. Inform client contacts that medication is provided by the health department for both treatment and prophylaxis (first visit).

6. Instruct client to schedule rest and activity to avoid fatigue while maintaining endurance (first visit).

7. Instruct client in respiratory isolation procedures if necessary; suggest provision of a well-ventilated room supplied with disposable supplies and utensils and a waterproof bag for disposal (first visit).

8. Instruct client to cover nose and mouth when coughing or sneezing and in proper disposal of tissues and other used supplies (first visit).

9. Instruct client in proper handwashing technique and in when to perform procedure (first visit).

10. Instruct client in administration (including names, times, side effects, dose, and food/drug/alcohol interactions) of isoniazid, ethambutol, rifampin, and streptomycin (and possibly pyrazinamide, ethionamide, cycloserine, and kanamycin); instruct client to avoid over-the-counter or nonprescribed drugs (first visit; reinstruct on second visit).

11. Instruct client contacts in administration and side effects of isoniazid (first visit).

12. Instruct client and family contacts to comply with scheduled appointments with private physician or public health department for follow-up testing and medication (each visit).

13. Inform client to report hypersensitivities (e.g., rash, urticaria), pruritus, difficulty in breathing, jaundice, urinary changes, peripheral neuritis, or changes in visual or hearing acuity (first visit).
14. Encourage client to be tested for human immunodeficiency virus (HIV) because the incidence of TB is high among persons with HIV infection (first visit).
15. Initiate referral to public health agencies and social services and to self-help and support groups (first visit).
16. Refer HHA to assist when necessary (first visit).

CLIENT AND FAMILY/CAREGIVER INTERVENTIONS

1. Client administers prescribed medications correctly using check-off sheet, labeled tablet compartments, or another method as a reminder.
2. Client secures medication in advance from public health services or home nurse to facilitate compliance.
3. Caregiver and family comply with diagnostic procedures (skin testing and x-ray films, with return for test reading) and with prophylactic medication regimen as prescribed for family contacts.
4. Client notifies health care provider of pregnancy.
5. Client performs ADL according to needs, resting before and after to avoid fatigue; secures physician permission to return to usual activities and work patterns.
6. Client avoids drinking alcohol, smoking, and taking any non-prescribed drugs.
7. Caregiver washes hands after each contact with client and used supplies and disposes of used supplies and utensils in a sealed, waterproof bag.
8. Client notifies physician of untoward or toxic reactions to medications.
9. Client and caregiver use community resources.

CARDIOVASCULAR SYSTEM

❋ *Angina Pectoris/Coronary Artery Disease*

Coronary artery disease (CAD), also known as arteriosclerotic heart disease, is the narrowing or obstruction of the arteries of the heart by atherosclerotic plaque, causing a decrease in blood flow. It leads to a decrease in oxygen supply to the heart (i.e., ischemia), resulting in retrosternal or substernal chest pain or pressure that may extend to the left arm or jaw with varying degrees of severity and frequency. Typically, the pain is precipitated by exertion and is relieved by a smooth muscle relaxant or a vasodilator. Predisposing or risk factors include hypertension, elevated lipid panel, obesity, cigarette smoking, sedentary lifestyle, and diabetes mellitus.

Home care is primarily concerned with the teaching of medication regimens to prevent or control attacks and the control of risk factors by compliance with exercise and dietary regimens.

> Primary Diagnoses:
> Angina Pectoris—ICD code: 413.9
> Chronic Ischemic Heart Disease—ICD code: 414.9
> Coronary Artery Disease—ICD code: 414.00

NURSING DIAGNOSIS CHRONIC PAIN

▌*Related Factors:* Biologic injuring agents

▌*Defining Characteristics:* Verbalization of pain descriptors (dullness, crushing, tightness, choking, pressing feeling in chest); grimace; holding or guarding chest or arm; clenched fist over sternum; pain with activity and awakening from sleep; elevated pulse and blood pressure

OUTCOMES

Short Term

Absence of pain, as evidenced by client's statement that pain is relieved or controlled by measures to prevent discomfort; relaxed posture and expressions (expected in 1 to 7 days)

Long Term

Optimal comfort level and freedom from anginal pain, as evidenced by continued absence of pain and compliance with medication regimen related to anticipatory need and activity restrictions (expected in 1 month)

NURSING INTERVENTIONS/INSTRUCTIONS

1. Assess and instruct client to assess pain and characteristics and precipitating and alleviating factors, with emphasis on early recognition of onset; have client maintain a diary with a record of each pain episode and characteristics (first visit).
2. Monitor pain for type, location, intensity, and duration to establish individual anginal pattern, and instruct client to report to physician any aberration in established pattern (each visit).
3. Instruct client in administration of sublingual nitroglycerin for use at onset of pain (first visit):
   - Use at first sign of an attack (relate to pain diary).
   - Administer prescribed dose in tablet form under the tongue or in the buccal pouch and allow to dissolve; avoid swallowing the tablet.
   - Repeat dosage up to three times at 5-minute intervals if pain is not relieved.
   - Notify physician, call ambulance, and go to emergency room if total of three tablets taken over a 15-minute period does not relieve pain.
4. Instruct client in alternative form and route of antianginal medications if prescribed (first visit).
5. Instruct client to rest during acute episode and to maintain supine or semi-Fowler's position to reduce oxygen requirement (first visit).

CLIENT AND FAMILY/CAREGIVER INTERVENTIONS

1. Client maintains pain diary; identifies trends and reports to physician when necessary.

2. Client administers and records medication to prevent or treat angina.
3. Client uses positions of comfort and takes rest periods as needed.
4. Client schedules medication regimen around activities.
5. Client calls physician and/or ambulance if three doses of nitroglycerin are ineffective.
6. Client adapts lifestyle to reduce stress as necessary to prevent pain episodes.

NURSING DIAGNOSIS ACTIVITY INTOLERANCE

■*Related Factors:* Imbalance between oxygen supply and demand

■*Defining Characteristics:* Abnormal response (changes in pulse, blood pressure; difficulty breathing; pain) to activity; electrocardiogram (ECG) changes reflecting arrhythmias or ischemia; known presence of CAD

OUTCOMES

■Short Term
Increase in activity tolerance and endurance, as evidenced by client's statement that stressors have been avoided and pain episodes associated with activity have decreased (expected in 1 to 7 days)

■Long Term
Optimal activity and self-care achieved with adaptation to established limitations in functioning (expected in 2 weeks)

NURSING INTERVENTIONS/INSTRUCTIONS

1. Assess lifestyle, participation in activities of daily living (ADL), and effects of activity on angina (first visit).
2. Identify activities that increase oxygen consumption and cause pain (first visit).
3. Assist client in planning a progressive daily self-care schedule, and instruct him or her to refrain from any activity that precipitates symptoms, including exposure to cold, exertion after a meal, and exertion from sexual intercourse (first visit).

4. Advise client that activity may be continued by modifying it so that no symptoms of angina are elicited and that nitroglycerin may be prescribed for prophylactic use before activity is to be performed (first visit).

5. Initiate referral to physical, occupational, or sex therapist as indicated (any visit).

CLIENT AND FAMILY/CAREGIVER INTERVENTIONS

1. Client maintains activity and rest schedule as planned.
2. Client progresses in ADL and endurance level without angina response.
3. Client ceases activity and rests when angina occurs.
4. Client seeks assistance to increase activity and sexual activity tolerance if needed.

NURSING DIAGNOSIS ANXIETY

■ *Related Factors:* Threat of death; threat to or change in health status

■ *Defining Characteristics:* Verbalization of fear of death from heart attack; increased tension and apprehension; feeling of uncertainty with lifestyle changes; fear of unspecific consequences

OUTCOMES

■ *Short Term*
Decrease in anxiety, as evidenced by client's statement expressing reduction in and control of anxiety to manageable level (expected in 1 week)

■ *Long Term*
Continuing manageable level of anxiety with optimal psychologic and emotional functioning, as evidenced by resumption of daily living pattern with modifications to prevent angina episodes (expected in 2 weeks)

NURSING INTERVENTIONS/INSTRUCTIONS

1. Establish rapport with and allow time and supportive environment for client to communicate concerns and fears (each visit).

2. Provide information about all tests and treatments to monitor and control condition (first visit).
3. Allow time for questions, and answer in understandable terms and with honesty (each visit).
4. Reaffirm positive lifestyle changes (each visit).
5. Refer client to counseling if anxiety becomes chronic (last visit).
6. Teach relaxation techniques if client is agreeable (first visit or when needed).

CLIENT AND FAMILY/CAREGIVER INTERVENTIONS

1. Client inquires about condition and methods to control anxiety.
2. Client initiates necessary lifestyle changes.
3. Client contacts self-help groups or counseling.
4. Client uses relaxation techniques to control anxiety.

NURSING DIAGNOSIS DEFICIENT KNOWLEDGE

▎**Related Factors:** Lack of information about medical regimen

▎**Defining Characteristics:** Request for information about medications, disease process, nutritional and activity restrictions, and health measures to prevent complications and decrease risks

OUTCOMES

▎**Short Term**
Adequate knowledge, as evidenced by client's ability to describe signs and symptoms and progression of the condition, compliance with exercise and dietary controls, and reduction in known stressors and smoking (expected in 1 week)

▎**Long Term**
Functional knowledge of and compliance with medical regimen, as evidenced by client's meeting the requirements of a changed lifestyle to achieve optimal level of wellness and functioning (expected in 1 month and ongoing)

NURSING INTERVENTIONS/INSTRUCTIONS

1. Assess lifestyle and ability to adapt, dietary patterns, learning and coping abilities and interest, and family participation and support in the medical regimen (first visit).

2. Assess cardiovascular status (see Cardiovascular System Assessment, p. 12, for guidelines) and note blood pressure; pulse changes; angina pain patterns; history of chronic illness; and use of caffeine, alcohol, and tobacco. Assess for more distant heart sounds; fourth heart sound; more diffuse apical pulse; and presence of nausea, diaphoresis, cool extremities, and vertigo during acute episodes of angina (each visit).

3. Instruct client to maintain an activity diary and relate activities to angina episodes; teach from the known to the unknown; and allow client to verbalize signs and symptoms, precipitating factors, and first indication of onset (first visit; reinforce on second visit).

4. Instruct client to identify stressors, including heavy meals, exertion, exposure to cold, emotional upsets, or any combination of these (first visit).

5. Instruct client to closely follow prescribed health regimen for any chronic condition such as hypertension or diabetes mellitus (first visit).

6. Advise client to stop smoking, and refer client to support group if needed (first visit).

7. Instruct client to maintain a food diary; instruct client in lowering caloric intake for reducing weight if indicated, avoiding foods high in saturated fats and cholesterol and limiting low-fat foods that contain monounsaturated and polyunsaturated fats; include low sodium–intake instructions if recommended, and supply client with food lists and sample menus during teaching sessions (first visit; reinforce when needed).

8. Advise client to follow a paced, incremental walking program (first week).

9. Instruct client in administration of long-acting nitrites, β-adrenergic–blocking agents, calcium channel blockers, antilipemic medications, and prophylactic antiplatelet agents, including dose, route, frequency, side effects, and food/drug/alcohol interactions; instruct client to avoid skipping doses or abruptly discontinuing medications and to avoid over-the-counter (OTC) drugs unless advised by a physician (first visit).

10. Instruct client in administration of antianginal medications/ nitroglycerin before or during angina attack and to note vertigo, syncope, or headache with initial dose and tolerance to drug (first visit).

11. Advise client to carry medication at all times (away from body heat), to store it in a dark container, and to replace tablets every 3 months (first visit).
12. Instruct client to report any aberration in anginal pattern and pain that is not relieved by medication (first visit).
13. Instruct client to carry or wear identification information indicating condition and medications being taken (first visit; check for compliance on second visit).
14. Inform client of available social services, community agencies, resources, and groups for information and support (first visit).

CLIENT AND FAMILY/CAREGIVER INTERVENTIONS

1. Client administers medication appropriately and accurately.
2. Client avoids identified stressors and manages anginal episodes quickly and effectively.
3. Client complies with dietary and exercise programs as instructed.
4. Client limits alcohol intake and reduces or ceases cigarette smoking.
5. Client notifies physician of medication side effects, unrelieved pain, or changes in vital signs.
6. Client uses social services, nutritionist, or physical therapist as needed.

✳ *Congestive Heart Failure*

Congestive heart failure (CHF) is a chronic, progressive syndrome characterized by the inability of the heart to act as a pump. The result is a cardiac output that is inadequate to meet the body's metabolic requirements. CHF results from myocardial infarction (MI), CAD, inflammatory diseases of the heart, hypertension, valvular disorders, or any other condition that strains the heart over a long period. The compensatory mechanisms of increased heart rate and cardiac dilation and hypertrophy are adaptive responses to diminished cardiac output. The cause determines whether hypertrophy occurs on the left or right side or involves both sides. Treatment is directed at management of specific etiologic and pathophysiologic factors, reversal of compensatory mechanisms, and elimination of contributing factors.

Home care is primarily concerned with assessment and with teaching the client about the disorder, the medical regimen designed to prevent the occurrence of heart failure, and measures to treat this chronic condition.

Primary Diagnosis:
Congestive Heart Failure—ICD code: 428.0

NURSING DIAGNOSIS: DECREASED CARDIAC OUTPUT

■ **Related Factors:** Mechanical factors causing alteration in preload and afterload; inotropic changes in the heart; structural factors

■ **Defining Characteristics:** Alterations in hemodynamic readings (e.g., pulse, blood pressure); fatigue; dyspnea; rales; cyanosis; pallor; oliguria; left-sided heart failure, with overlapping of symptoms of fluid excess as condition progresses

OUTCOMES

Short Term
Adequate cardiac output, as evidenced by reduction in signs and symptoms of lowered cardiac output; compliance with medical regimen, resulting in return of vital signs to baseline ranges (expected in 2 to 7 days)

Long Term
Optimal cardiac status within disease limitations, as evidenced by ability to resume and maintain adapted lifestyle without distress or complications (expected in 2 to 4 weeks)

NURSING INTERVENTIONS/INSTRUCTIONS

1. Assess circulatory status, noting rate and rhythm of apical and peripheral pulses; blood pressure; presence of cough or dyspnea; activity intolerance levels; and presence of S_3 or S_4 heart sounds, accentuated S_2, or summation gallop (S_3 with S_1) (see Cardiovascular System Assessment, p. 12, for guidelines) (each visit).
2. Perform complete physical assessment, including renal, hepatic, and neurologic systems, and note any stressors that increase

cardiac output, such as chronic inflammatory or infectious diseases, increased blood pressure, pulmonary emboli, arrhythmias, anemia, or thyrotoxicosis (first visit).

3. Assess lifestyle and relate it to contributing factors as a basis for teaching, noting tobacco use, excessive alcohol use, sodium and caffeine intake, stressors, or problems with excess weight (first visit).

4. Instruct client to monitor and record apical and radial pulses; stress alterations that should be reported to physician rather than absolute values (first visit).

5. Instruct client to keep a diary of activities and periods of exacerbations to recognize activities to avoid. Instruct client to avoid fatigue by pacing activities and rest periods; instruct to rest and sleep in semi-Fowler's position (first visit).

6. Instruct client in administration of vasodilators, and advise client to note side effects, implication of decreased blood pressure on position, resultant headaches, and altered renal function; instruct client to avoid OTC drugs unless approved by physician (first visit).

7. Instruct client in administration of cardiotonics; advise client to take pulse before administration and to withhold drug if pulse is lower than 60 beats/min; inform client of signs and symptoms of toxicity, including nausea, vomiting, anorexia, diarrhea, confusion, visual changes, and new or worsening pulse irregularities (first visit).

8. Instruct client to report deteriorating condition, including increasing fatigue with activity, dyspnea, pallor, diaphoresis, thready pulse or alteration in pulse baseline, persistent cough, feelings of suffocation, cyanosis, restlessness, anxiety, or panic (first visit).

CLIENT AND FAMILY/CAREGIVER INTERVENTIONS

1. Client monitors and records daily pulses, blood pressure, capillary refill, and skin for any change in color.

2. Client administers medications correctly and states implications and expected results.

3. Client avoids fatigue, stressors, and excessive activity.

4. Client lists signs and symptoms of digitalis toxicity and reports if present.

5. Client reports changes in vital signs that indicate change in cardiac output.

NURSING DIAGNOSIS EXCESS FLUID VOLUME

▌*Related Factors:* Compromised regulatory mechanisms

▌*Defining Characteristics:* Edema; unexplained weight gain; shortness of breath; orthopnea; change in respiratory pattern; oliguria; jugular vein distension; pulmonary effusion; congestion on x-ray films; abnormal breath sounds (e.g., crackles); right-sided failure with overlapping symptoms of decreased cardiac output as condition progresses

OUTCOMES

▌*Short Term*
Fluids in balance, as evidenced by intake and output returned to baselines, weight maintained, and edema reduced or absent (expected in 3 to 4 days)

▌*Long Term*
Fluid and electrolytes in balance, as evidenced by normal serum electrolyte values, optimal weight, and achievement of optimal renal and pulmonary function for lifestyle requirements (expected in 1 month)

NURSING INTERVENTIONS/INSTRUCTIONS

1. Assess fluid requirements; calculate for age and weight (usually approximately 2 L/day unless restricted) (first visit).
2. Measure height and abdominal girth; instruct client to take daily weight at same time, on same scale, and wearing same clothing, and to record and report weight gains (first visit).
3. Monitor for discrepancies between estimated intake and output and for pedal and ankle swelling, increasing fatigue, abdominal fullness, ascites, oliguria, and weight gain (each visit).
4. Assess chest sounds for crackles and changes in respiration (each visit).
5. Monitor and instruct client in diuretic therapy and potassium levels when they are available; encourage foods high in potassium, including citrus fruits, bananas, poultry, potatoes, and raisins; administer potassium replacement if prescribed (first visit).
6. Monitor and instruct client in dietary sodium intake and in compliance with restrictions (first visit).

7. Instruct client to inform physician of edema, breathing changes or difficulties, or weight gain (first visit).

CLIENT AND FAMILY/CAREGIVER INTERVENTIONS

1. Client monitors weight and fluid intake and urinary output estimations.
2. Client properly administers diuretics and electrolyte replacement and observes for side effects.
3. Client complies with sodium restriction.
4. Client reports weight gains, edema, or any other symptoms of fluid retention.

NURSING DIAGNOSIS FATIGUE

▌**Related Factors:** Increased energy requirements; overwhelming physical and psychologic demands

▌**Defining Characteristics:** Verbalization of lack of energy; fatigue; inability to maintain usual routine; poor oxygenation of tissues; bed rest causing deconditioning

OUTCOMES

▌**Short Term**
Decreasing fatigue, as evidenced by client's statement of increased energy and endurance and by participation in paced activities (expected in 1 week)

▌**Long Term**
Energy and endurance returned to baseline levels, as evidenced by achievement of self-care and mobility for optimal functioning within condition limitations (expected in 1 to 2 months)

NURSING INTERVENTIONS/INSTRUCTIONS

1. Assess lifestyle, ADL abilities, and limitations imposed by illness (first visit).
2. Identify activities that elicit symptoms and deplete energy reserves (first visit).
3. Assist client in progressive planning for daily care; instruct client to avoid any activity that precipitates symptoms, to pace activities, and to allow for rest periods (first visit).

4. Use energy-saving devices and techniques for ADL (each visit).
5. Inform client to avoid strenuous activity or exercise (first visit).
6. Refer home health aide (HHA) to assist with ADL (first visit).
7. Refer to occupational therapy for counseling in energy conservation as indicated (first visit).

CLIENT AND FAMILY/CAREGIVER INTERVENTIONS

1. Client identifies physical and mental stressors and avoids them when possible.
2. Client progresses in ADL in established limits.
3. Client satisfies rest and sleep needs.
4. Client implements occupational therapy instructions.

NURSING DIAGNOSIS | INEFFECTIVE COPING

Related Factors: Multiple life changes; inadequate coping methods

Defining Characteristics: Verbalization of inability to cope or ask for help, inability to solve problems, chronic worry and anxiety; inappropriate use of defense mechanisms

OUTCOMES

Short Term
Improved coping, as evidenced by client's statement of understanding of need for adaptations in lifestyle and positive coping strategies (expected in 1 week)

Long Term
Optimal coping, as evidenced by adaptations in lifestyle and by compliance with medical regimen to achieve health and optimal functioning (expected in 1 to 2 months)

NURSING INTERVENTIONS/INSTRUCTIONS

1. Assess mental and emotional status, coping abilities, use of defense mechanisms, and problem-solving skills (first visit).
2. Provide an accepting environment for expression of concerns (each visit).
3. Assist client in identifying goals and positive coping mechanisms (each visit).

4. Allow client to participate in planning and managing care and to practice effective problem-solving skills (each visit).
5. Initiate referral to medical social worker or psychotherapist for counseling if indicated (any visit).

CLIENT AND FAMILY/CAREGIVER INTERVENTIONS

1. Client develops and uses effective coping mechanisms.
2. Client shares concerns with family members and requests assistance and support when needed.
3. Client plans care and solves problems that arise from inadequate care.
4. Client manages care effectively and maintains a positive attitude.

NURSING DIAGNOSIS DEFICIENT KNOWLEDGE

▌*Related Factors:* Lack of information about condition

▌*Defining Characteristics:* Request for information about disease and its effect and compliance with daily medical regimen

OUTCOMES

▌Short Term
Adequate knowledge, as evidenced by client's description of disease process, signs and symptoms, complications, and effect of disease on body systems and general health (expected in 3 days)

▌Long Term
Functional knowledge, as evidenced by compliance with the medical regimen to meet requirements of a changed lifestyle for achievement of an optimal level of health and functioning (expected in 1 month)

NURSING INTERVENTIONS/INSTRUCTIONS

1. Assess lifestyle and ability to adapt, learning abilities and interest, and family participation and support (first visit).
2. Outline a program to teach disease process and preventive measures (first visit):

   · Medication administration, with complete information for accuracy and desired effects

- Oxygen therapy and safety precautions
- Signs and symptoms of disease and of complications
- Activity and rest program
- Bowel hygiene and prevention of change in normal pattern
- Diet for weight reduction, low in sodium, fats, and cholesterol
- Cessation of smoking; limitations on caffeine and alcohol
- Review of laboratory tests and changes needed
- Foods to avoid and include in dietary regimen

3. Instruct client to comply with physician and laboratory appointments and to check with physician for results and possible changes in therapy (first visit).
4. Instruct client to carry or wear medical identification information (first visit).
5. Refer client to agencies and support groups to assist in compliance with medical regimen if needed (any visit).

CLIENT AND FAMILY/CAREGIVER INTERVENTIONS

1. Client follows medical regimen as taught.
2. Client reports known signs and symptoms of complications if present.
3. Client administers medications safely, with awareness of side effects or untoward effects to report.
4. Client manages care with assistance of agency or group if needed.
5. Client verbalizes understanding that measures to maintain cardiac status are lifelong.

✳ *Coronary Bypass Surgery*

Coronary bypass is a surgical procedure that circumvents obstructed coronary arterial vessels through a process of myocardial revascularization. The resulting unobstructed blood flow oxygenates previously ischemic heart muscle. Autogenous blood vessels commonly used to bridge the occluded areas are the internal mammary arteries or the saphenous veins. The clinical profile of a surgical candidate includes a history of arteriosclerotic heart disease and CAD, notably unstable angina pectoris and localized rather than

diffuse disease. Some controversy exists about the surgical procedure because, although it offers dramatic relief from pain and other
symptoms, it may not necessarily positively affect the prognosis of
the disease.

Home care is primarily concerned with assessment and postoperative teaching of the medical regimen to prevent complications and with lifestyle changes that will promote wellness within
limitations imposed by the procedure and the underlying heart
condition.

> Primary Diagnoses:
> Vary according to underlying disease process
> Coronary Bypass Surgery—ICD code: 36.10

NURSING DIAGNOSIS INEFFECTIVE COPING

■ *Related Factors:* Multiple life changes; personal vulnerability

■ *Defining Characteristics:* Verbalization of inability to cope,
meet role expectations, solve problems; inappropriate use of
defense mechanisms; alterations in societal participation; chronic
worry and anxiety about outcome of surgery

OUTCOMES

■ Short Term
Improved coping behaviors, as evidenced by statement of feeling
more able to handle stressors and by use of appropriate and effective coping and defense mechanisms (expected in 1 to 2 weeks)

■ Long Term
Adequate and positive coping, as evidenced by progression from
sick-role behaviors to relaxation and adaptive behaviors and by
resumption of ADL and other activities within limitations imposed
by convalescence (expected in 1 to 2 months)

NURSING INTERVENTIONS/INSTRUCTIONS

1. Establish rapport and provide an accepting environment for
   expression of concerns and questions (each visit).
2. Assess mental status, ability to adapt, use of coping mechanisms,
   and internal resources; and explore with client the most effective
   coping mechanisms and selection of positive options (first visit).

3. Assess client's interest in and participation in activities and resumption of role and place in family (first visit).
4. Allow client to actively participate in plan of health care regimen (first visit).
5. Arrange for contact with support group (any visit).
6. Refer to medical social worker for assistance with coping strategies as indicated (any visit).

CLIENT AND FAMILY/CAREGIVER INTERVENTIONS

1. Client expresses feelings and concerns.
2. Client identifies and uses coping mechanisms that are the most effective and develops coping skills as needed.
3. Client participates in own health care planning.
4. Client uses support group and social services for information and help.

NURSING DIAGNOSIS DEFICIENT KNOWLEDGE

■ *Related Factors:* Lack of information about postoperative care

■ *Defining Characteristics:* Request for information regarding medications, cardiac rehabilitation, dietary restrictions, lifestyle changes, sexual function, and signs and symptoms to report to physician

OUTCOMES

■ Short Term
Adequate knowledge of follow-up care, as evidenced by client's ability to describe the condition, risk factors, and required lifestyle adaptations and by compliance with medication, diet, and rehabilitation program (expected in 1 week)

■ Long Term
Functional knowledge, as evidenced by client's complying with postoperative recommendations to achieve optimal level of health and functioning without complications (expected in 1 month and ongoing)

NURSING INTERVENTIONS/INSTRUCTIONS

1. Review physician's postoperative health regimen, amount and type of teaching done, and reinforcement needed so that home care becomes a continuum of previous teaching (first visit).

2. Facilitate establishment of an environment that is conducive to learning and free of outside distractions, in which client is free of pain and excessive anxiety, and teach care based on identified needs for information and demonstration (each visit).

3. Assess cardiovascular and respiratory status (see Cardiovascular System Assessment, p. 12, and Pulmonary System Assessment, p. 8, for guidelines); note vital signs (compare with baselines), point of maximal impulse (PMI), and presence of irregularities or pain (each visit).

4. Instruct client to monitor and record pulse daily for 1 full minute after a 5-minute quiet period and to notify physician of changes or deviation from usual pulse rate and regularity (first visit).

5. Instruct client to take weekly weights at same time, with same clothing, and on same scale and to report unexplained gains or losses to physician (first visit).

6. Instruct client in need for rest and to plan activities around rest periods; suggest 8 hours of sleep per night or more; and inform client of importance of following cardiac rehabilitation program without exception (first visit).

7. Inform client that activity progression will be determined by results of rehabilitation participation, and advise that sexual activity may begin 6 to 8 weeks after surgery, based on physician recommendation and feelings of client and spouse (first visit).

8. Assess for incisional healing; discomfort at operative area; or change in wound, including redness, swelling, or drainage (each visit).

9. Assess for presence of chest pain, and differentiate between preoperative and postoperative pain (anginal or cardiac); instruct client in administration of analgesics (each visit).

10. Evaluate exercise tolerance, and advise against driving or sitting for long periods, abruptly changing positions from lying to sitting or sitting to standing, or lifting heavy objects (first visit).

11. Instruct client in administration and implications of antihypertensive, antiarrhythmic, cardiotonic, diuretic, anticoagulant, and analgesic medications (first visit; reinforce on second visit).

12. Instruct client to continue prescribed regimen for control of chronic conditions such as hypertension or diabetes mellitus (first visit).

13. Instruct client in low-calorie, low-cholesterol, low-fat, low-sodium diet; instruct client to avoid caffeine and alcohol except in small amounts (first visit; reinforce on second visit).

14. Instruct client to avoid Valsalva maneuver during bowel elimination and to take stool softeners to prevent constipation (first visit).

15. Remind client that smoking should be reduced and preferably eliminated, and suggest group support to assist in cessation (first visit).

16. Instruct client to report signs and symptoms of complications or regression to preoperative profile, including erratic pulse, chest pain, activity intolerance, fatigue, or unexplained anxiety and restlessness (first visit).

17. Instruct client to carry or wear identifying information about condition and medications (first visit).

18. Inform client of importance of compliance with medical regimen that includes cardiac rehabilitation and of follow-up appointments with physician and laboratory (first visit).

19. Monitor changes in medical orders and laboratory results when applicable (each visit).

20. Initiate referral to social worker, HHA, and other support personnel and groups as appropriate (any visit).

CLIENT AND FAMILY/CAREGIVER INTERVENTIONS

1. Client monitors and records pulse daily and notifies physician of changes.

2. Client monitors weight weekly and reports significant gains or losses.

3. Client integrates rest periods with increasing activities; tries to get 8 hours of sleep per night.

4. Client participates in cardiac rehabilitation program and has a monitored walking program between sessions.

5. Client resumes sexual activity.

6. Client manages incisional discomfort with medication; provides care for incisional site (handwashing, bathing, dressing).

7. Client avoids sitting for extended periods, lifting heavy objects, or participating in strenuous exercises or sports.

8. Client administers prescribed medications as instructed.

9. Client continues medical regimens for treating chronic conditions.

10. Client maintains diet that promotes ideal weight.
11. Client prepares and eats diet with restrictions in sodium, cholesterol, and fat; limits caffeine and alcohol intake.
12. Client maintains bowel elimination based on individual pattern.
13. Client identifies signs and symptoms of incisional infection, return to preoperative heart abnormalities, or complications of surgical procedure, and reports to physician.
14. Client wears or carries medical identification at all times.
15. Client complies with follow-up physician and laboratory appointments.
16. Client participates in self-help or support groups, contacts community agencies for information, and uses nutritionist or therapist as needed.

✳ *Hypertension*

Hypertension can be defined as sustained arterial blood pressure of more than 140 mm Hg systolic and 90 mm Hg diastolic. It causes arterial walls to become thickened, to lose elasticity, and to resist blood flow, which results in decreased blood supply to tissue and increased cardiac workload. The etiology of essential, or primary, hypertension is unknown. It can be treated and controlled but not cured. Secondary hypertension is associated with disorders of the kidney, adrenal glands, central nervous system, or great vessels or with the use of medications. In the absence of complications, essential hypertension is asymptomatic. Clinical manifestations are nonspecific and result from vascular changes in the heart, brain, or kidneys.

Home care is primarily concerned with the teaching of medication regimens to control the condition and preventive measures to control complications and risk factors.

Primary Diagnoses:
Hypertension—ICD code: 401.0
Hypertensive Heart Disease—ICD codes: 429.0-429.3

NURSING DIAGNOSIS DEFICIENT KNOWLEDGE

▌*Related Factors:* Lack of information about medical regimen

▌*Defining Characteristics:* Request for information about medications, dietary and exercise program, and disease and its effects and complications

OUTCOMES

▌*Short Term*
Adequate knowledge, as evidenced by client's ability to describe disease process and effects, signs and symptoms, risk factors, and lifestyle modification requirements; familiarity and compliance with medication regimen (3 to 7 days)

▌*Long Term*
Functional knowledge, as evidenced by meeting requirements of modified lifestyle to control condition and achieve optimal health and functioning (expected in 2 weeks)

NURSING INTERVENTIONS/INSTRUCTIONS

1. Assess lifestyle, learning and adaptation abilities, interest level, and family participation and support (first visit).
2. Assess all systems for effect of long-term hypertension; note history for predisposing factors or disorders that relate to secondary hypertension (first visit).
3. Assess and instruct client in monitoring blood pressure and pulse (first visit).
4. Inform client of high-risk factors associated with condition, including smoking; obesity; high-sodium, high-fat, and high-cholesterol intake; stress; and sedentary lifestyle. Include family members in teaching because heredity plays a role in predisposition to increased blood pressure (first visit).
5. Advise client about lifestyle changes, methods of stress management, and dietary changes and to have regular screening for blood pressure and circulatory and visual changes (first visit).
6. Instruct client to take blood pressure three times per week; emphasize sitting quietly for 5 minutes before taking pressure, using the right size cuff, applying cuff smoothly and snugly and

fastening securely, and positioning arm at heart level; instruct client to report repeated and unexplained elevations to physician (first visit; reinforce when needed).

7. Instruct client in administration of diuretics, antihypertensive agents, antilipemic medications, potassium replacement, and vasodilators, including doses; route; frequency; side effects; and food, drug, or alcohol interactions. Caution client not to alter doses or abruptly stop taking medication and to avoid OTC drugs unless recommended by physician (first visit; reinforce second visit).

8. Encourage client to participate in full range of previous activity as long as blood pressure is controlled; include an exercise program of walking, swimming, and biking, with 8 hours of sleep per night (first visit).

9. Advise client about weight reduction if needed; instruct client to maintain a food diary for 1 week, and offer a list of foods to avoid (ones that are high in cholesterol and saturated fats); encourage a more liberal intake of fruits and vegetables, whole grains, fish, and poultry (first and second visits).

10. Instruct client in sodium restriction (usually 2 g/day); advise client not to add salt to foods and to avoid cured, processed, or convenience foods, and suggest use of herbs and spices for flavoring (first visit).

11. Inform client with diuretic therapy regimen about foods that are high in potassium, including a list of those to include and avoid, especially if potassium supplement is not given (first visit).

12. Suggest that client reduce or stop smoking and limit or avoid alcohol intake and hot baths or hot tub (first visit).

13. Instruct client to rise slowly from lying position to avoid orthostatic hypotension (first visit).

14. Instruct client to carry or wear identification information about condition and medications (first visit).

15. Emphasize importance of keeping appointments with physician for monitoring condition and therapy changes if needed, and for laboratory testing (first visit).

16. For information and support or counseling, initiate referral to community agencies and groups, including American Heart Association and smoking and weight-control groups (first visit).

CLIENT AND FAMILY/CAREGIVER INTERVENTIONS

1. Client monitors blood pressure as instructed and recommended and records in log to review with physician.
2. Client administers medications correctly and records any side effects.
3. Client participates in an exercise program that is ongoing and progressive as appropriate.
4. Client avoids excessive alcohol and tobacco intake; reduces frequency of use.
5. Client complies with dietary restriction of sodium, fat, and cholesterol.
6. Client monitors weight weekly if on reduction diet and adjusts caloric intake accordingly.
7. Client wears or carries identification information.
8. Client maintains laboratory and physician appointment schedules.
9. Client uses support groups and counseling services if needed.

NURSING DIAGNOSIS RISK FOR INJURY

■ *Related Factors:* Internal factor of complication of hypertension

■ *Defining Characteristics:* Failure to comply with medical regimen; sustained elevated blood pressure; cardiovascular and central nervous system symptomatology (e.g., hypertensive crisis, heart attack, cerebrovascular accident)

OUTCOMES

■ *Short Term*
Absence of signs and symptoms of complication, as evidenced by compliance with medication regimen (expected in 1 week)

■ *Long Term*
Optimal cardiovascular, neurologic, and renal system function, as evidenced by lifestyle modification and ongoing compliance with medical regimen to achieve health and wellness without complications (expected in 1 month and ongoing)

NURSING INTERVENTIONS/INSTRUCTIONS

1. Assess for behaviors that indicate resistance to or inability to comply with prescribed treatment regimen (first visit).
2. Reinforce instruction in diet, exercise, and medication programs and limitations on stress, alcohol and tobacco intake, and weight gain (first visit).
3. Assess for markedly elevated blood pressure, headache, visual disturbance, nausea, vomiting, palpitations, restlessness, confusion, tachycardia, arrhythmias, chest pain, or dyspnea, and instruct client in noting and reporting such signs and symptoms (each visit).
4. Encourage client to participate in plan and take control of care (each visit).
5. Assist client with compliance by writing out plan and expectations (first visit).
6. Encourage client to ask questions, seek information, and participate in discussions about condition; praise compliance and accomplishments (each visit).
7. Inform client of importance of lifestyle changes that maintain blood pressure status and prevent complications (each visit).

CLIENT AND FAMILY/CAREGIVER INTERVENTIONS

1. Client complies with lifestyle changes and medical regimen.
2. Client reports signs and symptoms of complications immediately to physician.
3. Client supports all attempts at management of care and prevention of complications.
4. Client secures and reads information about condition and consequences of poor control of hypertension.

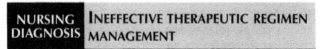

NURSING DIAGNOSIS **INEFFECTIVE THERAPEUTIC REGIMEN MANAGEMENT**

▌**Related Factors:** Complexity of therapeutic regimen

▌**Defining Characteristics:** Inappropriate choices of daily living for meeting the goals of a treatment or prevention program; failure to achieve weight loss and lower cholesterol level; inaccurate or inconsistent medication administration; observation of client smoking; reduction in exercise program; verbalization that action has not been taken to reduce risk factors for prevention of complications

OUTCOMES

▐ Short Term
Verbalization of and specific plans and behaviors for therapeutic regimen, as evidenced by intention of following recommended dietary, exercise, and medication regimens with commitment (expected in 1 week)

▐ Long Term
Compliance with management of therapeutic regimen, as evidenced by active participation in therapy and by demonstration of behaviors consistent with goals of therapy to achieve optimal health and to prevent complications (expected in 1 month and ongoing)

NURSING INTERVENTIONS/INSTRUCTIONS

1. Assess reasons for client's disregarding therapeutic regimen and with which aspect client is having difficultly complying (first visit).
2. Provide client with detailed written instructions and a plan for specific behaviors, such as medications taken via oral route, and include a simplified method if several medications are taken per day; regimen should be tailored to client lifestyle in peak action and scheduling where possible (first and second visits).
3. Inform client of consequences of smoking, and assist him or her to develop a plan to quit smoking, to cope with withdrawal symptoms, to deal with the possibility of a relapse, and to use available resources and community programs (first visit).
4. Assist client in planning realistic dietary modifications; inform client of benefits of the diet and the effects of noncompliance (first and second visits).
5. Inform client that behavior changes take time, and suggest methods to reinforce behavior changes and environmental changes to accommodate daily routines (first visit).
6. Instruct client in monitoring behavior(s) regularly, recording for analysis, and the need for alternative behaviors or strengthening of existing behaviors (first and second visits).

CLIENT AND FAMILY/CAREGIVER INTERVENTIONS

1. Client demonstrates accurate performance of specific health behavior(s) consistent with goals of therapeutic regimen.
2. Client verbalizes and adheres to a plan to follow diet, to quit smoking, to follow exercise program, and to take medications as prescribed.
3. Client establishes a system to administer medications accurately and to manage the medication regimen for optimal effects in accordance with lifestyle.
4. Client uses resources and support groups to assist with compliance.
5. Client modifies lifestyle to fit management of therapeutic regimen and changes when needed.

❋ *Myocardial Infarction*

An MI results from a partial or complete occlusion of a coronary artery. It is caused by atherosclerotic buildup in the artery, resulting in narrowing of the artery, a thrombus in the artery, or arterial spasm, leading to ischemia and necrosis of the heart tissue. The location of the infarct may vary, but most occur in the area of the left ventricle. Management is directed at preventing further damage, preventing recurrence or complications, and controlling symptomatology.

Home care is primarily concerned with assessment and with the teaching of a medication regimen, control of risk factors to prevent recurrence, and measures to allow the heart to heal.

Primary Diagnosis:
Acute Myocardial Infarction—ICD code: 410.9

NURSING DIAGNOSIS ACUTE PAIN

▮ **Related Factors:** Biologic injuring agents

▮ **Defining Characteristics:** Verbalization of pain descriptors (deep, crushing, squeezing chest pain in varying degrees of intensity); chest pain radiating to left arm, jaw, or neck (substernal or visceral); changes in vital signs; arrhythmias; chest holding; dyspnea; nausea; vomiting; sense of impending doom; diaphoresis; restlessness

OUTCOMES

▍*Short Term*

Reduced pain, as evidenced by client's statement that pain has been relieved; relaxed facial expressions and posturing; and participation in ADL without pain (expected in 1 week)

▍*Long Term*

Absence of pain, as evidenced by progression to optimal level of health and performance of ADL without pain recurring (expected in 2 weeks)

NURSING INTERVENTIONS/INSTRUCTIONS

1. Assess pain location, severity, and type; precipitating factors; and effect of medication on pain (each visit).
2. Instruct client in medication (e.g., nitrites) administration to relieve pain (first visit).
3. Instruct client to notify physician if pain returns or is not controlled and to have emergency numbers available (first visit).
4. Instruct client about various types of referred pain and other symptoms associated with an MI (first visit).
5. Instruct client to stay calm and to rest in semi-Fowler's position or with head elevated until emergency assistance arrives (first visit).

CLIENT AND FAMILY/CAREGIVER INTERVENTIONS

1. Client administers medications correctly and effectively.
2. Client reports complaints of pain and other MI symptoms to physician.
3. Client maintains calm environment and reduces stressors when pain occurs.
4. Client calls on emergency services if pain and associated symptoms that indicate a heart attack occur.

NURSING DIAGNOSIS ACTIVITY INTOLERANCE

■*Related Factors:* Imbalance between oxygen supply and demand

■*Defining Characteristics:* Verbal report of fatigue or weakness; abnormal heart rate or blood pressure or dyspnea in response to activity; reduced energy and endurance level

OUTCOMES

■*Short Term*
Increased activity and endurance, as evidenced by performance of ADL and other activities and by progressive moderate exercising and ambulation (expected in 2 to 3 weeks)

■*Long Term*
Participation and independence in ADL and mobility to achieve optimal level of health and functioning with progressive increase in endurance (expected in 1 to 2 months)

NURSING INTERVENTIONS/INSTRUCTIONS

1. Review results of discharge treadmill exercise test if done (first visit).
2. Assess for and encourage participation in ADL and diversional activities (each visit).
3. Encourage gradual increase in an individualized daily exercise and/or walking program based on absence of symptoms, results of treadmill exercise test, and physician recommendation; relate activities to age, general condition, cardiac status, interests, and lifestyle (each visit).
4. Instruct client to rest before and after exercise program; to avoid heavy lifting, stress, large meals, extremes in temperature, and stimulants (caffeine) or any combination of these; and to avoid isometric exercises (first visit; reinforce on second visit).
5. Instruct client to cease activity and notify physician if activity intolerance occurs, including unwarranted fatigue, shortness of breath, diaphoresis, weakness, pulse not reverting to baseline in 5 minutes after rest, change in pulse trends, or chest pain (first visit).

6. Encourage client to enroll and participate in a formal cardiac rehabilitation program, with prescription from physician (first visit).
7. Refer HHA to assist in ADL (first visit).

CLIENT AND FAMILY/CAREGIVER INTERVENTIONS

1. Client participates in planned activities with progressive increases.
2. Client schedules rest periods with activities and plans diversional activities.
3. Client refrains from cardiac stressors and extreme exertion or activities.
4. Client adjusts work to activity tolerance.
5. Client reports new or recurrent symptoms of activity intolerance.

NURSING DIAGNOSIS DECREASED CARDIAC OUTPUT

Related Factors: Electrical factor of alteration in rate, rhythm, and conduction

Defining Characteristics: Changes in hemodynamic readings and ECG; arrhythmias

OUTCOMES

Short Term

Adequate cardiac output, as evidenced by vital signs returning to baseline determinations (expected in 2 to 3 days)

Long Term

Cardiac output maintained, as evidenced by vital signs and cardiac status returning to level to achieve optimal functioning without complications (expected in 2 weeks)

NURSING INTERVENTIONS/INSTRUCTIONS

1. Assess circulatory status, noting blood pressure, PMI, pulse rate and rhythm, capillary refill time, skin color and temperature, presence of pain or edema, fatigue, weakness, nausea, vomiting, or unexplained restlessness or anxiety (see Cardiovascular System Assessment, p. 12, for guidelines) (first visit and ongoing).

2. Instruct client to monitor vital signs and record in a log, noting any changes to report to physician or ask physician about (first visit).
3. Instruct client in administering and assessing response to medications (e.g., vasodilators, β-adrenergic–blocking agents, calcium channel blockers, antihypertensive medications, diuretics, inotropic agents, low-dose aspirin), including dose; route; frequency; side effects; food, drug, or alcohol interactions; and implications for self care. Emphasize compliance with regimen and avoidance of OTC drugs, and caution against altering, omitting, or abruptly stopping any of the prescribed medications (first visit; reinforce on each visit).

CLIENT AND FAMILY/CAREGIVER INTERVENTIONS

1. Client administers all prescribed medications correctly and monitors for desired effects.
2. Client monitors vital signs daily as instructed, in different positions and at different times, and records findings; identifies changes to report.
3. Client reports signs and symptoms of reduced cardiac output.

NURSING DIAGNOSIS SEXUAL DYSFUNCTION

Related Factors: Altered body function caused by disease process

Defining Characteristics: Verbalization of the problem; actual or perceived limitations imposed by disease; fear of heart attack and death

OUTCOMES

Short Term
Improved sexual adequacy, as evidenced by client's statement of awareness that sexual activity is allowed and that options with intimacies are being explored (expected in 1 week)

Long Term
Optimal sexual relationship with significant partner achieved with required adaptations (expected in 2 months)

NURSING INTERVENTIONS/INSTRUCTIONS

1. Assess sexual history and concerns, beliefs, and attitude about sexual activity after MI; assess activity tolerance and results of treadmill exercise test and two-flight stair-climb test; review drug profile and relate to persistent problems with decreased libido or impotence (first visit).
2. Provide written information about sexual activity after MI to client and partner (first visit).
3. Encourage expression of concerns and questions after initial assessment, and include partner in all discussions (each visit).
4. Encourage nonsexual activities that promote intimacy, including participating in activities together and talking together (first visit).
5. Advise client about sexual options that minimize cardiac workload (first visit):
   - Rest before sexual activity, or engage in activity after a night's rest.
   - Take prophylactic nitrite, if prescribed, before activity.
   - Use side-to-side or less taxing positions.
   - Avoid activity after eating a large meal or drinking alcoholic beverages.
   - Avoid extremes of temperature, stress, and fatigue.
   - Avoid anal intercourse.
6. Instruct client to cease activity and to notify physician if intolerance to sexual activity occurs, including persistent increase in pulse and respirations after activity, chest pain at any time, or extreme protracted fatigue following activity (first visit).
7. Refer client to sex therapist if appropriate (any visit).

CLIENT AND FAMILY/CAREGIVER INTERVENTIONS

1. Client verbalizes concerns and inquires about sexual activity.
2. Client communicates concerns with partner.
3. Client promotes intimacy through both nonsexual and sexual approaches.
4. Client structures sexual activity to minimize stressors and distractors.
5. Client verbalizes effect of fear and certain medications on sexual activity, desire, or performance.
6. Client sees therapist with partner if needed.

NURSING DIAGNOSIS DEFICIENT KNOWLEDGE

▌*Related Factors:* Lack of information about post-MI medical regimen

▌*Defining Characteristics:* Request for information about medications, dietary and fluid needs, need for lifestyle changes, and follow-up requirements; denial of condition

OUTCOMES

▌**Short Term**
Adequate knowledge, as evidenced by client's ability to describe signs and symptoms of condition, management of risk factors, and compliance with medical regimen (expected in 1 week)

▌**Long Term**
Functional knowledge, as evidenced by client's meeting requirements of adapted lifestyle to achieve optimal health and functioning without complications (expected in 1 month)

NURSING INTERVENTIONS/INSTRUCTIONS

1. Assess lifestyle, ability to adapt, coping and learning abilities, and family participation and support (first visit).
2. Assess for precipitating or risk factors associated with the condition, including family history, previous MI, hypertension, diabetes mellitus, obesity, sedentary lifestyle, hyperlipidemia, and personality response to stress; adapt teaching to data (first visit).
3. Instruct client in circulatory assessment, to monitor resting pulse for 1 full minute daily, and to withhold inotropic agent if pulse is less than 60 beats/min; inform client of signs and symptoms of cardiac complications to report, including changes in pulse or blood pressure, chest pain, edema, changes in skin color, fatigue, weakness, nausea, vomiting, or restlessness (first visit).
4. Instruct client in administration of medications (e.g., vasodilators, β-adrenergic–blocking agents, calcium channel blockers, antihypertensive agents, diuretics, anticoagulants, antilipemic medications, inotropic agents, low-dose aspirin), and prepare a written schedule with administration instructions for client (first visit).
5. Instruct client to weigh weekly on same scale, at same time of day, and wearing same clothing (first visit).

6. Assess nutritional status and caloric requirements, and instruct client in reduction diet to maintain ideal weight and in low-cholesterol, low-fat, sodium-restricted diet as prescribed (first visit; reinforce on second visit).

7. Instruct client to avoid smoking, stress, and intake of alcohol and stimulating beverages (first visit).

8. Inform client of importance of compliance with exercise and cardiac rehabilitation program (each visit).

9. Instruct client in bowel program and to avoid straining at defecation (first visit).

10. Assist client in identifying stressors, and teach relaxation techniques and stress management (each visit).

11. Offer food list and sample menus of food, and fluid inclusions and restrictions (first visit).

12. Instruct client to maintain fluid intake, to monitor intake and output for balance, and to compare with weight gains or losses and presence of edema (first visit).

13. Instruct client to avoid high altitudes; inform client of possible limitation of air travel (first visit).

14. Instruct client to notify physician of deteriorating condition or complications, including erratic pulse, dyspnea, unexplained anxiety, feelings of confusion or impending doom, persistent or recurrent chest pain, or fever (first visit).

15. Encourage client to comply with physician and laboratory appointments (first visit).

16. Advise client to carry or wear identification and information regarding health status (first visit).

17. Initiate referral to counseling, community agencies and groups for smoking cessation and weight loss, and the American Heart Association for literature and support (first visit).

CLIENT AND FAMILY/CAREGIVER INTERVENTIONS

1. Client administers all medications safely as instructed.
2. Client monitors vital signs and reports changes.
3. Client balances work, rest, exercise, and diversional activities.
4. Client avoids smoking, stressful situations, and alcohol intake.
5. Client maintains ideal weight.
6. Client prepares and consumes special diet of calculated calories that is low in sodium, cholesterol, and fat.
7. Client maintains bowel pattern of soft, formed stool.

8. Client reports to physician symptoms of condition change or inquires if unsure about changes.
9. Client complies with physician and laboratory appointments.
10. Client wears medical identification at all times.
11. Client contacts support or self-help groups as needed.

✳ *Pacemaker Implantation*

A permanent pacemaker is an electric device, inserted into the chest wall, that maintains a normal rhythm of myocardial contractions by delivering an electrical stimulus to the myocardium. A pacemaker may stimulate the heart at a constant and fixed rate (i.e., asynchronous, competitive) or it may deliver a stimulus on demand (i.e., synchronous, noncompetitive) when the heart does not contract at a set rate. A transvenous approach is commonly taken, in which the electrode (lead) is inserted percutaneously through the right cephalic, jugular, or subclavian vein and positioned in the right ventricle. The distal end of the electrode is attached to the pulse generator (pacemaker), which is placed in a subcutaneous pocket in the upper chest. The pacemaker contains circuitry and battery programs for a heart rate generally between 50 and 100 beats/min. The pacemaker regulates the heart rate, which results in an adequate cardiac output. Permanent pacemakers are inserted into clients with heart block, arrhythmias, or conduction defects.

Home care is primarily concerned with the teaching of the medical regimen that is followed and the monitoring of pacemaker functioning and heart rate to prevent complications.

> Primary Diagnoses:
> Pacemaker Problem—ICD code: 996.01
> Pacemaker, Cardiac—ICD code: 37.80

NURSING DIAGNOSIS RISK FOR INFECTION

▮**Related Factors:** Invasive procedure of pacemaker insertion

▮**Defining Characteristics:** Redness, swelling, pain, fluid collection at the site of insertion; temperature elevation

OUTCOMES

▌ *Short Term*

Absence of infection, as evidenced by clean and dry insertion site, with healing in progress and edges of incision well approximated (expected in 3 days)

▌ *Long Term*

Skin integrity maintained at incisional site, as evidenced by completely healed incision without irritation, discomfort, or disruption of skin (expected in 4 to 6 weeks)

NURSING INTERVENTIONS/INSTRUCTIONS

1. Assess, and instruct client to assess, vascular (cutdown) access and pacemaker insertion sites for local heat, erythema, edema, tenderness or pain, drainage, or disruption of suture edges (each visit).
2. Instruct client in handwashing technique and clean wound and skin care (first visit; reinforce on second visit).
3. Monitor temperature and instruct client to take temperature and note chilling or flushing and to report these changes and elevations above 100° F to physician (first visit).
4. Instruct client in antibiotic prophylactic therapy if prescribed (first visit).

CLIENT AND FAMILY/CAREGIVER INTERVENTIONS

1. Client monitors temperature and condition of sites.
2. Client verbalizes signs and symptoms of infection to report.
3. Client provides clean wound care; performs handwashing before giving any care to wounds.
4. Client administers full course of antibiotic therapy.
5. Client uses positions that prevent pressure on sites and that promote comfort.

NURSING DIAGNOSIS ANXIETY

▌ *Related Factors:* Change in health status; fear of death

▌ *Defining Characteristics:* Verbalization of fear of pacemaker malfunction and consequences; feeling of helplessness caused by dependence on pacemaker; increased apprehension and uncertainty

OUTCOMES

▌*Short Term*
Reduction in anxiety, as evidenced by client's statement that anxiety has decreased, that muscles and posturing have relaxed, and that pacemaker function and limitation imposed on lifestyle are understood (expected in 2 to 3 days)

▌*Long Term*
Anxiety controlled and managed, as evidenced by lifestyle changes made to achieve level of health commensurate with pacemaker and medical regimen (expected in 2 weeks)

NURSING INTERVENTIONS/INSTRUCTIONS

1. Assess mental and emotional status and effect of stress on pacemaker function (see Psychosocial Assessment, p. 52, for guidelines) (first visit).
2. Assess for inner personal resources, ability to cope, and responses to presence of pacemaker (first visit).
3. Provide an accepting environment, and allow for expression of fears and concerns regarding pacemaker function (each visit).
4. Instruct client in relaxation techniques, and help client identify and avoid stressful situations (first and second visits).
5. Provide continuing information about condition, improvements, tests, and treatments, and answer all queries honestly and in understandable language (each visit).
6. Initiate referral for counseling for stress and anxiety reduction as indicated (any visit).

CLIENT AND FAMILY/CAREGIVER INTERVENTIONS

1. Client verbalizes and vents concerns regarding pacemaker, restrictions, and knowledge needed to prevent complications.
2. Client inquires about pacemaker and its function and about changes in lifestyle expected.
3. Client uses relaxation and diversional techniques to decrease anxiety.
4. Client consults physician if unable to control anxiety and if it affects daily activities.

NURSING DIAGNOSIS DEFICIENT KNOWLEDGE

▌*Related Factors:* Lack of knowledge about pacemaker

▌*Defining Characteristics:* Request for information about function and monitoring of pacemaker, malfunction of pacemaker battery, failure to capture or sense, or malpositioning or malfunctioning of pacing catheter

OUTCOMES

▌Short Term

Adequate knowledge of pacemaker, as evidenced by client's ability to describe type of pacemaker, why it is needed, how it functions, and symptoms and signs of pacemaker failure or complications and consequences; pulse maintained at set rate and regularity (expected in 3 days)

▌Long Term

Functional knowledge of safe, appropriate pacemaker functioning, as evidenced by meeting requirements of pacemaker monitoring and functioning and associated medical regimen to achieve optimal level of cardiac function and general health (expected in 2 to 4 weeks)

NURSING INTERVENTIONS/INSTRUCTIONS

1. Assess lifestyle, abilities for ADL, ability to learn and adapt, interest in learning pacemaker functioning, and family participation and support (first visit).
2. Assess cardiovascular status; note blood pressure, pulse rate, and rhythm of apical and peripheral pulses (see Cardiovascular System Assessment, p. 12, for guidelines) (each visit).
3. Review pacemaker instruction manual and note implications for client teaching (first visit).
4. Instruct client in administration of medications for underlying conditions and cardiac medications prescribed (first visit).
5. Instruct client to take and record radial pulse daily; stress the need to rest for 5 minutes before taking pulse and to monitor pulse for 1 full minute; instruct client to report to physician any significant deviation from pacer setting or any change that reflects prepacemaker condition (first visit; reinforce on second visit).

6. Instruct client in normal function of the heart and how the pacemaker performs to maintain heart rate (first visit).

7. Monitor client for signs and symptoms of decreased cardiac output, including fatigue, vertigo, decreased blood pressure, slow or erratic pulse, shortness of breath, diminished peripheral pulses, altered mental status, or chest pain, and instruct client to notify physician if any of these occur (first visit).

8. Inform client of range of activities, such as sexual activity, allowed or when they may be resumed according to physician recommendations; instruct client to avoid contact sports, constrictive clothing around pacemaker, jerky or exaggerated movements on pacemaker side, or toying with insertion sites (first visit).

9. Inform client of sources of electromagnetic interference and implications for pacemaker (first visit).

   · Ground all home appliances (electric and battery operated), and maintain them in good working order.
   · Light switches, radios, television, and most household convenience appliances may be used, as long as none are held over the insertion site.
   · Avoid proximity to microwave ovens (stay at least 6 feet away if in use); avoid large electrical generators.
   · Move away from any field that interferes with pacemaker function, and normal function will resume.
   · Always inform other professionals (dentist, technician, physician) about presence of pacemaker before having any procedure or testing performed.
   · When traveling by air, inform security personnel before passing through metal detector because pacemaker will trigger alarm.

10. Instruct client in telephone pacemaker check (done every 3 months) and to keep physician appointments for monitoring and evaluating pacemaker at least twice a year (first visit).

11. Inform client of need for battery change and unit replacement, and instruct client to schedule evaluation before and near "expiration date" (first visit).

12. Instruct client in range-of-motion (ROM) exercises on side of pacemaker if needed (first visit).

13. Instruct client to carry pacemaker history at all times, with information that includes type, manufacturer, model and serial number, programmed rate, location of pulse generator,

implant date, medications being taken, and name and number of attending physician (first visit; reinforce on second visit).

14. Instruct client to have emergency numbers on hand at all times (first visit).

15. Provide list of agencies and groups that can assist with information and support (first visit).

CLIENT AND FAMILY/CAREGIVER INTERVENTIONS

1. Client monitors pulse daily as instructed.
2. Client administers medications safely and effectively.
3. Client reports to physician signs and symptoms of pacemaker malfunction.
4. Client reports to physician signs and symptoms indicating change in cardiac output as a result of malfunction.
5. Client engages in full range of activities, with adaptations to minimize injury or electromagnetic interference.
6. Client monitors pacemaker function periodically by telephone or by clinic or hospital visit.
7. Client carries pacemaker information at all times.
8. Client complies with instruction to avoid complication of pacemaker dysfunction.
9. Client complies with appointments and schedules for evaluation and battery change.
10. Client uses community resources for information and support.

✳ *Peripheral Vascular Disease*

Peripheral vascular disease (PVD) refers to a condition characterized by interference with blood flow to or from the extremities; the condition may involve either arteries or veins of the extremities. It may be caused by atherosclerosis or arteriosclerosis resulting in narrowing of the arteries, inflammation (as in thrombosis or thromboangiitis obliterans), or in vasospasms (as in Raynaud's disease or varicose veins). Whether PVD is caused by inefficient cardiac pump actions or obstructed, damaged, inflamed, or infected vessels, the defining characteristic is a decreased peripheral blood flow resulting in ischemia.

Home care is primarily concerned with assessment and teaching of a medical regimen that enhances circulatory status in the extremities and prevents complications associated with impaired peripheral circulation.

Primary Diagnoses:
Peripheral Vascular Disease—ICD code: 443.9
Venous Insufficiency—ICD code: 459.81
Ulcer, Lower Extremity—ICD code: 707.1

NURSING DIAGNOSIS | INEFFECTIVE TISSUE PERFUSION, PERIPHERAL

Related Factors: Interruption of arterial flow; venous congestion

Defining Characteristics: Arterial flow: intermittent claudication, absent or weak peripheral pulses, decreased capillary filling time, cold feet, pallor on elevation, rubor when dependent, delayed healing, atrophy of skin, hair loss; venous flow: aching, heavy sensation, unilateral edema, deep muscle tenderness and cramping pain, warmth and increased pigmentation of area, prominent superficial veins, stasis ulcer

OUTCOMES

Short Term
Improved circulation to extremities, as evidenced by return to baseline lower-extremity color, temperature, size, and peripheral pulse; absence of discomfort in extremities (expected in 1 week)

Long Term
Adequate perfusion of extremities, as evidenced by return of circulation to baseline with optimal use and functional ability of extremities (expected in 1 to 2 months)

NURSING INTERVENTIONS/INSTRUCTIONS

1. Assess circulatory status and effect on extremities (see Cardiovascular System Assessment, p. 12, for guidelines) (first visit).

2. Review history for age at onset of circulatory problem, cardiac status, number of pregnancies, chronic disease, familial tendency toward circulatory problems, trauma, infections, use of tobacco and alcohol, or weight problem (first visit).
3. Differentiate between arterial and venous deficiency or dysfunction (first visit).
4. Assess peripheral pulses, capillary refill time, skin color and integrity, temperature, pain in extremities, paresthesia, degree of motion and sensation, and calf measurement (each visit).
5. Instruct client to protect extremities against chilling, to avoid use of constrictive hose or clothing and accessories, to avoid prolonged standing or leg crossing, and to avoid use of heating pad or hot water bottle (first visit).
6. Instruct client in a walking program and elevation of legs above heart level when sitting to reduce venous congestion (first visit; reinforce on second visit).
7. Instruct client in measures to increase arterial flow, including elevating head using a foam-rubber wedge, resting with legs below heart level, performing postural exercises, and walking as prescribed (first visit; reinforce on second visit).

CLIENT AND FAMILY/CAREGIVER INTERVENTIONS

1. Client protects extremities from temperature extremes, burns, or trauma.
2. Client avoids application of heat, constriction of circulation to extremities, and prolonged sitting or standing.
3. Client rests and exercises daily as prescribed to promote circulation and prevent pain.
4. Client performs ROM, Buerger-Allen, and walking exercises as prescribed.

NURSING DIAGNOSIS **RISK FOR IMPAIRED SKIN INTEGRITY**

▌*Related Factors:* Internal factor of altered circulation

▌*Defining Characteristics:* Skin discoloration, thickening, scarring; dermatitis; altered sensation; ischemic lesion; stasis ulcer

OUTCOMES

▌*Short Term*
Absence of skin breakdown, as evidenced by intact skin and
absence of irritation, excoriation, and trauma (expected in 2 days)

▌*Long Term*
Skin integrity maintained, as evidenced by intact skin and
improved circulation, allowing for optimal health and use of
extremities (expected in 1 month)

NURSING INTERVENTIONS/INSTRUCTIONS

1. Assess skin for breakdown areas and deviations from baseline
   condition (see Integumentary System Assessment, p. 39, for
   guidelines) (first visit).
2. Instruct client to monitor skin on extremities for trauma or any
   disruptions and to notify physician of changes (first visit).
3. Instruct client to avoid injury (first visit).

   · Examine feet and legs daily for skin breakdown.
   · Avoid scratching or rubbing extremities.
   · Wear sturdy, well-fitting shoes with clean, loose-fitting white
     cotton stockings.
   · Bathe in tepid water with a neutral soap and dry thoroughly.
   · Trim nails straight across.
   · Apply lotion to skin on extremities.

4. Instruct client in application of antiembolic stockings or elastic
   bandages (first visit; reinforce on second visit).
5. Inform client that bed cradle may be used to keep linens off
   extremities (first visit).
6. Apply Unna's boot or compression bandages or dressings on
   leg ulcer as ordered (any visit).
7. Refer to podiatrist or perform routine foot care to treat ingrown
   nails, corns, and calluses (first visit).

CLIENT AND FAMILY/CAREGIVER INTERVENTIONS

1. Client monitors skin daily and reports abnormalities to physician.
2. Client avoids conditions or trauma that injure skin on extremities.
3. Client wears support stockings and proper shoes and socks.
4. Client maintains skin integrity in presence of circulatory disorder.

5. Client uses podiatrist for foot care if needed.
6. Client provides daily foot and skin care on both extremities.

NURSING DIAGNOSIS DEFICIENT KNOWLEDGE

■ *Related Factors:* Lack of information about circulatory disorder

■ *Defining Characteristics:* Request for information about disease and its effects, measures to prevent symptoms and complications of disorder, and mobility requirements and restrictions

OUTCOMES

■ *Short Term*
Adequate knowledge, as evidenced by client's statement of signs and symptoms of circulatory deficiency and escalating condition, compliance with medical regimen, and adaptive lifestyle behaviors (expected in 4 to 7 days)

■ *Long Term*
Functional knowledge, as evidenced by client's meeting requirements to achieve optimal level of health and functioning within limitations imposed by chronic circulatory condition; absence of complications (expected in 1 to 2 months)

NURSING INTERVENTIONS/INSTRUCTIONS

1. Assess lifestyle, adapting abilities, learning interest and ability, and family participation and support (first visit).
2. Assess mobility status, including ability to walk without pain or discomfort, claudication, or aching extremities with increased ambulation, and instruct client to rest when pain occurs (first visit).
3. Instruct client to cease or reduce smoking and give rationale (first visit).
4. Instruct client to reduce weight or to maintain desired body weight, and assist client in planning low-fat, low-cholesterol diet (first visit).
5. Instruct client in medication administration, including vasodilators, β-adrenergic-blocking agents, and analgesics, and instruct client to avoid OTC drugs without physician advice (first visit; reinforce on second visit).

6. Assess client's knowledge of condition and its signs and symptoms, and instruct client to notify physician of deteriorating condition or worsening symptoms indicating complications, including severe pain with or without activity, decrease in or loss of sensory or motor function, and changes in skin appearance or temperature (first visit).

7. Instruct client to get adequate rest, including 8 hours of sleep per night; to maintain proper positioning of extremities based on arterial or venous insufficiency; to follow only the prescribed activity and exercise regimen; and to stop activity when pain occurs (first visit).

8. Instruct client in stress-management techniques, or inform client of availability of assistance from counseling (any visit).

9. Refer client to support group for weight reduction or smoking cessation (first visit).

CLIENT AND FAMILY/CAREGIVER INTERVENTIONS

1. Client administers medications safely and monitors effects.
2. Client notifies physician if signs and symptoms of circulatory compromise are present.
3. Client participates in programs to reduce weight and to stop smoking.
4. Client maintains weight-reduction diet and restricts intake of fat and cholesterol.
5. Client maintains rest and exercise programs.
6. Client avoids stressful situations; practices stress-reducing exercises.
7. Client reconciles pain with activity needs.

✳ *Thrombophlebitis*

Thrombophlebitis refers to a venous thrombus accompanied by venous inflammation, usually occurring in the lower extremity. Symptoms may vary; they depend in part on location and on which vessels are affected. The causes of thrombophlebitis include venous stasis, venous trauma, and increased blood coagulation. The condition may be complicated by vessel obstruction by the clot or by movement of the clot into the circulation (i.e., embolus).

Home care is primarily concerned with the control of factors that contribute to thrombus formation and the prevention of chronic venous insufficiency or pulmonary emboli by teaching the client the medical regimen and the importance of compliance with instruction.

Primary Diagnosis:
Venous Thrombosis—ICD code: 453.8

NURSING DIAGNOSIS ACUTE PAIN

▌*Related Factors:* Biologic injuring agents

▌*Defining Characteristics:* Verbalization of pain descriptors; pain, warmth, redness, unilateral edema of calf; protective behavior of affected leg

OUTCOMES

▌*Short Term*
Decreased pain, as evidenced by client's statement of pain reduction, relaxed posture and absence of guarding behavior, decrease in inflammation of calf, and resumption of physical activity (expected in 1 week)

▌*Long Term*
Absence of pain, as evidenced by independence in ADL and by activity to achieve optimal level of health and functioning without discomfort (expected in 2 to 4 weeks)

NURSING INTERVENTIONS/INSTRUCTIONS

1. Assess pain, including type, location, severity, and influence of position and activity (each visit).
2. Encourage periods of rest with leg elevated and supported; perform ROM exercises (active or passive) as prescribed (each visit).
3. Instruct client to avoid any constriction of popliteal space on affected leg (first visit).
4. Apply warm soaks or compresses to affected leg, and teach client to perform procedure (first visit).
5. Encourage client to perform as many ADL as possible, and instruct client in ambulation as allowed (first visit).

6. Instruct client in application of antiembolic stockings if prescribed (first visit).
7. Instruct client in administration of analgesics, and take special note of any interactions with anticoagulant therapy (first visit).
8. Refer HHA to assist with ADL (first visit).

CLIENT AND FAMILY/CAREGIVER INTERVENTIONS

1. Client engages in activity and rest with progressive increases daily.
2. Client administers medications and heat treatments as instructed.
3. Client uses aids in ambulation as needed.
4. Client participates in ADL and progresses until independence is achieved.
5. Client reports return of pain to physician.
6. Client uses physical therapist if appropriate.

NURSING DIAGNOSIS DEFICIENT KNOWLEDGE

▌**Related Factors:** Lack of information about medical regimen and preventive measures

▌**Defining Characteristics:** Request for information about risk factors for recurrence or complication of condition, activity and weight restrictions, and normal peripheral perfusion

OUTCOMES

▌**Short Term**
Adequate knowledge, as evidenced by client's statement of effects of activity and weight on condition; compliance with medication regimen; and adequate perfusion of extremity (expected in 2 to 3 days)

▌**Long Term**
Functional knowledge, as evidenced by client's meeting requirements to achieve optimal functioning of extremity without complications or recurrence of condition (expected in 1 month)

NURSING INTERVENTIONS/INSTRUCTIONS

1. Assess for knowledge of disease and history or lifestyle that includes risk factors for the condition, including use of

contraceptives, past surgeries and injuries, use of tobacco, tendency toward being overweight, and blood pressure problems (first visit).

2. Assess extremities for integrity, color, warmth, size (take calf measurements bilaterally), motion, pain, presence of peripheral pulses, capillary refill time, and paresthesia (each visit).

3. Instruct client in calf assessment and to report asymmetry caused by edema (first visit).

4. Instruct client in weight reduction, including reducing calories in diet and following exercise program when appropriate (first visit; reinforce on second visit).

5. Instruct client in leg exercises, ROM exercises, and a progressive walking program with or without aids (each visit).

6. Suggest reduction in or cessation of smoking; refer client to support group for assistance (first visit).

7. Instruct client to avoid constrictive clothing, prolonged sitting or standing, or leg crossing while sitting or resting; to elevate the legs above heart level when sitting; and to position the legs to avoid popliteal compression by use of pillows under the knees (first visit).

8. Measure and smoothly apply elastic antiembolic stockings from toes to knees or to groin area; instruct client in application and how to avoid bunching or rolling down of stockings; instruct to remove for sleep (first visit).

9. Suggest use of bed cradle or other device to keep covers off leg (first visit).

10. Instruct client to avoid rubbing or massaging extremity (first visit).

11. Instruct client in administration of anticoagulants, including dose; frequency; side effects; and food, drug, or alcohol interactions; to avoid OTC drugs that contain aspirin or other medications (nonsteroidal antiinflammatory drugs) that interfere with platelet function; and to comply with laboratory testing for prothrombin time as prescribed (first visit; reinforce on second visit).

12. Instruct client in signs and symptoms of effects of anticoagulant therapy, including bleeding of gums, ecchymoses, and epistaxis and blood in urine, stool, or sputum, and to report such incidents to physician (first visit).

13. Instruct client to report any change in integrity of skin of extremity, such as stasis dermatitis or ulceration, and to report

any signs and symptoms of pulmonary emboli, including anxiety, restlessness, breathlessness, syncope, increased pulse and respirations, cough, or pleuritic pain (first visit).

14. Instruct client to carry or wear identification indicating medications being taken (first visit).

15. Refer client to podiatrist if appropriate (any visit).

CLIENT AND FAMILY/CAREGIVER INTERVENTIONS

1. Client monitors extremities, including skin characteristics, daily for signs and symptoms to report.
2. Client complies with leg exercises, activity program, and dietary program as instructed.
3. Client avoids circulatory compromise in clothing, positioning, movement, pressure, or massage.
4. Client reduces smoking and alcohol and caffeine intake.
5. Client engages in weight-reduction program if needed.
6. Client wears antiembolic hose properly; removes every 8 hours for skin and leg assessment.
7. Client administers anticoagulant therapy correctly, based on periodic prothrombin time testing.
8. Client avoids trauma, medication, or straining that increases the risk of bleeding and reports bleeding from any orifice, skin, or mucous membrane; reports the presence of blood in any excretions or secretions.
9. Client complies with laboratory testing and physician appointments.
10. Client wears identifying information.
11. Client uses podiatrist for foot care.

NEUROLOGIC SYSTEM

✳ *Alzheimer's Disease*

Alzheimer's disease is a progressive, dementia-type degenerative disease of the brain that is characterized by a large loss of cells from the cerebral cortex and other areas. It results in behavior changes, memory loss, and impaired intellectual functioning. The brain changes include atrophy with wide sulci, senile plaques, and neurofibrillary tangles. The exact cause is unknown, but the disease is believed to be associated with genetic, viral, autoimmune disease and choline O-acetyltransferase–deficiency etiologies. The degree of severity of the dementia is a clinical judgment; diagnosis of Alzheimer's disease is made after years of evaluation of the presenting signs and symptoms.

Home care is primarily concerned with the teaching of safety, the medical regimen, and the preservation of cognitive, social, physical, and psychologic function.

Primary Diagnoses:
Alzheimer's Disease—ICD code: 331.0
Dementia, Alzheimer's—ICD codes: 294.10, 249.11

NURSING DIAGNOSIS: DISTURBED THOUGHT PROCESSES

▌**Related Factors:** Physiologic changes

▌**Defining Characteristics:** Cognitive dissonance; memory deficit or problems; impaired ability to make decisions, grasp ideas, solve problems, reason, and conceptualize; altered attention span; disorientation to time, place, person, circumstances, and events; hallucinations; inappropriate or non–reality-based thinking

OUTCOMES

▋*Short Term*

Preservation of cognitive and intellectual function, as evidenced by an ability to maintain reality within disease limitations (expected in 2 weeks, depending on stage of illness)

▋*Long Term*

Optimal cognitive and intellectual functioning within parameters established for the stage of the disease (expected to be ongoing)

NURSING INTERVENTIONS/INSTRUCTIONS

1. Assess short-term–memory deficits; orientation to time, place, and person; effect of medications on cognitive function; reactions to stimulation; aggressive, abusive behavior (each visit).
2. Instruct family or caregiver to provide orientation-based stimulation, including keeping clocks, calendars, and familiar objects in reach, and to repeat or correct misunderstood or confusing interactions and to provide time to encourage reminiscence (first visit).
3. Instruct family to approach client calmly and quietly in a non-threatening manner; to treat client with dignity and respect; and to avoid hostility and criticisms when behavior is unacceptable (first visit).
4. Instruct family to allow client time for accomplishing tasks, to set up a schedule for care and events, and to allow for time to respond to client's questions (first visit).
5. Instruct family to limit stimulation to what client can manage without confusion and agitation and to reduce environmental stimulation such as noise and excessive lighting (first visit).

CLIENT AND FAMILY/CAREGIVER INTERVENTIONS

1. Caregiver orients client to time, place, and person and helps client maintain a realistic thought process when appropriate.
2. Caregiver modifies environment to enhance cognitive ability; permits hoarding, pictures of past life, and use of a telephone.
3. Caregiver maintains a supportive, nonjudgmental environment.
4. Caregiver allows client time to accomplish tasks, to communicate, and to process thinking to reduce frustration and agitation.
5. Caregiver avoids actions that cause overstimulation or sensory overload.

NURSING DIAGNOSIS RISK FOR INJURY

▌*Related Factors:* Internal biochemical regulatory function of brain

▌*Defining Characteristics:* Integrative dysfunction; sensory dysfunction; wandering; unsafe environment; restlessness; balance and coordination problems; lack of awareness; disorientation; forgetfulness

OUTCOMES

▌*Short Term*
Reduction in risk for physical trauma, as evidenced by absence of environmental hazards and accidental injury (expected in 1 week)

▌*Long Term*
Absence of injury, as evidenced by adjustment of environment and provision of assistance necessary for safe ambulation and activities-of-daily-living (ADL) practices (expected in 1 to 2 weeks and ongoing)

NURSING INTERVENTIONS/INSTRUCTIONS

1. Assess for instability in gait, for muscle weakness, and for sensory perceptual dysfunction; assess environment for hazards to be corrected (first visit).
2. Instruct family or caregiver in environmental changes to be made, such as clearing pathways; removing or moving furniture; removing small rugs; making slippery floors safe; removing matches from accessibility and remaining with client when he or she is smoking; and making other adjustments, such as providing hand bars and assistive aids for walking (first visit).
3. Instruct family to secure and install a signaling device that will sound an alarm when client wanders past a certain point or out the door (first visit).
4. Provide assistance with and incorporate an appropriate amount of assistance and appropriate frequency of ambulation into daily activity plan (first visit; reinforce on second visit).
5. Instruct family to reorient client to environment when necessary, to orient client to anything new in the immediate surroundings, to place articles for frequent use in reach, and to maintain same placement of articles and furniture (first visit).

6. Instruct family to avoid applying hot articles to the skin, offering food that is hot, or allowing hot water for bathing; burns can result (first visit).

7. Instruct family to store medications in a safe, locked cabinet (first visit).

8. Inform family that low-heeled, nonskid shoes should be worn by client for walking; instruct client to use a wide base stance when standing or ambulating (first visit).

CLIENT AND FAMILY/CAREGIVER INTERVENTIONS

1. Caregiver identifies and eliminates or controls hazards in the environment.

2. Caregiver prevents falls or other injuries or trauma.

3. Caregiver provides identification bracelet or alarm device to prevent wandering away and reduce risk for injury.

4. Caregiver assists and supervises activities based on client's cognitive and mentation status.

5. Caregiver incorporates ambulation and diversional activities into client's daily schedule.

NURSING DIAGNOSIS BATHING/HYGIENE, DRESSING/GROOMING, FEEDING, TOILETING SELF-CARE DEFICIT

▌*Related Factors:* Perceptual or cognitive impairment; motor deficits

▌*Defining Characteristics:* Inability to perform ADL; inability to recognize need for daily personal care; inability to use assistive devices or utensils; inability to dress and undress; inability to distinguish what is appropriate from what is inappropriate in dressing, grooming, and toileting

OUTCOMES

▌*Short Term*

Self-care maintained within limitations imposed by disease, as evidenced by personal appearance and care being adequate and appropriate (expected in 1 to 2 weeks)

▌ *Long Term*

Appropriate pattern of ADL achieved, as evidenced by cleanliness and adequate hygiene, grooming, dressing, eating, and toileting with or without assistance or assistive aids (expected in 1 month and ongoing)

NURSING INTERVENTIONS/INSTRUCTIONS

1. Assess areas of self-care deficits and their causes, client's need for assistance or supervision and assistive aids (see Functional Assessment, p. 55, for guidelines) (each visit).

2. Instruct family or caregiver to verbally remind or use cues for client to perform specific activity, to give only the assistance that is needed, and to avoid expectations of task performance that may be frustrating (each visit).

3. Provide and instruct client and family in use of assistive aids and devices for eating, including using large or padded handles on utensils, using a plate guard, placing food in view, and removing items not needed for meal (first visit).

4. Provide and instruct client and family in use of aids for toileting, including raised toilet seat and commode, hand bar for holding, and undergarments that are easy to remove and replace; instruct caregiver to offer toileting opportunity or to remind client to use toilet (first visit).

5. Provide and instruct client and family in use of aids for bathing, dressing, and grooming, including Velcro closures, zippers, large neck openings, elastic waistbands, and keeping articles in reach; suggest possibility of purchasing several articles of clothing that are the same if client likes to wear the same things every day; suggest that caregiver lay out clothing daily in order of application and demonstrate use of articles if needed (each visit).

6. Provide client with and instruct in the use of a stool in the shower or hand bars to get in and out of the tub; supervise client in regulating the water temperature (first visit).

7. Refer home health aide (HHA) to assist with ADL as needed (first visit).

8. Initiate referral to occupational therapist as indicated (first visit).

CLIENT AND FAMILY/CAREGIVER INTERVENTIONS

1. Caregiver assists in ADL as needed.
2. Caregiver supervises self-care activities without impinging on independence and causing frustration; avoids rushing client to complete a task.
3. Caregiver provides assistive aids to enhance client's self-care in ADL.
4. Caregiver recognizes client's capabilities and assists in areas of self-care deficits.
5. Client maintains adequate personal care, grooming, hygiene, and appearance.
6. Client and caregiver use services of occupational therapist and HHA.

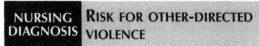

NURSING DIAGNOSIS **RISK FOR OTHER-DIRECTED VIOLENCE**

▌*Related Factors:* Brain abnormalities

▌*Defining Characteristics:* Restlessness; irritability; combative behavior; fear; bewilderment; agitation; outbursts when unable to complete tasks; lack of rest and sleep; frustration

OUTCOMES

▌*Short Term*
Minimal other-directed violence, as evidenced by reduction in agitation, frustration, and combative behavior (expected in 1 to 2 weeks)

▌*Long Term*
Absence of other-directed violence, as evidenced by lack of agitation, frustration, and combative behavior (expected to be ongoing)

NURSING INTERVENTIONS/INSTRUCTIONS

1. Assess possible sensory overload, reactions to events and precipitating factors, depression, coping mechanisms used, misinterpretation of environment, and sleep and rest patterns (each visit).
2. Note behaviors indicating suspiciousness, fear, irritability, agitation, or combativeness (each visit).

3. Provide for verbalization of feelings to avoid suppressed feelings that lead to frustrations; instruct family or caregivers to avoid assigning tasks or having expectations that cause frustrations (each visit).

4. Promote a calm environment, and instruct family or caregiver to reduce stimuli, to avoid distressing client, and to provide diversion to diffuse a situation that does distress client (first visit).

5. Instruct family or caregiver to approach client slowly and in a calm manner, to use slow gestures, and to keep hands where client can see them (first visit).

6. Instruct family or caregiver (and reinforce regularly) to avoid giving care or bothering client when the client is agitated; to limit client's intake of foods and beverages containing caffeine (chocolate, coffee); to face client when present during client's upsets or combative periods; and to protect self from possible injury from client (each visit).

7. Instruct family to avoid allowing client to nap excessively and to offer daily activities, remind client when bedtime approaches, and fulfill rituals before sleep; if client is awakened during night, reassure him or her with a quiet, calm voice that it is night and time for sleep (first visit).

8. Refer client and family to counseling or social worker for coping strategies as indicated (any visit).

CLIENT AND FAMILY/CAREGIVER INTERVENTIONS

1. Caregiver identifies cause of agitation and combative behavior and takes measures to prevent violence and frustration.

2. Caregiver responds to client's emotions and provides a calm, reassuring environment.

3. Caregiver allows for open expression of anxiety, frustrations, and feelings with an accepting attitude.

4. Caregiver allows client as much control over environment as possible.

5. Caregiver provides for rest and sleep needs as determined by previous patterns.

6. Caregiver eliminates or minimizes stimuli or expectations that agitate client.

7. Caregiver uses social services.

NURSING DIAGNOSIS — WANDERING

■ **Related Factors:** Pathologic brain changes; cognitive impairment

■ **Defining Characteristics:** Frequent movement from place to place; persistent locomotion; locomotion resulting in unintended leaving of a premise; getting lost

OUTCOMES

■ **Short Term**

Protected wandering behavior in a safe environment, as evidenced by increased environmental security without fear of injury or possibility of becoming lost (expected in 1 week)

■ **Long Term**

Minimized wandering behavior, as evidenced by reduced restlessness, agitation, and frustration (expected to be ongoing)

NURSING INTERVENTIONS/INSTRUCTIONS

1. Assess for possible behavioral disturbances, including wandering, restlessness, and hyperactivity; determine level of motor activity; note gait disturbances (see Psychosocial Assessment, p. 52, for guidelines) (each visit).
2. Assess environmental safety and security; determine level of supervision and assistance available to client (see Environmental Assessment, p. 57, for guidelines) (first visit).
3. Instruct family or caregiver to provide a safe and secure environment; to eliminate clutter; to maintain low-glare lighting; and to provide night lights in bathroom and bedroom, out-of-reach locks on doors, and consistent supervision. Teach caregiver to ensure that client wears identification bracelet at all times and to make a plan of what to do in case client becomes lost (first visit).
4. Instruct family to reduce stressors by maintaining a structured, consistent environment; preserving familiar objects; maintaining consistent daily routines; and minimizing noise and disruptions (each visit).
5. Assist family in developing communication strategies such as diversion, reality orientation, and validation therapy to maintain

calmness and promote orientation; assist family in planning a schedule of activities to foster activity during the day and sleep at night (ongoing).
6. Initiate referrals to social service as indicated (each visit).
7. Inform client and family about resources provided by the Alzheimer's Association, including the Safe Return Program (first visit).

CLIENT AND FAMILY/CAREGIVER INTERVENTIONS

1. Family and caregiver develop and maintain a safe and secure environment, including a secure walking area that has good lighting and is clutter free.
2. Client wears identification at all times and is consistently supervised by family or caregiver.
3. Caregiver takes client for walks daily; a daily routine is maintained.
4. Caregiver communicates in a calm, soft-spoken manner; client receives positive reinforcement for desired behavior.
5. Caregiver maintains a calm, consistent, distraction-free environment with familiar objects and reduced noise and disruptions.
6. Caregiver uses social services, Alzheimer's Association, and other community resources as needed.

NURSING DIAGNOSIS INTERRUPTED FAMILY PROCESSES

▌*Related Factors:* Situational crisis of progressive degeneration of brain function of family member

▌*Defining Characteristics:* Family system unable to meet physical and emotional needs of family and ill family member; family unable to express or accept feelings and security needs of members; family unable to accept change or deal with traumatic experience of caring for ill member

OUTCOMES

▌*Short Term*

Progressive adaptation to care of family member, as evidenced by family's statement of decreased anxiety and fatigue and by effective use of coping mechanisms (expected in 1 to 2 weeks)

▌*Long Term*

Optimal adjustment and adaptation to care of ill member, as evidenced by satisfactory physical, social, and psychologic health of family members (expected in 1 month and ongoing)

NURSING INTERVENTIONS/INSTRUCTIONS

1. Assess family interventions, family dynamics, supportive behaviors, past patterns of social and diversional activities, past roles, and overall health status of caregiver(s) (see Family Assessment, p. 59, for guidelines) (first visit).
2. Inform family that disorder is progressive, that no cures are available, and that care is supportive (first visit).
3. Include all family members or significant persons in all teaching and planning of care, while scheduling and incorporating into daily routines (each visit).
4. Discuss possible hired help or respite care, a day care program, or other useful programs to assist in care and supervision of client to give family relief from constant attendance to client needs (any visit).
5. Inform and instruct family in relaxation and coping techniques and in strategies to manage their own behavior caused by unrelieved responsibilities (first and second visits).
6. Instruct family or caregivers to monitor their own health needs, and help them identify problem areas for referral and evaluation if needed; emphasize the need to maintain their physical and emotional health (first and second visits).
7. Inform family of the importance of continuing or maintaining social and diversional activities and of the availability of social supports to participate in care (first visit).
8. Discuss anxiety produced by role reversal and feeling of powerlessness in caring for parent (any visit).
9. Instruct family in, and encourage them to discuss, methods to deal with client behavior and reactions (first visit).
10. Refer family to social services for assistance with finances or to consultation with legal advisor if needed for client who has changes in cognitive ability and competence (any visit).
11. Refer family or caregiver to family counseling or individual counseling as appropriate (any visit).
12. Suggest and discuss local and national resources, such as Alzheimer's Disease and Related Disorders Association and

Children of Aging Parents, for information and support (first visit).

13. Discuss the need for long-term placement in the future as disease progresses or if family resources become exhausted (any visit).

CLIENT AND FAMILY/CAREGIVER INTERVENTIONS

1. Family verbalizes feelings and concerns.
2. Family identifies problems in family and how family solves those problems together.
3. Family resolves lifestyle changes together.
4. Family seeks out and participates in support group activity.
5. Family uses respite day care assistance.
6. Family maintains family health: physical, emotional, and social.
7. Family consults with social worker, financial counselor, and legal advisor for assistance.
8. Family considers and begins to adapt to future long-term custodial care.

NURSING DIAGNOSIS CAREGIVER ROLE STRAIN

▌Related Factors: Unpredictable illness course or instability in care receiver's health; psychologic or cognitive problems in care receiver; lack of respite for caregiver

▌Defining Characteristics: Report of not having enough resources (e.g., emotional and physical strength, help from others) to provide care; worry about the receiver's health and emotional state or about having to place care receiver in an institution; feeling that caregiving interferes with other roles

OUTCOMES

▌Short Term
Caregiver role strain identified, as evidenced by verbalization of difficulties encountered in performing care and concern about ability and conflicts in giving care and adapting to role (expected in 1 week)

▌Long Term
Adaptation to and reduction of strain in caregiver role, as evidenced by continued safe and appropriate care provided without

compromise to caregiver's own physical and emotional needs (expected in 1 month and ongoing)

NURSING INTERVENTIONS/INSTRUCTIONS

1. Assess demands and care needs of receiver and ability and desire of caregiver to perform role; assess participation of family members in care (first visit).
2. Assess relationship between care receiver and caregiver before illness; assess stressors placed on relationship by progressive nature of disorder (first visit).
3. Assist caregiver in monitoring his or her continued ability to perform care and treatments and to provide for day-to-day needs; assist in monitoring how care receiver's behavior and needs change this ability; assess maintenance of routines and need for additional resources (e.g., aides, homemaker, respite care, friends, family) (each visit).
4. Discuss role performance and whether expectations are realistic; discuss flexibility of role and decision-making process (first visit).
5. Initiate referral to HHA, social services, or psychologic counseling, and suggest other community resources to contact for assistance with economic, mental health, or physical health needs (any visit).

CLIENT AND FAMILY/CAREGIVER INTERVENTIONS

1. Caregiver develops coping strategies for the caregiving role and flexibility in day-to-day functioning.
2. Caregiver explores financial, legal, emotional, and physical assistance sources and considers referral to these services.
3. Caregiver maintains own health and well-being in caregiver role.
4. Caregiver uses respite care and assistance from others for relief from stress of constant caregiving.
5. Caregiver maintains ongoing caregiving and treatment regimen.

NURSING DIAGNOSIS	DEFICIENT KNOWLEDGE

■ *Related Factors:* Lack of information about disease and care

■ *Defining Characteristics:* Request for information about medication administration, measures to prevent acute or chronic illness, prognosis, and progression of disease

OUTCOMES

▌*Short Term*
Adequate knowledge, as evidenced by family or caregiver's statement of correct medication scheduling and administration and methods to identify health problems (expected in 1 week)

▌*Long Term*
Functional knowledge, as evidenced by optimal health and function in disease limitations (expected to be ongoing)

NURSING INTERVENTIONS/INSTRUCTIONS

1. Instruct family or caregiver in assessment for presence of urinary tract infection, upper respiratory tract infection, or other physical manifestations that might arise when client is unable to communicate symptoms; instruct family in taking temperature and recognizing changes in vital signs, urine or stool characteristics, or expressions (nonverbal) of pain in any area and to report them to the physician (each visit).
2. Instruct family in administration of cholinesterase inhibitors, tranquilizers, antidepressants, and sedatives, including dose, action, frequency, side effects to report, when to discontinue the drug, and food and drug interactions (first visit; reinforce second visit).
3. Inform family that it is important to prevent exposure to infections and that health maintenance measures are important to prevent hospitalization, which would be traumatic for the client and might hasten progression of the disease (first visit).
4. Instruct family in daily nutritional, fluid, and elimination needs, and provide written lists of high-calorie foods that can be managed successfully, even if finger foods; instruct caregiver in client's need for a daily intake of 8 glasses of fluid per day if appropriate; use of stool softeners or suppository to prevent constipation and fecal impaction; and regularity in elimination pattern for urination and defecation (first visit).

CLIENT AND FAMILY/CAREGIVER INTERVENTIONS

1. Caregiver manages daily elimination needs; provides for basic nutritional and fluid needs.
2. Caregiver takes preventive measures to ensure health of client.

3. Caregiver correctly administers medications and reports untoward effects.
4. Caregiver assesses and reports changes in physical health status.

✳ *Amyotrophic Lateral Sclerosis*

Amyotrophic lateral sclerosis (ALS) is a motor neuron disease in which the presenting symptoms are associated with the part of the nervous system most affected. ALS is characterized by progressive degeneration of the corticospinal tracts and the anterior horn cells or bulbar efferent neurons. This degeneration causes muscle weakness and atrophy, beginning in the hands and spreading to the forearms and legs, that may eventually become generalized. In some cases, chewing, talking, and swallowing are affected. Muscle fasciculations are also commonly apparent. The exact cause is unknown, and treatment is based on symptomatic relief.

Home care is primarily concerned with the assessment, maintenance, and teaching aspects of preservation of muscle function and independence in and control of therapy and care.

Primary Diagnosis:
Amyotrophic Lateral Sclerosis—ICD code: 335.20

NURSING DIAGNOSIS: IMPAIRED PHYSICAL MOBILITY

▌**Related Factors:** Neuromuscular impairment

▌**Defining Characteristics:** Inability to purposefully move in physical environment, including bed mobility, transfer, and ambulation; decreased muscle strength, control, or mass

OUTCOMES

▌**Short Term**
Preservation of physical mobility, as evidenced by ambulation and participation in ADL within limitations imposed by disease (expected in 1 week and ongoing)

■*Long Term*

Optimal continued ability to perform gross- and fine-motor activities to achieve and maintain functioning (expected to be ongoing)

NURSING INTERVENTIONS/INSTRUCTIONS

1. Assess degree of mobility, range of motion (ROM), weakness of upper extremities, muscle wasting, and fasciculations (see Musculoskeletal System Assessment, p. 31, for guidelines) (each visit).
2. Assess client's ability to wash body parts, put on or take off clothing, get to and use toilet, bring food from receptacle to mouth, and difficulty in chewing and swallowing (first visit).
3. Instruct client in strengthening exercises to maintain function for as long as possible (first and second visits).
4. Instruct client in use of assistive devices for ambulation and ADL, and help client obtain necessary equipment to maintain independence, such as lift, hospital bed, wheelchair, and spring seats (first visit).
5. Instruct client in positioning, transferring, and turning techniques (first visit; reinforce as needed).
6. Initiate referral to physical and occupational therapists to address aforementioned interventions (any visit).
7. Refer HHA to assist with ADL (first visit).

CLIENT AND FAMILY/CAREGIVER INTERVENTIONS

1. For as long as possible, client performs ADL and walking activities with or without use of assistive aids, as disease progression allows.
2. Client uses techniques to assist in turning, positioning, and transferring.
3. Client maintains function within disease limitations as long as possible, with as much independence as possible.
4. Client complies with physical and occupational therapy schedule and practices activities as instructed.

NURSING DIAGNOSIS INEFFECTIVE COPING

■*Related Factors:* Personal vulnerability; multiple life changes; consequences of fatal chronic illness

■ *Defining Characteristics:* Verbalization of inability to cope or ask for help; chronic worry and anxiety; chronic fatigue; chronic depression; emotional tension; inability to meet basic needs and role expectations

OUTCOMES

■ Short Term
Adequate coping, as evidenced by client's statement of need for lifestyle changes, expectations of disease and prognosis, and need for improved coping mechanisms (expected in 1 week)

■ Long Term
Optimal coping, as evidenced by progressive grieving throughout illness, with reduction in anxiety and worry about prognosis and debilitation (expected in 3 months and ongoing)

NURSING INTERVENTIONS/INSTRUCTIONS

1. Establish rapport; provide an accepting environment for expression of concerns and questions (each visit).
2. Assess mental status, ability to adapt, use of coping mechanisms, and internal resources, and explore with client the most effective coping mechanisms and selection of positive options (first visit).
3. Help client identify goals and positive coping mechanisms (each visit).
4. Allow client to participate in care and care planning, and practice effective problem-solving skills (each visit).
5. Instruct client to avoid events that produce stress or prevent use of constructive coping mechanisms or behavior (first visit).
6. Instruct client in coping, communication, and problem-solving skills if able (first and second visits).
7. Instruct client in relaxation techniques and in diversional techniques such as music, muscle relaxation, and reading (first visit).
8. Refer to medical social worker for assistance with coping strategies (any visit).

CLIENT AND FAMILY/CAREGIVER INTERVENTIONS

1. Client develops effective use of coping mechanisms.
2. Client avoids stress-provoking events.
3. Client engages in relaxation and diversional activities.

4. Client requests assistance when needed.
5. Client reduces and/or controls anxiety level, expresses feelings and concerns.
6. Client adapts to change in lifestyle to comply with medical regimen.

NURSING DIAGNOSIS RISK FOR POWERLESSNESS

▌*Related Factors:* Illness-related regimen

▌*Defining Characteristics:* Expressions of uncertainty about fluctuating energy levels, resentment, anger, guilt, passivity, dependence on others; verbal expressions of having no control

OUTCOMES

▌*Short Term*
Improved perception of control over current situation, as evidenced by expressions of increased input into care (expected in 1 week)

▌*Long Term*
Optimal perception of ability to affect care outcome, as evidenced by participation in planning care

NURSING INTERVENTIONS/INSTRUCTIONS

1. Assess mental and emotional status; expressions of degree of control over situation; behavioral changes indicating resentment, anger, guilt, passivity, or frustration; and use of defense mechanisms and coping and problem-solving skills (first visit).
2. Provide an accepting environment to promote expressions of frustrations and concerns (all visits).
3. Encourage client to participate in administering and planning of care; provide choices in areas of client's control (all visits).
4. Initiate referral to social services, support groups, counseling, or psychotherapy as indicated (any visit).
5. Inform client about the National Amyotrophic Lateral Sclerosis Foundation (first visit).

CLIENT AND FAMILY/CAREGIVER INTERVENTIONS

1. Client expresses feelings about ability to control the situation.
2. Client participates in the planning and administration of care.

3. Client makes choices in areas of control.
4. Family and caregiver allow and encourage participation of client.
5. Client uses social services, support groups, and counseling as appropriate.

NURSING DIAGNOSIS	IMBALANCED NUTRITION: LESS THAN BODY REQUIREMENTS

■ *Related Factors:* Inability to ingest food

■ *Defining Characteristics:* Dysphagia; decreased gag reflex; weight loss; muscle wasting; inability to chew food

OUTCOMES

■ Short Term
Adequate nutrition, as evidenced by intake of nutrients via mouth, nasogastric tube, or total parenteral nutrition (expected in 1 week)

■ Long Term
Adequate nutritional intake by appropriate method and route to maintain sustenance for as long as disease permits (expected to be ongoing)

NURSING INTERVENTIONS/INSTRUCTIONS

1. Assess nutritional status, caloric and vitamin and mineral needs, ability to chew and swallow, presence of choking episodes, weight loss, and ideal weight (see Gastrointestinal System Assessment, p. 22, for guidelines) (each visit).
2. Instruct client to weigh weekly at same time, on same scale, and wearing the same clothing and to compare with ideal weight (first visit).
3. Assess for feeding method, presence of nasogastric tube, gastrostomy, esophagostomy, or right atrial catheter and feeding provided (first and second visits).
4. Instruct caregiver to offer high-protein, high-calorie soft foods, such as casseroles, that can be easily managed for oral feeding; client should avoid intake of liquids after chewing food (first visit).

5. Instruct caregiver to offer foods that are hot or cold to stimulate mouth receptors; avoid semisolid foods and milk (first visit).
6. Instruct client to position himself or herself upright with neck flexed during feedings or meals (first visit).
7. Refer to speech-language pathologist and nutritionist as indicated (any visit).

CLIENT AND FAMILY/CAREGIVER INTERVENTIONS

1. Client maintains nutritional status via oral, intravenous, or gastrostomy route.
2. Client maintains actual weight, or as close to it as possible with consideration of muscle wasting; weighs weekly.
3. Client calculates caloric intake and compares with weight loss.
4. Client minimizes the risk of choking and aspiration of food.
5. Client prepares and ingests foods that are easy to chew and swallow.

NURSING DIAGNOSIS DEFICIENT KNOWLEDGE

▌*Related Factors:* Lack of information about disease

▌*Defining Characteristics:* Request for information about medical regimen, safety precautions to prevent trauma, and measures to maintain function

OUTCOMES

▌Short Term
Adequate knowledge, as evidenced by client's ability to describe progressive characteristics of the disease, the medical regimen, and precautions to be taken to maintain function for as long as possible (expected in 1 week)

▌Long Term
Adequate knowledge, as evidenced by compliance with treatments for optimal preservation of abilities for functioning (expected to be ongoing based on disease progression)

NURSING INTERVENTIONS/INSTRUCTIONS

1. Assess lifestyle, extent of disease and its effects, learning and adaptation abilities, interest level, and family participation and support (first visit).

2. Inform client of disease process, prognosis, reason for loss of neuromuscular function, and the primary symptoms of the disease (first visit).
3. Inform client of and stress need for continuing activity and socialization; offer suggestions for diversional activities to support cognitive abilities; emphasize continuing need for self-care and independence for as long as possible (each visit).
4. Suggest use of a companion, ways to change lifestyle, and methods to manage stress and anxiety (first visit).
5. Assist client with compliance with medical regimen by writing out plan of care and activities and realistic expectations (first visit; reinforce or revise on second visit).
6. Instruct client in medication administration, including dose, time, frequency, action of drug, side effects, and food and drug interactions (first visit).
7. Instruct client in skin care, massage and protective padding of bony areas, and importance of changing positions every 2 to 4 hours; report any breakdown or skin changes that do not disappear (first visit).
8. Refer to speech pathologist if client is still able to speak or is having a problem with swallowing; suggest a microphone for amplification or an electrolarynx for phonation; if client is unable to speak, use environmental-control system activated by pictures or slight movements (eye opening or closing) (first visit).
9. Instruct client that risk for infection, especially respiratory tract infection, is high; to avoid people with upper respiratory tract infections or other illnesses; and to dispose of tissues properly. Instruct caregiver to use proper handwashing technique before giving care and to report any respiratory changes to the physician (first visit).
10. Inform client of, instruct in, and provide mechanical ventilator assistance if client is at end stage and is remaining at home and family or caregiver is able to manage this care (each visit).
11. Refer client and family to community agencies or social worker for assistance and support (any visit).

CLIENT AND FAMILY/CAREGIVER INTERVENTIONS

1. Client supports all care and treatments and prevents complications.

2. Client adapts to and complies with the medical regimen.
3. Client manages lifestyle changes and supports independence in functional activities.
4. Client maintains cognitive abilities with activities that provide stimulation.
5. Client reports complications when appropriate.
6. Client secures assistance with physical, economic, or psychologic referral as needed.

✳ *Cerebrovascular Accident*

Cerebrovascular accident (CVA) is the cerebral inefficiency or hemorrhage resulting from blood flow disturbance caused by infarction or rupture of a blood vessel. The blood flow interruption may be caused by a thrombosis or an embolism, and the hemorrhage may be caused by a congenital aneurysm, trauma, or hypertension. Transient ischemic attacks are temporary disturbances that may precede a CVA. Both types of CVA may have abrupt onsets, with the hemorrhagic type having the most acute and destructive onset. The extent of neurologic deficits and their permanence depend on the person's age and health status and on the site and size of the lesion.

Home care is primarily concerned with teaching of the medical regimen that is used to treat the underlying condition and with rehabilitation and aftercare to maximize the health and wellness potential of the client. The nature of the home care required depends on the severity and extent of the neurologic deficit.

Primary Diagnoses:
Cerebral Vascular Accident (CVA)—ICD code: 436
CVA with Dysphasia—ICD code: 436 or 784.5
CVA with Hemiplegia—ICD code: 436 or 342.90
CVA with Aphasia—ICD code: 784.3
Transient Ischemic Attacks—ICD code: 435.9

NURSING DIAGNOSIS IMPAIRED PHYSICAL MOBILITY

▌*Related Factors:* Neuromuscular impairment

▌*Defining Characteristics:* Hemiplegia; hemiparesis; inability to purposely move in physical environment, including bed mobility, transfer, and ambulation; immobility

OUTCOMES

▌*Short Term*

Progressive return of physical mobility, as evidenced by ambulation in limitations imposed by condition (expected in 1 week)

▌*Long Term*

Optimal continued return of mobility, as evidenced by maximal level of ability to ambulate, transfer, and perform other activities (expected to be ongoing)

NURSING INTERVENTIONS/INSTRUCTIONS

1. Assess degree and type of mobility impairment; ROM; ability to transfer and change positions; and muscle flaccidity, spasticity, and reflexes (see Musculoskeletal System Assessment, p. 31, for guidelines) (each visit)

2. Perform and instruct client in passive ROM exercises, with progress to active ROM exercises as appropriate in affected extremities (each visit).

3. Instruct client to position affected extremities using pillows, trochanter roll (for hip), or other aids (e.g., footboard) and to place affected side with joint at higher level than joint proximal to it (first visit).

4. Instruct client to support limbs when repositioning (first visit).

5. Instruct client to elevate head of bed 15 degrees when in supine position and to use hard devices to support hand and soft devices to support leg (first visit).

6. Instruct client to limit turning to and lying on affected side for 1 hour at a time and to avoid allowing the affected arm to rest on chest when in side-lying position (first visit).

7. Instruct client in exercises and movements, such as sitting up in bed or at side of bed, using head and body supports to

prevent falling out of bed, moving to sitting position from lying position, moving from bed to chair, and moving from sitting position to standing position (first visit; reinforce each visit).

8. Initiate referral to physical and/or occupational therapists, and inform client of importance of compliance with exercises taught and use of aids to maximize self-mobility (first visit).

CLIENT AND FAMILY/CAREGIVER INTERVENTIONS

1. Client performs exercises and ambulation with or without aids.
2. Client uses techniques to assist in turning, positioning, and transferring.
3. Client maintains ambulation within limitations.
4. Client prevents contractures, maintains circulation, and maintains tone of muscles.
5. Client complies with physical rehabilitation schedule and practices activities as instructed.

NURSING DIAGNOSIS

BATHING/HYGIENE, DRESSING/GROOMING, FEEDING, TOILETING SELF-CARE DEFICIT

■ *Related Factors:* Perceptual impairment; paralysis; urinary and/or bowel incontinence

■ *Defining Characteristics:* Inability to wash body parts, put on or take off clothes, get to and use toilet or be aware of urge to eliminate, and/or bring food from receptacle to mouth; inadequate nutritional intake; inability to swallow

OUTCOMES

■ Short Term
Progressive return to self-care, as evidenced by participation in feeding, toileting, bathing, personal hygiene, dressing, and grooming (expected in 1 week)

■ Long Term
Optimal return of functional abilities, as evidenced by maximal level of ability to perform ADL with or without assistance or assistive aids (expected in 2 to 3 months and ongoing)

NURSING INTERVENTIONS/INSTRUCTIONS

1. Assess client's ability to perform self-care, to swallow and eat, to get on and off bedpan or use commode, and to use one hand if hemiplegic; assess client's neurologic impairment (tactile, visual, auditory, kinesthetic) and response to stimuli (see Functional Assessment, p. 55, for guidelines) (each visit).
2. Instruct family or caregiver to provide assistance or supervision as needed for performance of ADL (first visit).
3. Provide and instruct client in use of assistive aids and devices for eating, including using large, swivel, or padded handles on utensils; using a plate guard; placing food in view; and removing items not needed for meal (first visit).
4. Provide and instruct client in use of aids for toileting, including raised toilet seat and commode, hand bar for holding, and undergarments that are easy to remove and replace (first visit).
5. Provide and instruct client in use of aids for bathing, dressing, and grooming, including Velcro closures, zippers, large neck openings, elastic waistbands, and keeping articles in a holder or stuck to wall or counter (first visit).
6. Initiate referral to occupational therapist for instruction and practice in ADL and suggestions for other assistive aids for performance of aforementioned interventions as appropriate (any visit).
7. Refer HHA for assistance with ADL (first visit).

CLIENT AND FAMILY/CAREGIVER INTERVENTIONS

1. Caregiver assists with ADL while encouraging independence.
2. Client uses assistive aids and devices in performing ADL.
3. Client maintains functional abilities in daily activities.
4. Client complies with occupational rehabilitation schedule and practices activities as instructed.

NURSING DIAGNOSIS IMPAIRED VERBAL COMMUNICATION

▌*Related Factors:* Physical barrier of decreased circulation in brain

▌*Defining Characteristics:* Inability to speak (i.e., aphasia); dysarthria

OUTCOMES

▌*Short Term*

Adequate communication, as evidenced by ability to communicate needs effectively (expected in 1 week)

▌*Long Term*

Return to communication patterns, as evidenced by optimal speech or development of an effective method of communication (expected in 2 to 3 months and ongoing)

NURSING INTERVENTIONS/INSTRUCTIONS

1. Determine communication deficits and remaining strengths or positive features (first visit).
2. Instruct family or caregiver to speak to client in short simple statements, to ask questions that need a yes or no answer, to speak slowly and in a normal tone, and to allow time for a response (first visit).
3. Instruct client to use gestures, paper and pencil, slate board, pictures, or cards and to reinforce established communication techniques if appropriate (first visit).
4. Instruct client in oral and facial exercises to improve muscular integrity (first and second visits).
5. Initiate referral to speech-language pathologist for therapy (any visit).

CLIENT AND FAMILY/CAREGIVER INTERVENTIONS

1. Caregiver speaks to client slowly and clearly and in a normal tone.
2. Caregiver avoids interrupting client, forcing client to communicate, or criticizing client's speech.
3. Client uses facial expressions or pantomime to communicate.
4. Client uses pencil and paper, slate board, pictures, cards, or any other effective method to communicate.
5. Caregiver maintains a quiet environment, positions speaker in front of client, and decreases distractions.
6. Caregiver anticipates needs if client is unable to express them.
7. Client complies with speech-language pathologist's schedules and instructions.

NURSING DIAGNOSIS RISK FOR TRAUMA

▌*Related Factors:* Weakness; balancing difficulties; reduced temperature and/or tactile sensation; neurologic deficit

▌*Defining Characteristics:* Hemiparesis; hemiplegia; loss of muscle tone; visuospatial misperception; inability to orient self and movement in the environment; unsteady gait; lack of safety precautions in the environment; neurosensory impairment (tactile)

OUTCOMES

▌*Short Term*
Minimal possibility of trauma, as evidenced by absence of falls or injury and by client's statement of safety precautions (expected in 1 week and ongoing)

▌*Long Term*
Absence of trauma, as evidenced by safe environment maintained to accommodate neurologic deficits (expected in 1 month and ongoing)

NURSING INTERVENTIONS/INSTRUCTIONS

1. Assess sensory perception of heat and cold, sharpness and dullness; awareness of body parts; visual or auditory deficits; presence and degree of paralysis; ability for ambulation and movement; and disorientation or change in mentation (each visit).

2. Instruct client and family to adjust environment to reduce possibility of falls and trauma by arranging furniture for holding, providing clear pathways, removing door to accommodate wheelchair, removing small rugs, and providing proper lighting and to use assistive aids when walking, or refer to occupational therapist for this assistance (first visit).

3. Provide and instruct family or caregiver to provide a consistent approach when assisting with ambulation and ADL (first visit).

4. Instruct client to turn head and scan environment; instruct caregiver to approach on affected side and to place objects on affected side if visual-field impairment is present (first visit).

5. Instruct client to protect affected limbs from extremes of hot or cold or from hot or cold applications to limbs if tactile perception is affected (first visit).

6. Instruct family or caregiver to supervise all activities if judgment of position, distance, or rate of movement is impaired (first visit).
7. Instruct family or caregiver in skin care if tactile perception is affected, including assessment and protection, massage of pressure points, frequent changes of position (every 2 hours), and cleansing and application of an emollient to the skin (first and second visits).

CLIENT AND FAMILY/CAREGIVER INTERVENTIONS

1. Caregiver allows as much independence as possible.
2. Caregiver protects client from falls and from trauma to skin and affected limbs.
3. Caregiver promotes visual-field enhancement.
4. Client and caregiver adapt environment to deficits and for safe mobility.

NURSING DIAGNOSIS DEFICIENT KNOWLEDGE

Related Factors: Lack of information about disease and treatments

Defining Characteristics: Request for information about medication, medical regimen, and rehabilitation program

OUTCOMES

Short Term
Adequate knowledge, as evidenced by client's statement of nutritional, fluid, elimination, and medication regimen and rehabilitation needs (expected in 3 days)

Long Term
Adequate knowledge, as evidenced by compliance with medical regimen and achievement of optimal health and functioning (expected in 1 to 3 months)

NURSING INTERVENTIONS/INSTRUCTIONS

1. Assess lifestyle, learning and adaptation abilities, interest level, and family participation and support (first visit).

2. Assess all systems for effect of long-term hypertension; note history for predisposing factors or disorders that relate to secondary hypertension (first visit).

3. Assess and instruct client in monitoring blood pressure and pulse (first visit).

4. Advise client about lifestyle changes, methods of stress management, and dietary changes; to have regular screening for blood pressure, circulatory, and visual changes; and to have laboratory testing if warfarin sodium (Coumadin) therapy is prescribed (first visit).

5. Instruct client in administration of antihypertensive agents, anticoagulant medications, diuretics, stool softeners, and vitamin and/or mineral supplements, including dose, route, frequency, side effects, and food and drug interactions (first visit).

6. Instruct client in constipation program to include increased fluid intake (8 to 10 glasses/day), increased bulk in diet, and daily activity and exercise program (first visit).

7. Instruct client to include in his or her diet foods that he or she prefers that are textured for easy swallowing; to use thickeners; to place foods on unaffected side of mouth; to allow plenty of time for meals; and to avoid milk and foods that are too thin and smooth (first visit).

8. Instruct client in urinary bladder rehabilitation by offering elimination opportunity every 2 hours; scheduling voiding at certain times with fluid intake; and using temporary measures such as pads or waterproof undergarments (first and second visits).

9. Inform client of importance of compliance with physical, occupational, and speech therapy regimens (first visit).

10. Instruct client to report to the physician changes such as headache or vertigo, changes in mentation, or visual disturbances (first visit).

11. Inform client that emotional lability is common and of the possibility of becoming depressed and the need for counseling services if appropriate (any visit).

12. Inform client of agencies such as American Heart Association to contact for information, assistive devices, and support services (first visit).

CLIENT AND FAMILY/CAREGIVER INTERVENTIONS

1. Client adapts to lifestyle changes to accommodate medical regimen.

2. Client verbalizes nutritional, fluid, and elimination measures to ensure optimal function.
3. Client complies with medication and rehabilitation schedules and carries out safe interventions as instructed.
4. Client verbalizes signs and symptoms to report indicating possible recurrence of stroke.
5. Client uses community agencies for assistance and support.

NURSING DIAGNOSIS COMPROMISED FAMILY COPING

▌*Related Factors:* Prolonged disease or disability that exhausts the supportive capacity of significant people

▌*Defining Characteristics:* Expression of concern or complaint about client's health problem; lack of information about residual damage from stroke

OUTCOMES

▌*Short Term*
Improved coping, as evidenced by acknowledgment of disabling effects of disease and required lifestyle changes and by cooperation and participation in treatment regimen (expected in 1 week)

▌*Long Term*
Optimal level of participation and support by family members to facilitate changes in client's lifestyle and improvement in health status (expected in 1 to 2 months)

NURSING INTERVENTIONS/INSTRUCTIONS

1. Assess family interactions and coping abilities, strengths of individual members, level of participation and support, and resources available and used by family (see Family Assessment, p. 59, for guidelines) (first visit).
2. Provide accurate information to family about treatment regimen and deficits that cannot be changed; allow time for questions or clarifications (each visit).
3. Encourage family to discuss strengths and options for change and to identify coping mechanisms used (each visit).
4. Include family members in teaching and realistic planning of care (each visit).

5. Inform client and family that full or partial recovery may take a long time (first visit).
6. Inform client and family of government and community agencies available for support and assistance (first visit).
7. Initiate referral to social services, and encourage family to contact counselor if appropriate (any visit).

CLIENT AND FAMILY/CAREGIVER INTERVENTIONS

1. Family verbalizes concerns and feelings about burden of care of family member with chronic disorder.
2. Family seeks assistance if needed.
3. Family participates in planning and implementing care.
4. Family adapts to limitations of client and integrates them into family activity.
5. Family copes with client's response to the losses.
6. Family continues family activities and open communication.

✳ *Head Injury*

Head injury is penetration of the skull or traumatic impact to the skull that damages the brain tissue at the point of impact. The injury may be a concussion, cerebral contusion, laceration, or brainstem trauma and may result in edema or hemorrhage, causing increased intracranial pressure, amnesia, hemiplegia, impaired consciousness, breathing impairment, or coma. Head injury is usually the result of an accident.

Home care depends on the extent and severity of the injury and is primarily concerned with teaching of the medical regimen and treatment of the residual effects to facilitate restoration of normal function.

Primary Diagnosis:
Head Injury—ICD code: 959.01

NURSING DIAGNOSIS   RISK FOR INJURY

▌*Related Factors:* Internal regulatory function; physical function; psychologic function

■*Defining Characteristics:* Inability to purposefully move about; unsteady gait; sensory and/or perceptual deficits; disorientation; change in consciousness; visual disturbances; seizure activity

OUTCOMES

■*Short Term*
Improved function within limitations imposed by condition, as evidenced by mental alertness; return of thought processes; orientation to time, place, and person; and resumption of mobility and ADL without injury (expected in 1 week or as practical)

■*Long Term*
Progressive return to optimal health and functioning without injury, with awareness of residual deficits (expected in 3 to 6 months)

NURSING INTERVENTIONS/INSTRUCTIONS

1. Assess for presence of reflexes, mentation changes, motor- or sensory-function changes, paralysis, visual impairment, and cognitive ability (each visit).
2. Inform client of possible changes in judgment, emotional control, and social restraint in association with this condition (first visit).
3. Instruct family or caregiver to adjust environment to prevent trauma from falls or other injury, to reorient client as needed, to provide supervision and/or assist with ambulation and ADL as needed, and to provide assistive aids as needed (each visit).
4. Instruct family or caregiver in measures to protect client from injury during seizure activity, including staying with client, turning client on side, avoiding restraining client, and placing pillow under client's head (first visit).
5. Refer HHA to assist with ADL as needed (first visit).
6. Consult with home care rehabilitation specialist (any visit).
7. Refer to physical therapist as indicated (any visit).

CLIENT AND FAMILY/CAREGIVER INTERVENTIONS

1. Caregiver provides assistance with ambulation and ADL with or without aids.
2. Caregiver maintains safe environment with clear pathways and lighted rooms; makes sure client has proper shoes and eyeglasses.

3. Caregiver prevents injury during seizure activity with protective measures.
4. Caregiver notes and reports changes in mentation or behavior.
5. Caregiver uses services of therapist and HHA as needed.

NURSING DIAGNOSIS DEFICIENT KNOWLEDGE

▪**Related Factors:** Lack of knowledge about consequences of injury

▪**Defining Characteristics:** Request for information about injury, effects, prognosis, and medication and rehabilitation regimens

OUTCOMES

▪**Short Term**
Adequate knowledge, as evidenced by client's ability to describe cause and effects of the injury and the medication and rehabilitative regimens (expected in 1 week)

▪**Long Term**
Adequate knowledge, as evidenced by compliance with medical regimen to achieve optimal health and functioning and progressive recovery (expected in 1 to 6 months)

NURSING INTERVENTIONS/INSTRUCTIONS

1. Assess lifestyle, learning and adaptation abilities, interest level, cognitive deficits, and family participation and support (first visit).
2. Inform family that time and patience are needed to deal with the deficits or problems and that the appearance of client may not be an indication of level of recovery if any (first visit).
3. Instruct family or caregiver in administration of anticonvulsant medications, anticoagulant agents, and muscle relaxants, including dose, action, frequency, side effects, and food and drug interactions, and instruct not to skip doses or discontinue without advice of physician (first visit).
4. Instruct family or caregiver in performing neurologic checks and assessing mentation and in changes in consciousness to report (each visit).

5. Inform client that recovery may take 6 months, including rehabilitation to treat specific residual deficits of posttraumatic stage (first visit).
6. Instruct family in appropriate interaction patterns to avoid family dysfunction and that client should avoid intake of alcohol, driving, use of hazardous equipment, and unsupervised smoking (first visit).
7. Inform family of importance of keeping appointments with rehabilitation team and with agencies that assist with economic, psychologic, and physical support (any visit).

CLIENT AND FAMILY/CAREGIVER INTERVENTIONS

1. Client adapts to changes in lifestyle to include rehabilitation.
2. Caregiver participates in and supports client's recovery from chronic problems and mental and emotional sequelae.
3. Client administers medications correctly and reports side effects or ineffective response from medications.
4. Caregiver provides a safe environment, in which client is encouraged to avoid consuming alcohol, smoking alone, using guns and hazardous machinery or appliances, driving a car, and using over-the-counter (OTC) drugs.
5. Client maintains rehabilitation schedule as prescribed.

✳ *Multiple Sclerosis*

Multiple sclerosis (MS) is a chronic, slowly progressive central nervous system (CNS) disease causing demyelination in the brain and spinal cord. It is associated with an immunologic abnormality causing an inflammatory process that is responsible for the loss of the myelin sheath from the axon cylinders of the nerves, primarily in the white matter. The disease is characterized by remissions and exacerbations of symptoms, which include transient weakness, stiffness and fatigue of a limb, gait disturbances, vertigo, loss of bladder and bowel control, visual disturbances, emotional lability, and lack of judgment.

Home care is primarily concerned with the teaching of safety and the medical regimen and with the preservation of physical and mental function.

Primary Diagnoses:
Multiple Sclerosis—ICD code: 340
Muscle Atrophy (Disuse)—ICD code: 728.2

NURSING DIAGNOSIS · SITUATIONAL LOW SELF-ESTEEM

Related Factors: Biophysical, psychosocial factors

Defining Characteristics: Verbal responses to change in body function; self-negating verbalizations; expression of shame (e.g., regarding incontinence); inability to deal with illness; hesitancy to change lifestyle; inability to perform ADL; depression

OUTCOMES

Short Term
Improved self-esteem, as evidenced by client's statement of ability to cope with long-term debilitation and changes in lifestyle associated with dysfunction (expected in 1 week)

Long Term
Progressively more positive attitude about prolonged illness, with participation in treatment regimen to achieve optimal health and functioning within limitations of disease (expected in 2 to 3 months and ongoing)

NURSING INTERVENTIONS/INSTRUCTIONS

1. Assess client for behavioral changes and emotional status, including anxiety and depression, feelings of powerlessness, and use and effectiveness of coping mechanisms (each visit).
2. Focus on remaining abilities, and instruct family to maintain a positive attitude and support (each visit).
3. Discuss effect of illness on self-concept (any visit).
4. Encourage client to participate in treatments and ADL; instruct family to assist when needed but to allow for independence when possible (first visit).
5. Allow for expression of feelings and concerns about neurologic functioning and effect on lifestyle (each visit).

6. Refer client to counseling and social services as indicated (any visit).

CLIENT AND FAMILY/CAREGIVER INTERVENTIONS

1. Client sets goals and participates in treatments.
2. Client identifies and uses effective coping mechanisms.
3. Client uses a planned program for entire day to deal with boredom and anxiety.
4. Client maintains independence and uses measures to reduce embarrassment caused by changes in function.
5. Client expresses feelings during nurse's visits.
6. Client accepts and participates in counseling services if needed.

NURSING DIAGNOSIS RISK FOR POWERLESSNESS

Related Factors: Illness-related regimen

Defining characteristics: Expressions of uncertainty about fluctuating energy levels, resentment, anger, guilt, passivity, dependence on others; verbal expressions of having no control

OUTCOMES

Short Term
Improved perception of control over current situation, as evidenced by expressions of increased input into care (expected in 1 week)

Long Term
Optimal perception of ability to affect care outcome, as evidenced by participation in planning care (expected to be ongoing)

NURSING INTERVENTIONS/INSTRUCTIONS

1. Assess mental and emotional status; expressions of degree of control over situation; behavioral changes indicating resentment, anger, guilt, passivity, or frustration; and use of defense mechanisms and coping and problem-solving skills (first visit).
2. Provide an accepting environment to promote expressions of frustrations and concerns (all visits).
3. Encourage client to participate in administering and planning care. Provide choices in areas of client's control (all visits).

4. Initiate referral to social services, support groups, counseling, or psychotherapy as indicated (any visit).
5. Inform client about the National Multiple Sclerosis Society (first visit).

CLIENT AND FAMILY/CAREGIVER INTERVENTIONS

1. Client expresses feelings about ability to control the situation.
2. Client participates in the planning and administration of care.
3. Client makes choices in areas of control.
4. Family and caregiver allow and encourage participation of client.
5. Client uses social services, support groups, and counseling as appropriate.

NURSING DIAGNOSIS IMPAIRED URINARY ELIMINATION

■ *Related Factors:* Sensorimotor impairment

■ *Defining Characteristics:* Urgency, frequency, dribbling, incontinence, retention, or spastic or flaccid bladder, depending on site of lesion

OUTCOMES

■ Short Term
Progressive absence of urinary elimination impairment, as evidenced by reduction in incontinence episodes and by retention with residual less than 150 ml (expected in 1 to 2 weeks)

■ Long Term
Urinary continence and absence of retention, as evidenced by establishment of urinary elimination pattern for optimal functioning (expected in 2 to 3 months and ongoing)

NURSING INTERVENTIONS/INSTRUCTIONS

1. Assess for presence of spastic bladder (incontinence); flaccid bladder (retention); suprapubic distension; or cloudy, foul-smelling urine (first visit).
2. Instruct client and family in administration of cholinergic or anticholinergic medications to relieve bladder symptoms, including action, dose, frequency, side effects, precautions, and food and drug interactions (first visit).

3. Instruct client and family in fluid needs (8 to 10 glasses/day), and assess for possible urinary bladder infection if residual is present (first visit).
4. Perform Credé's maneuver or reflex stimulation manually, and instruct client in use of these methods if retention is present (first and second visits).
5. Instruct client or family to perform catheterization intermittently if ordered to treat retention (any visit).
6. Instruct client in protection methods to prevent embarrassment from incontinence (first visit).
7. Refer client to bladder training program if appropriate (any visit).

CLIENT AND FAMILY/CAREGIVER INTERVENTIONS

1. Client maintains fluid intake of 3000 ml/day.
2. Client participates in methods to stimulate or control urinary elimination.
3. Client correctly administers medications to relieve bladder symptoms.
4. Client monitors intake and output; assesses for presence of urinary tract infection.
5. Client uses garment protectors and waterproof underwear.
6. Client participates in bladder training program.

NURSING DIAGNOSIS IMPAIRED PHYSICAL MOBILITY

Related Factors: Neuromuscular impairment

Defining Characteristics: Inability to purposefully move in physical environment, including bed mobility, transfer, and ambulation; weakness; muscle pain and spasms; unsteady gait; limb stiffness; vertigo; paresthesias; inability to perform ADL

OUTCOMES

Short Term

Adequate mobility and activity performance, as evidenced by preservation of ability to ambulate and participate in ADL within limitations imposed by disease (expected in 1 to 2 weeks)

▊*Long Term*

Optimal ability to perform gross- and fine-motor activities to achieve and maintain present functioning (expected in 1 to 2 months and ongoing)

NURSING INTERVENTIONS/INSTRUCTIONS

1. Assess mobility status; presence and duration of muscle spasms; risk for injury related to altered mobility, paralysis, or paresthesia; need for wheelchair (see Musculoskeletal System Assessment, p. 31, for guidelines) (each visit).
2. Instruct client and family in administration of antispasmodics to decrease spasticity, including dose, time, frequency, precautions, side effects, and food and drug interactions (first and second visits).
3. Emphasize and instruct client in daily exercises, including stretching and stride increasing by walking with feet farther apart (for gait training) (first visit).
4. Instruct client to apply ice to spastic muscle (or use warm bath) before exercising and to rest between exercises (first visit).
5. Instruct client in use of assistive devices for self-care; instruct family to assist while encouraging independence (each visit).
6. For a safe environment, and especially to prevent falls, instruct family to clear pathways, remove small rugs, and provide rails or assistive aids for ambulation (first visit).
7. Initiate referral to physical and occupational therapists as indicated (first visit).
8. Refer client to HHA and durable medical equipment and homemaker services as needed.

CLIENT AND FAMILY/CAREGIVER INTERVENTIONS

1. Client administers medications correctly and reports side effects; avoids driving and hazardous activities, use of alcohol, and abrupt discontinuation of medications.
2. Client meets needs for ADL with or without assistance and use of aids.
3. Client relieves muscle spasticity, increases coordination, and uses nonaffected muscles for impaired ones if possible.
4. Client participates in physical therapy with water exercises, massage, and occupational therapy as needed.
5. Family provides safe environment for functioning.

6. Client uses HHA and homemaker services to assist with ADL, meal preparation, and shopping; uses any other services that are needed.

NURSING DIAGNOSIS DEFICIENT KNOWLEDGE

▌Related Factors: Lack of information about disease and manifestations

▌Defining Characteristics: Request for information about changes in lifestyle to promote functional maintenance and to maintain general health

OUTCOMES

▌Short Term
Adequate knowledge, as evidenced by client's statement of precautions and treatments to implement and methods to ensure health and functioning (expected in 1 week)

▌Long Term
Optimal knowledge, as evidenced by maintenance of general health and functioning and by compliance with medical regimen and instructions (expected in 1 to 2 months)

NURSING INTERVENTIONS/INSTRUCTIONS

1. Assess lifestyle, learning and adaptation abilities, interest level, and family participation and support (first visit).
2. Inform client and family of cause of disease and reason for neurosensory and neuromuscular dysfunction (first visit).
3. Inform client and family of and stress need for long-term physical therapy and maintenance of mobility and independent functioning (first visit).
4. Advise client to avoid fatigue, extremes of heat and cold, and any exposure to people with illness or infections; instruct client to balance rest and activity (first visit).
5. Instruct client to avoid constipation by increasing dietary intake of fiber and fluids, including items from the basic four food groups, and eating well-balanced, nutritious meals (first and second visits).

6. Inform client that tinnitus or decreased auditory acuity and visual changes such as blurred vision or patches of blindness are caused by CNS involvement; suggest use of large print and other aids available for visual or auditory deficits (first visit).
7. Instruct client and family in skin care if client is confined to wheelchair or bed (first and second visits).
8. Review and instruct client in administration of all medications (e.g., antineoplastic and immunosuppressive drugs), and instruct client to avoid OTC drugs unless advised by physician (first and second visits).
9. Inform client of eventual possible sexual dysfunction, impotence in males, decreased libido, and decreased vaginal lubrication in women, and suggest resources (any visit).
10. Instruct client and family in grieving process and reason for behaviors that are normal and, perhaps, predictable as function is lost (each visit).
11. Inform client and family that signs and symptoms of disease and changes in behavior (e.g., anger, depression) may be initiated by fatigue, infection, or physical or emotional stress or trauma (any visit).
12. Refer client and family to social services, National Multiple Sclerosis Society, and local agencies for information and support (any visit).

CLIENT AND FAMILY/CAREGIVER INTERVENTIONS

1. Client describes health measures to prevent complications and maintain function.
2. Client avoids stress, fatigue, formation of contractures, and skin breakdown by complying with physical therapy protocol.
3. Client participates in goal setting and decision making regarding care schedule.
4. Client maintains nutritional status needed for health and functioning; includes daily intake of vitamins, fiber, and fluid (3000 ml/day).
5. Client avoids exposure to or involvement in activities that predispose to infections.
6. Client seeks out assistance for sexual dysfunction with counseling or sex therapy and alternate sexual expression.
7. Client safely and appropriately adapts to and complies with complete medical regimen.
8. Client contacts and uses social services and community agencies for information and support.

� *Parkinson's Disease*

Parkinson's disease is a chronic, progressive CNS disorder characterized by muscular rigidity, a slow decrease in movement, and tremors. It involves the degeneration of the brain centers that control movement and is associated with low concentrations of dopamine, which account for the symptoms of the disease. The incapacitation that occurs from this disease may take years to develop.

Home care is primarily concerned with the teaching of medication administration and self-care activities to ensure meeting basic needs, depending on symptomatic effects of the disease.

> Primary Diagnoses:
> Parkinson's Disease—ICD code: 332.0
> Parkinson's Disease, Secondary—ICD code: 332.1

NURSING DIAGNOSIS IMPAIRED PHYSICAL MOBILITY

Related Factors: Neuromuscular impairment; decreased strength and endurance

Defining Characteristics: Inability to purposefully move in physical environment, including poor ambulation, bradykinetic tremor, contractures, deformities, unsteady gait, muscle rigidity

OUTCOMES

Short Term
Preservation of physical mobility, as evidenced by ambulation and participation in ADL within limitations imposed by disease (expected in 1 week and ongoing)

Long Term
Continued optimal ability to perform gross- and fine-motor activities to achieve or maintain present functioning throughout illness (expected to be ongoing)

NURSING INTERVENTIONS/INSTRUCTIONS

1. Assess degree of mobility, ROM, presence of contractures or bradykinesia, ability to stand from sitting position, and need for

assistive aids (see Musculoskeletal System Assessment, p. 31, for guidelines) (first visit).

2. Assess client's ability to wash body parts, put on or take off clothing or fasten clothing, bring food to mouth to feed self, and perform personal hygiene and grooming activities (see Functional Assessment, p. 55, for guidelines) (first visit).

3. Instruct client in daily ambulation and active or passive ROM and other exercises in all extremities, head, and neck; include stretching, stride increasing, and facial exercises (first and second visits).

4. Instruct client to use straight chair for sitting and how to get up using arm rests, to carry object in hand or place hand in pocket to reduce tremors, to change positions to avoid resting tremor, to lift toes when stepping and step over imaginary or real lines, and to step backward once and forward with two steps to correct akinesia or freezing (first visit; reinforce when needed).

5. Instruct client in application of hot packs and use of massage to reduce muscle rigidity (first visit).

6. Encourage and instruct client in use of assistive aids for ADL, and provide assistance by referring HHA when needed (any visit).

7. Initiate referral to physical and occupational therapists as appropriate (first visit).

CLIENT AND FAMILY/CAREGIVER INTERVENTIONS

1. Client performs ambulation and exercises, ADL, and other activities within limitations imposed by disease.
2. Client makes use of measures to facilitate mobility, reduce tremor, and change positions.
3. Client uses aids to facilitate ADL and maintain independence.
4. Client participates in physical and occupational therapy.
5. Client makes use of measures to reduce muscle rigidity.

NURSING DIAGNOSIS RISK FOR FALLS

■ *Related Factors:* Physical illness (Parkinson's disease)

■ *Defining Characteristics:* Impaired physical mobility; impaired balance; gait difficulty

OUTCOMES

▌*Short Term*
Reduced risk for falls, as evidenced by increased environmental safety features (expected in 1 week)

▌*Long Term*
Minimal risk for falls, as evidenced by demonstration of safety precautions to prevent falls (expected in 1 month)

NURSING INTERVENTIONS/INSTRUCTIONS

1. Assess degree of physical mobility, balance, and gait; assess caregiver's knowledge and ability to assist client with mobility to prevent falls and to assist client in case of a fall (first visit).
2. Assess environment for safety features, including devices and features to assist with mobility, balance, and gait; assess environment for hazards, including dim lighting, scatter rugs, and general clutter (first visit).
3. Initiate referral to physical therapist (first visit).
4. Instruct client and caregiver to eliminate environmental hazards including scatter rugs (first visit).
5. Instruct client about adding environmental aids, such as grab bars in bathroom, as indicated (first and second visit).
6. Instruct caregiver in how to safely assist client when ambulating and transferring and in measures to take in case of a fall (expected to be ongoing).

CLIENT AND FAMILY/CAREGIVER INTERVENTIONS

1. Client participates in physical therapy.
2. Client/family eliminate environmental hazards.
3. Client/family incorporate safety features in home to aid client mobility.
4. Caregiver safely assists client when transferring or ambulating and ensures that client wears supportive footwear to prevent falls.

NURSING DIAGNOSIS ▌INEFFECTIVE COPING

▌*Related Factors:* Personal vulnerability; multiple life changes

▌*Defining Characteristics:* Verbalization of inability to cope, inability to meet basic needs, alteration in societal participation, change in usual communication patterns, chronic anxiety, depression, loss of control

OUTCOMES

▌*Short Term*
Adequate coping, as evidenced by progressive participation in treatment program and use of coping and problem-solving skills (expected in 1 week)

▌*Long Term*
Optimal coping, as evidenced by attitude and lifestyle changes indicating achievement of optimal physical and emotional functioning (expected in 3 months and ongoing)

NURSING INTERVENTIONS/INSTRUCTIONS

1. Assess for verbalization of behavioral changes indicating anxiety, lability, depression, social isolation, or body image disturbance; assess use and effectiveness of coping mechanisms (see Psychosocial Assessment, p. 52, for guidelines) (each visit).
2. Discuss self-concept, including appearance and loss of neurologic and musculoskeletal functioning (e.g., drooling, tremor, slurred speech); discuss adjustment to and acceptance of the disease (each visit).
3. Instruct client to use typewriter, slate, or paper and pencil to assist in communication (first visit).
4. Inform client and family of need for socialization and of agencies and groups in the community that perform services and provide information and support (first visit).
5. Assist client in establishing realistic goals for functioning, and instruct client in coping and problem-solving skills to achieve these goals (first and second visits).
6. Initiate referral to social services for counseling as appropriate (any visit).

CLIENT AND FAMILY/CAREGIVER INTERVENTIONS

1. Client uses a planned program for entire day to deal with anxiety and depression.
2. Client identifies and uses coping skills that are effective.
3. Client sets realistic goals and participates in treatments.
4. Client maintains independence and uses measures to reduce embarrassment from changes in functioning.

5. Client expresses feelings and concerns; accepts counseling if needed.
6. Client improves self-concept with adjustment to the disease and its problems.

NURSING DIAGNOSIS   DEFICIENT KNOWLEDGE

▌*Related Factors:* Lack of information about disease

▌*Defining Characteristics:* Request for information about disease's cause, effects, and prognosis; medication administration; fluid, nutritional, and activity regimen; preservation of abilities; and prevention of injury

OUTCOMES

Short Term
Adequate knowledge, as evidenced by client's description of disease's cause and progressive nature, medical regimen, and precautions for preventing complications (expected in 1 week)

Long Term
Functional knowledge, as evidenced by compliance with medical regimen for optimal preservation of functional abilities (expected in 1 month and ongoing)

NURSING INTERVENTIONS/INSTRUCTIONS

1. Inform client of disease process and cause of and reason for loss of neurologic and musculoskeletal functioning (first visit).
2. Inform client of and stress need for continuing activity and socialization and need for self-care and independence in ADL to maintain functioning (first visit).
3. Instruct client to take frequent rest periods throughout the day (first visit).
4. Instruct client and family in nutritional needs, including small, frequent high-calorie, high-protein meals with a selection of high-fiber foods and fluid intake of up to 3000 ml/day, to maintain nutrition and prevent constipation; inform client and family that accidents involving food and drinks are common and need to be ignored and treated with kindness; suggest eating slowly and chewing foods thoroughly (first and second visits).

5. Instruct client and family in administering medications, including dose, action, frequency, side effects, precautions, and signs and symptoms resulting from medication to report to physician; discuss use of stool softeners and antiparkinsonian drugs (dopaminergic, anticholinergic), and instruct client to avoid taking OTC drugs unless advised by physician (first visit and any visit as needed).

6. Instruct client and family in safety measures, including removal of small rugs and furniture from pathways and use of elevated chair and toilet seat (first visit).

7. Inform client that exercises to strengthen muscles used for speaking, chewing, and swallowing should be included in daily physical therapy and refer to speech pathologist if appropriate (first visit).

8. Inform client and family of and direct them to community resources, including The American Parkinson Disease Association, for information and support (first visit).

CLIENT AND FAMILY/CAREGIVER INTERVENTIONS

1. Client adapts to and complies with medical regimen.

2. Client correctly administers medications as prescribed and reports untoward effects.

3. Client participates in activity, rest, and fluid and nutritional program within limitations or restrictions imposed by disease.

4. Client establishes and maintains adequate bowel elimination, weight, and nutritional status.

5. Client and family institute measures to prevent falls and to encourage independence.

6. Client and family contact and use community agencies for information and support.

✳ *Seizure Disorders*

Seizures are recurrent paroxysmal disorders of cerebral function that are characterized by altered consciousness, sensory phenomena, altered motor activity, or changes in behavior. Any recurrent seizure pattern is known as epilepsy. Seizures are classified as partial or generalized and may be caused by cerebral or systemic disorders, such as acute infections (e.g., CNS infections), cerebral hypoxia, cerebral fracture, brain lesions or tumors, toxic agents, congenital brain defects, cerebral edema, cerebral trauma, cerebral hemorrhage, cerebral infarct, and anaphylaxis. Seizure activity resulting from any cause may be transient and may not recur after the disorder is corrected or ends.

Home care is primarily concerned with the teaching of medication administration to control seizures and with prevention of physical and psychologic trauma that may result from seizure activity.

Primary Diagnosis:
Seizure Disorder—ICD code: 780.39

NURSING DIAGNOSIS RISK FOR INJURY

Related Factors: Internal regulatory function (sensory, integrative dysfunction)

Defining Characteristics: Musculoskeletal trauma from falls; oral tissue trauma from biting; soft tissue bruising; lack of safety precautions; uncontrolled movements

OUTCOMES

Short Term
Minimal injury or absence of injury, as evidenced by mouth, tongue, bone, or soft tissue damage being controlled or absent during and after seizure activity (expected within time frame of seizure)

Long Term
Absence of injury, as evidenced by mucous membranes, bones, or absence of breaks in skin, as seizures are controlled (expected to be ongoing)

NURSING INTERVENTIONS/INSTRUCTIONS

1. Assess for type and frequency of seizure activity, loss of consciousness, loss of muscle tone, tongue biting, falling to the floor, weakness or paralysis, and presence of aura (first visit).

2. Instruct caregiver to allow client to slide to floor; place client in side-lying position; avoid restricting any movement, jerking, or stiffening; loosen constricting clothing (first visit; reinforce on second visit).

3. Instruct caregiver to remain with client during entire seizure and to place small pillow under client's head or place client's head in lap (first visit).

4. Instruct client and family to remove harmful objects from the immediate environment (first visit).

5. Instruct client and caregiver to note if aura is present, how seizure began, how it progressed, and how long lasted, and to report presence of cyanosis, excessive saliva, incontinence, and post-seizure sleep period (first visit).

6. Instruct client to prevent seizure activity by avoiding emotional and physical stress or stimulation (e.g., noise, lights, drugs) that triggers seizure (first visit).

CLIENT AND FAMILY/CAREGIVER INTERVENTIONS

1. Caregiver performs measures to prevent trauma during seizure activity.

2. Caregiver provides safe environment during seizure activity.

3. Caregiver assesses aspects of seizure activity and reports to physician for evaluation.

4. Caregiver remains with and supports client during seizure activity.

5. Client avoids actions and stimuli that cause seizure activity.

NURSING DIAGNOSIS ANXIETY

■*Related Factors:* Threat to self-concept; threat of change in health status

■*Defining Characteristics:* Verbalized apprehension and uncertainty about unpredictable seizure activity; social withdrawal; feelings of inadequacy; stigma attached to presence of disorder

OUTCOMES

■*Short Term*

Reduced anxiety, as evidenced by client's statement that anxiety is at manageable level, embarrassment is controlled, and social and family interactions are improved (expected in 1 to 2 weeks)

▌*Long Term*

Anxiety level at optimal level for achievement of health and functioning, with self-concept enhanced (expected in 2 to 3 months)

NURSING INTERVENTIONS/INSTRUCTIONS

1. Assess anxiety level, social interactions and how condition impacts lifestyle and self-esteem, and perception of how others view disease (first visit and as needed).
2. Allow client to express feelings about diagnosis of epilepsy (each visit).
3. Assist client in developing coping strategies to reduce anxiety, and instruct client in relaxation techniques, including reading, music, imagery, and relaxation exercises (first and second visits).
4. Inform client of importance of maintaining social relationships and recreation and occupational activities (each visit).
5. Initiate referral to counseling if appropriate (any visit).

CLIENT AND FAMILY/CAREGIVER INTERVENTIONS

1. Client discusses feelings, anger, and anxiety regarding condition.
2. Client develops coping skills to reduce anxiety.
3. Client uses relaxation techniques to reduce anxiety.
4. Client maintains relationships and activities for optimal functioning.
5. Client adapts to lifestyle that includes stigma or misconception of the disease by others.
6. Client participates in counseling services if needed.

NURSING DIAGNOSIS — DEFICIENT KNOWLEDGE

▌*Related Factors:* Lack of information about disorder

▌*Defining Characteristics:* Request for information about medication administration and compliance and cause, treatment, and prognosis of disorder

OUTCOMES

▌*Short Term*

Adequate knowledge, as evidenced by client's ability to discuss cause, treatment, prognosis, and medication regimen (expected in 1 week)

▌*Long Term*

Optimal knowledge, as evidenced by compliance with medical regimen to achieve optimal health and functioning (expected in 1 month)

NURSING INTERVENTIONS/INSTRUCTIONS

1. Assess lifestyle, learning and adaptation abilities, interest level, and family participation and support (first visit).
2. Inform client of cause of seizure activity and of the importance of compliance with follow-up visits for laboratory testing and physician evaluation (first visit).
3. Instruct client in administration of anticonvulsant therapy, including dose, route, action, and side effects (e.g., gingival hypertrophy, visual disturbances, rashes, confusion) to assess and report; in food and drug interactions; not to discontinue medication without physician advice; and to avoid OTC drugs without physician advice (first and second visits).
4. Instruct client to have dental checkups every 6 months; instruct client in tooth care, including brushing and using dental floss to prevent oral infection (first visit).
5. Instruct client to report fever, sore throat, fatigue, or weakness, which may indicate agranulocytosis, and inform client of need to have a complete blood count evaluation every 6 months if ordered (first visit).
6. Instruct client to avoid late-night television, alcohol intake, fatigue, and stimulants known to cause seizure activity (first visit).
7. Inform client of immediate actions to take at onset of seizure and when to notify emergency service (first visit).
8. Suggest that client wears an identification bracelet or carries a card in a purse or wallet indicating condition, medication, physician, and physician's telephone number (first visit).
9. Inform client of antidiscrimination laws affecting work and other activities (first visit).
10. Inform client of National Epilepsy League and other agencies and groups available for support for people with the disorder (any visit).

CLIENT AND FAMILY/CAREGIVER INTERVENTIONS

1. Caregiver promotes independence and avoids overprotection.

2. Client complies with medication administration as instructed and maintains regimen unless advised to change by physician; keeps follow-up appointments.
3. Client manages lifestyle changes and adapts to changes brought about by disorder; uses resources available for information and support.
4. Client reports complications of condition when appropriate.
5. Client carries identification information.

✳ *Spinal Cord Injury*

Spinal cord injury is the contusion, compression, hemorrhage, laceration, or transection of the spinal cord, causing loss of neurologic function. The injury may be acute, in which all sensation and reflex activity below the injury level are lost, or partial, in which some motor and sensory loss occurs, depending on the tracts affected. The injury is usually the result of car or sports accidents, falls, wounds from guns or implements of war, or diseases of the spinal cord.

Home care depends on the extent of the injury and is primarily concerned with the teaching of the medical regimen and with rehabilitation and aftercare to maximize health and function.

> Primary Diagnoses:
> Spinal Cord Injury, Traumatic—ICD code: 952.9
> Spinal Cord Compression—ICD code: 336.9

NURSING DIAGNOSIS IMPAIRED PHYSICAL MOBILITY

Related Factors: Neuromuscular impairment; perceptual impairment

Defining Characteristics: Paraplegia; quadriplegia; immobility; inability to purposefully move in physical environment, including bed mobility, transferring, and ambulation; spasticity; muscle weakness

OUTCOMES

▌*Short Term*

Enhanced mobility, as evidenced by improved activity and movement, ability to transfer and change positions, and absence of contractures and muscle atrophy (expected in 1 to 2 weeks)

▌*Long Term*

Achievement of optimal mobility, movement, and activity for health and functioning within injury limitations (expected to be ongoing)

NURSING INTERVENTIONS/INSTRUCTIONS

1. Assess degree and type of injury and impairment; muscle strength; and presence of spasticity, muscle wasting, and sensorimotor deficits (see Musculoskeletal System Assessment, p. 31, for guidelines) (each visit).

2. Perform and instruct client in passive, assistive, or active ROM exercises, to be performed every 2 to 4 hours or as prescribed by physical therapist (first and second visits).

3. Instruct client and caregiver in positioning and position changes and for caregiver to provide any assistance needed; suggest prone position to relieve pressure on susceptible areas and use of fracture board under mattress to prevent sagging of mattress (first and second visits).

4. Instruct client in removal and application of hand or foot splints (or, for feet, to use tennis shoes with the toe cut out) to prevent contractures; instruct client to avoid use of footboard, which may promote development of plantar flexion (first visit).

5. Instruct client, and support physical therapy instructions, in methods to move and turn in bed and to transfer to chair, wheelchair, or elsewhere (any visit).

6. Instruct client to schedule rest periods to alternate with ROM and muscle-strengthening exercises and activities (first and second visits).

7. Inform client of comfort resulting from warm baths and massage and their role in preventing spasticity (first visit).

8. Initiate referral to physical and/or occupational therapists for rehabilitation to maximize function remaining and to obtain special equipment for ambulation and other activities (first visit).

9. Provide information for securing bed with trapeze, mechanical lift, transfer board, and other aids and protective devices (first visit).

CLIENT AND FAMILY/CAREGIVER INTERVENTIONS

1. Client performs exercises alternating with rest periods daily.
2. Client progresses in transfer techniques, movement, and activities, and improves in use of assistive aids and devices.
3. Client maintains optimal independence in mobility and activities within injury limitations.
4. Client secures necessary equipment and supplies for optimal movement.
5. Caregiver encourages and praises all attempts and accomplishments of client and goal achievement.
6. Client complies with rehabilitation regimen initiated by the physical and/or occupational therapists.
7. Client performs follow-up muscle- and joint-preservation measures.

NURSING DIAGNOSIS RISK FOR POWERLESSNESS

Related Factors: Illness-related regimen

Defining Characteristics: Expressions of resentment, anger, guilt, passivity, and depression; dependence on others; verbal expressions of having no control

OUTCOMES

Short Term
Improved perception of control over current situation, as evidenced by expressions of increased input into care (expected in 1 week)

Long Term
Optimal perception of ability to affect care outcome, as evidenced by participation in planning care (expected to be ongoing)

NURSING INTERVENTIONS/INSTRUCTIONS

1. Assess mental and emotional status; expressions of degree of control over situation; behavioral changes indicating resentment, anger, guilt, passivity, or frustration; and use of defense mechanisms and coping and problem-solving skills (first visit).

2. Provide an accepting environment to promote expressions of frustrations and concerns (all visits).
3. Encourage client to participate in administering and planning care based on physical ability; provide choices in areas of client's control (all visits).
4. Initiate referral to social services, support groups, counseling, or psychotherapy as indicated (any visit).

CLIENT AND FAMILY/CAREGIVER INTERVENTIONS

1. Client expresses feelings about ability to control the situation.
2. Client participates in the planning and administration of care.
3. Client makes choices in areas of control.
4. Family and caregiver allow and encourage participation of client.
5. Client uses social services, support groups, and counseling as appropriate.

NURSING DIAGNOSIS RISK FOR IMPAIRED SKIN INTEGRITY

■ *Related Factors:* External factors of pressure, physical immobilization, and excretions from urine and bowel incontinence; internal factors of altered sensation and nutrition

■ *Defining Characteristics:* Disruption of skin surface; redness at bony prominences; inability to change position

OUTCOMES

■ *Short Term*
Reduction in risk for breaks in skin integrity, as evidenced by intact skin and absence of reddened areas (expected in 1 week)

■ *Long Term*
Skin integrity maintained, as evidenced by absence of actual skin breakdown or injury or absence of signs and symptoms of beginning breakdown (expected to be ongoing)

NURSING INTERVENTIONS/INSTRUCTIONS

1. Assess skin at pressure areas for redness and perineal area for irritation or excoriation if client is incontinent of urine and/or feces (see Integumentary System Assessment, p. 39, for guidelines) (each visit).

2. Instruct client in proper positioning and position changes to relieve pressure and shearing forces on skin (first visit).
3. Instruct client in massage technique using lotion for hands, feet, and bony prominences in particular (first visit).
4. Instruct client in perineal care following elimination or incontinence, including washing with mild soap, rinsing with warm water, patting dry, and applying skin protector (first visit).
5. Instruct client to eliminate any crumbs or debris in bed, chair, or other area that comes into contact with skin (first visit).
6. Instruct client to avoid using hot water for bathing and to avoid applying heat to or spilling hot foods on areas deprived of sensation to prevent burns (first visit).
7. Perform decubitus care if break in skin is noted, and instruct client to assess and perform treatment appropriate for stage of pressure ulcer and to report poor response to treatment (any visit).

CLIENT AND FAMILY/CAREGIVER INTERVENTIONS

1. Client assesses skin condition daily and performs measures to prevent breakdown.
2. Client uses aids to prevent skin pressure.
3. Client avoids excessive heat or cold coming into contact with paralyzed area.
4. Client eliminates pressure and shearing or mechanical forces that injure skin.
5. Client performs movements and transfers without skin trauma, with or without assistance.

NURSING DIAGNOSIS | **BATHING/HYGIENE, DRESSING/GROOMING, FEEDING, TOILETING SELF-CARE DEFICIT**

▌*Related Factors:* Neuromuscular impairment; impaired mobility status

▌*Defining Characteristics:* Inability to wash body parts, put on or take off clothes, get to and use toilet or be aware of urge to eliminate, or bring food from receptacle to mouth; paralysis

OUTCOMES

▍*Short Term*
Ability to perform ADL, as evidenced by beginning participation in feeding, toileting, bathing, personal hygiene, dressing, and grooming, within limitations imposed by injury (expected in 1 to 2 weeks)

▍*Long Term*
Optimal participation in self-care for ADL with or without assistive aids or devices to achieve independence (expected in 2 to 3 months and ongoing)

NURSING INTERVENTIONS/INSTRUCTIONS

1. Assess client's ability to perform self-care (paraplegic, quadriplegic), including ability to feed, bathe, groom, and clothe self and ability to use bedpan, urinal, or commode (see Functional Assessment, p. 55, for guidelines) (each visit).
2. Provide assistance or supervision as needed for performance of ADL, and instruct client to ask for assistance when needed (each visit).
3. Suggest and instruct client in use of assistive aids and devices for eating, dressing, grooming, personal hygiene, and toileting, and inform client of clothing and utensils to purchase to enhance self-care (first visit).
4. Instruct client to allow time to perform activities without rushing, for best results (first visit).
5. Initiate referral to occupational therapist for instruction and support in ADL and for suggestions for other aids (any visit).
6. Refer HHA to assist with ADL as needed (first visit).

CLIENT AND FAMILY/CAREGIVER INTERVENTIONS

1. Client participates in ADL with progressive results, with or without the use of assistive aids or devices.
2. Client performs self-care independently with maximal rehabilitative potential.
3. Caregiver assists client to maintain functional abilities in daily activities.
4. Client complies with occupational rehabilitation schedule and practices activities as instructed.

NURSING DIAGNOSIS	INEFFECTIVE COPING

▋*Related Factors:* Multiple life changes; inadequate coping method

▋*Defining Characteristics:* Inability to cope, to meet role expectations, or to meet basic needs; chronic anxiety; poor self-esteem; feelings of fear and grief; negative feelings about body; change in sexual function; feelings of dependence and helplessness

OUTCOMES

▋*Short Term*

Improved individual coping, as evidenced by client's statement of realization of lifestyle changes that need to be made and willingness to adapt and learn effective coping mechanisms (expected in 1 to 2 weeks)

▋*Long Term*

Effective coping and adaptation to changed self-concept, as evidenced by achievement of requirements for optimal health and functioning within injury limitations, returning to employment, and retraining in sexual function and other life changes (expected in 3 months and ongoing)

NURSING INTERVENTIONS/INSTRUCTIONS

1. Assess for anxiety, depression, feelings about appearance and loss of neurologic functioning and effect on self-concept and body image, use and effectiveness of coping mechanisms, and behavioral and emotional changes and reasons for them (each visit).
2. Instruct client in developing new coping skills while maintaining current skills that are successful; assist client with problem-solving skills (first and second visits).
3. Include client in setting realistic goals for functioning and in developing the treatment plan and methods to evaluate progress (each visit).
4. Instruct client to avoid emotional and physical stress (first visit).
5. Show care, concern, and willingness to assist in coping with lifestyle changes (each visit).

6. Allow for expressions of feelings, concerns, and fears about the future, and inform client that this is acceptable behavior (each visit).
7. Refrain from using words such as "quad" or "cripple"; use words such as "disabled" (each visit).
8. Initiate referral to social services, psychotherapy, sexual therapy, occupational retraining, and rehabilitation as needed (any visit).

CLIENT AND FAMILY/CAREGIVER INTERVENTIONS

1. Client uses planned program during the entire day to meet goals and to prevent depression, boredom, and fatigue.
2. Client expresses feelings and grief as needed.
3. Client identifies and uses coping mechanisms that work; tries alternative methods to cope.
4. Client seeks counseling from appropriate referrals and rehabilitation resources; joins groups whose members have had similar experiences.

NURSING DIAGNOSIS BOWEL INCONTINENCE

Related Factors: Neuromuscular involvement

Defining Characteristics: Involuntary passage of stool; constipation; loss of voluntary function and urge to defecate

OUTCOMES

Short Term
Adequate elimination, as evidenced by reestablishment of regular, soft, formed stool pattern (expected in 1 to 2 weeks)

Long Term
Establishment of bowel elimination pattern without incontinence of stool or constipation (expected to be ongoing)

NURSING INTERVENTIONS/INSTRUCTIONS

1. Instruct client to have bowel evacuation at same time each day; instruct client to use gentle pressure on abdomen, gentle digital anal stimulation, and Valsalva maneuver to promote bowel movement (first and second visits).

2. Instruct client to drink 8 to 10 glasses of fluid per day and prune juice at bedtime (first visit).
3. Instruct client to add fiber to daily diet and suggest foods to include (first visit).
4. Instruct client to administer suppository 30 minutes before scheduled elimination during training for stool continence (first visit; reinforce on second visit).
5. Review and reinforce a total bowel regimen that includes fluids, diet, scheduling, stool softener, suppository, and digital stimulation (each visit).

CLIENT AND FAMILY/CAREGIVER INTERVENTIONS

1. Client maintains daily or every-other-day bowel-evacuation regimen.
2. Client prepares and ingests high-fiber diet and maintains fluid intake as instructed.
3. Client administers medication as appropriate to enhance elimination at scheduled times.

NURSING DIAGNOSIS REFLEX URINARY INCONTINENCE

Related Factors: Neurologic impairment (e.g., spinal cord injury)

Defining Characteristics: No awareness of bladder filling or fullness; no urge to void; uninhibited bladder contraction or spasm; neurogenic bladder; bladder distension; frequent voiding in small amounts; constant dribbling

OUTCOMES

Short Term
Improved bladder function, as evidenced by reduction in incontinence episodes with use of catheter or training program (expected in 1 to 2 weeks)

Long Term
Ability to maintain bladder function, with absence of infection, to achieve optimal urinary continence (expected to be ongoing)

NURSING INTERVENTIONS/INSTRUCTIONS

1. Instruct client in noting and reporting cloudy, foul-smelling urine (first visit).
2. Instruct client to increase fluid intake to 10 glasses/day, and suggest acid-ash juices such as cranberry juice (first visit).
3. Instruct client in use of indwelling catheter, if present, noting patency and using sterile technique in catheter and meatal care (first and second visits).
4. Instruct client in application and care of condom catheter if used (first visit).
5. Instruct client or family member in intermittent catheterization using sterile technique and care of catheters if procedure is appropriate (first and second visits).
6. Inform client of training program and instruct client in scheduling voiding and in performing Credé's maneuver if bladder is not distended, or refer client to a rehabilitation program if rehabilitation is possible (first visit).
7. Initiate referral to enterostomal therapist if appropriate (any visit).

CLIENT AND FAMILY/CAREGIVER INTERVENTIONS

1. Client or caregiver performs assessment for urinary bladder infection whether catheter is used or not.
2. Client or caregiver performs intermittent catheterization using sterile or clean technique as appropriate.
3. Client or caregiver maintains catheter patency and catheter care or condom catheter procedures.
4. Client participates in urinary control rehabilitation program if appropriate.

NURSING DIAGNOSIS   RISK FOR AUTONOMIC DYSREFLEXIA

▮**Related Factors:** Bladder distension; bowel distension

▮**Defining Characteristics:** Paroxysmal hypertension; bradycardia; diaphoresis above injured area; pallor below injured area

OUTCOMES

▮**Short Term**

Knowledge of risk for autonomic dysreflexia, as evidenced by verbalization of signs, symptoms, and prevention (expected in 1 week)

▌*Long Term*

Minimal risk for autonomic dysreflexia, as evidenced by absence of autonomic dysreflexia triggers including bowel and bladder distension (expected in 1 month)

NURSING INTERVENTIONS/INSTRUCTIONS

1. Assess for elimination patterns and other potential triggers such as drafts, heat, pain, and injury (first visit).
2. Teach client about autonomic dysreflexia, including signs and symptoms (e.g., hypertension, bradycardia, profuse sweating above level of injury) (first and second visits).
3. Teach client to avoid stressors, including bowel and bladder distension, heat, cold, pain, and injury; instruct in measures to take in case of occurrence (first visit and ongoing).

CLIENT AND FAMILY/CAREGIVER INTERVENTIONS

1. Client observes for sign and symptoms of autonomic dysreflexia, including monitoring blood pressure and pulse.
2. Client takes measures to avoid bowel and bladder distension and avoids other triggers.
3. Caregiver elevates head of client's bed and immediately notifies physician of appearance of signs and symptoms.

NURSING DIAGNOSIS DEFICIENT KNOWLEDGE

▌*Related Factors:* Lack of information about disability

▌*Defining Characteristics:* Request for information about medical and rehabilitation regimen and prevention of trauma or injury

OUTCOMES

▌*Short Term*

Adequate knowledge, as evidenced by client's statement of treatment regimen and potential for injury or complications (expected in 1 week)

▌*Long Term*

Optimal knowledge, as evidenced by achievement of requirements for optimal health and functioning within limitations imposed by injury (expected in 1 to 2 months and ongoing)

NURSING INTERVENTIONS/INSTRUCTIONS

1. Assess lifestyle, learning and adaptation abilities, interest level, and family participation and support (first visit).
2. Include all family members and caregivers in instructions (each visit).
3. Assist client in writing a plan to incorporate the medical regimen and rehabilitation schedules and instruction; revise daily as needed (each visit).
4. Instruct client to modify environment to prevent falls, to provide space needed for use of assistive aids such as a wheelchair, and to secure supplies and equipment that will ensure a safe home environment for ADL and other activities (first visit).
5. Instruct client to protect affected areas from excessively hot or cold applications or from trauma resulting from decreased sensory perception and motor deficits (first visit).
6. Instruct client in need to maintain fluid intake of up to 3000 ml/day and a diet high in calories, protein, and carbohydrates; offer food lists and sample menus to assist in planning meals (first visit).
7. Instruct client in signs and symptoms of respiratory tract infection and to report change in respiration, yellow or other color change in sputum, or temperature elevation (first visit).
8. Inform client of possible autonomic dysreflexia, signs and symptoms of disorder (e.g., hypertension, bradycardia, profuse sweating), actions to take to prevent this condition (i.e., prevent bowel and bladder distension), and actions to take if condition occurs (first and second visits).
9. Inform client of importance of compliance with physical, occupational, psychologic, and other therapy if applicable and to comply with scheduled visits to physician (first visit).
10. Inform client of stages of grieving and behavioral changes that can be expected to achieve stage of adjustment (each visit).
11. Inform client about availability of social services and other community resources (any visit).

CLIENT AND FAMILY/CAREGIVER INTERVENTIONS

1. Client identifies hazards and eliminates or modifies them.
2. Client uses assistive and supplemental aids.
3. Client maintains open communication during grieving process.

4. Client assesses for and reports complications.
5. Client maintains scheduled appointments for rehabilitative therapy.
6. Client uses agencies for assistance in transportation, information, support, food services, housekeeping services, and others.
7. Client complies with fluid, nutritional, rest, activity, and other regimens included in medical regimen with as much independence as possible.

NURSING DIAGNOSIS RISK FOR CAREGIVER ROLE STRAIN

Related Factors: Inexperience with caregiving; complexity or amount of caregiving tasks; duration of caregiving required; inadequate physical environment for providing care (e.g., housing, transportation, equipment, accessibility)

Defining Characteristics: Report of not having enough resources (e.g., emotional and physical strength, help from others) to provide care; difficulty in performing specific caregiving activities (e.g., bathing, cleaning up after urinary or bowel incontinence, moving and transferring, catheterization, managing discomforts and total care needs)

OUTCOMES

Short Term
Identification of potential for caregiver role strain, as evidenced by caregiver's verbalization of difficulties encountered in performing care and concern about ability and conflicts in giving care (expected in 1 week)

Long Term
Prevention of caregiver role strain, as evidenced by caregiver's providing of continued, progressive, and safe care without compromise to own physical and emotional needs (expected in 1 month and ongoing)

NURSING INTERVENTIONS/INSTRUCTIONS

1. Assess severity of disability and care needs of the receiver of care and ability of the caregiver to perform role (first visit).

2. Assess relationship between care receiver and caregiver before the illness and stressors placed on the relationship by the complexity of needs caused by the illness (first visit).
3. Assist caregiver in monitoring his or her continued ability to perform care and treatments, day-to-day needs that may need to be changed or learned, and changes in stressors and strains; assess maintenance of routines and need for additional resources (e.g., aides, friends, family) (each visit).
4. Discuss role performance, whether expectations are realistic, and flexibility of role and decision-making process (first visit).
5. Initiate referral to HHA, social services, or psychologic counseling to assist with economic or mental or physical health needs (any visit).

CLIENT AND FAMILY/CAREGIVER INTERVENTIONS

1. Caregiver develops ability to cope with caregiver role; incorporates flexibility into day-to-day functioning.
2. Caregiver explores financial, legal, and physical assistance sources, and considers a referral to these services.
3. Caregiver maintains own health and well-being in caregiver role.
4. Caregiver maintains ongoing care and treatment regimen for care receiver.

GASTROINTESTINAL SYSTEM

✳ *Cirrhosis of the Liver*

Cirrhosis of the liver is a chronic disease characterized by structural and degenerative changes, causing liver dysfunction and possible liver failure. Changes include the destruction of the liver parenchyma with the development of fibrous tissue that surrounds the hepatocytes and separates the lobules and, finally, the formation of nodules as the liver attempts to regenerate itself. Cirrhosis may be caused by chronic alcoholism, longstanding right-sided heart failure, alterations in the immune system, stasis of bile in the liver, or hepatic or other infections.

Home care is primarily concerned with ongoing assessment of the chronic symptoms of the disease, elimination of the underlying cause if possible, and the teaching involved in promoting maintenance of health status and prevention of further liver damage and complications.

Primary Diagnoses:
Cirrhosis, Liver—ICD code: 571.5
Cirrhosis, Liver, Alcoholic—ICD code: 571.2

NURSING DIAGNOSIS: IMBALANCED NUTRITION: LESS THAN BODY REQUIREMENTS

Related Factors: Inability to ingest food because of biologic factors; inability to digest foods because of biologic factors

Defining Characteristics: Anorexia; nausea; vomiting; inability to metabolize fats, proteins, and carbohydrates and to store nutrients; diarrhea or constipation; excessive fluid losses; weight loss; abdominal pain

OUTCOMES

Short Term

Adequate nutritional intake, as evidenced by compliance with a diet that facilitates appropriate weight maintenance for size, age, and frame; client's verbalization of foods to be included in a high-carbohydrate, moderately high-protein diet; abstinence from alcohol (expected in 3 days)

▌*Long Term*

Optimal nutrition, as evidenced by food consumption and weight maintained within expected requirements; continued abstinence from alcohol; achievement of optimal health and functioning within limitations imposed by disease (expected in 1 to 3 months and ongoing)

NURSING INTERVENTIONS/INSTRUCTIONS

1. Assess nutritional status and dietary inclusions and restrictions needed in presence of disease and in accordance with stage and symptoms of the disease (see Gastrointestinal System Assessment, p. 22, for guidelines) (first visit).
2. Instruct client to maintain a log of types and amounts of food eaten and likes and dislikes; review intake and use data as a basis for teaching diet; coordinate with dietitian (first, second, and third visits).
3. Assess alcohol intake and provide client with the rationale for avoiding all alcoholic beverages (each visit).
4. Assess for presence of anorexia, nausea, vomiting, malaise, fatigue, and muscle wasting; suggest a period of rest before meals (first visit).
5. Measure height and weight and calculate weight requirements (first visit).
6. Measure abdominal girth (each visit).
7. Assist client in planning and selecting foods for a high-carbohydrate, moderate-protein diet totaling approximately 2000 to 3000 calories per day; suggest supplemental feedings if needed; provide sample menu/diet plan (first visit; reinforce on second visit).
8. Instruct client to restrict fluids in presence of edema or ascites (any visit).
9. Instruct client to avoid salty and convenience foods and to restrict sodium intake to 200 to 500 mg/day in presence of edema or ascites; instruct client in how to read labels on foods to determine sodium content (first visit).
10. Instruct client in administration of vitamins and minerals, antiemetics, and other prescribed drugs; instruct client to

avoid over-the-counter (OTC) drugs unless advised by physician (first visit).

11. Instruct client to eat smaller, more frequent meals rather than three large meals per day (first visit).

12. Advise client to perform oral hygiene after meals and to use hard candy or sips of carbonated beverages or dry foods for nausea (first visit).

13. Initiate referral to nutritionist (first visit).

14. Refer home health aide (HHA) to assist with activities of daily living (ADL) and food preparation (first visit).

CLIENT AND FAMILY/CAREGIVER INTERVENTIONS

1. Client adheres to prescribed diet as instructed; maintains food diary.

2. Client limits sodium, fluids, or protein if indicated.

3. Client avoids alcohol intake.

4. Client weighs daily and reports any significant gains or losses.

5. Client administers medications and vitamin supplement.

6. Client eats six times per day in small amounts; adjusts intake if nausea or vomiting is present.

7. Client provides pleasant environment for meals.

8. Client maintains oral hygiene.

9. Client consults with nutritionist if needed.

NURSING DIAGNOSIS RISK FOR INFECTION

▌*Related Factors:* Inadequate secondary defenses; malnutrition

▌*Defining Characteristics:* Leukopenia; chronic inadequate nutritional intake and metabolism; elevated temperature; changes in breathing, urine characteristics, or any part of body

OUTCOMES

▌*Short Term*
Reduced risk for infection development, as evidenced by temperature and white blood cell count within normal ranges, lung fields clear, and skin intact (expected in 3 days)

▌*Long Term*
Absence of signs and symptoms of infection in any organ system (expected in 2 weeks)

NURSING INTERVENTIONS/INSTRUCTIONS

1. Assess skin for jaundice, pruritus, and evidence of scratches or excoriation (first visit).
2. Instruct client in relief measures for pruritus, including cool compresses, emollient baths, patting instead of rubbing skin dry, and use of mild soap and soft towel (first visit).
3. Instruct client to avoid scratching itchy areas and to keep fingernails short, clean, and well filed for smoothness (first visit).
4. Assess lungs for decreased breath sounds, cough, adventitious sounds, or change in respiratory rate, depth, or ease (first visit).
5. Instruct client to take temperature and notify physician of elevations or of changes in respiratory pattern or airway clearance (first visit).
6. Instruct client to avoid exposure to persons with infections (first visit).
7. Instruct client in antibiotic administration as prescribed (first visit).
8. Refer HHA to assist with bathing as indicated (first visit).

CLIENT AND FAMILY/CAREGIVER INTERVENTIONS

1. Client maintains personal hygiene; adjusts bathing, grooming, and dressing to enhance body image and protect jaundiced skin.
2. Client administers medications as instructed.
3. Client reports to physician signs and symptoms of infection if present.
4. Client monitors temperature if symptoms appear.
5. Client maintains absence of infection of skin, lungs, or any other organ.

NURSING DIAGNOSIS INEFFECTIVE PROTECTION

Related Factors: Abnormal blood profile

Defining Characteristics: Inability of liver to convert ammonia to urea, to produce coagulation factors, and to absorb vitamin K; leukopenia; ecchymoses; petechiae; bleeding from gums and mucous membranes

OUTCOMES

Short Term

Control of bleeding tendency, as evidenced by absence of bleeding from any site (expected in 3 days)

Long Term

Maintenance of blood profile within normal ranges within limitations imposed by severity of disease (expected in 2 to 4 weeks)

NURSING INTERVENTIONS/INSTRUCTIONS

1. Assess for bleeding, including petechiae, ecchymoses, and oozing or frank bleeding from any orifice or skin site; check hemoglobin and hematocrit levels if available; instruct client to report any bleeding to physician (each visit).
2. Instruct client to avoid trauma and constrictive clothing and to protect vulnerable areas from injury (first visit).
3. Instruct client in administration of vitamin K if appropriate (first visit).
4. Instruct client and HHA to avoid tooth brushing (use swabs instead) and taking temperature rectally (first visit).

CLIENT AND FAMILY/CAREGIVER INTERVENTIONS

1. Client identifies and reports signs and symptoms of bleeding.
2. Client administers prescribed medications.

NURSING DIAGNOSIS DISTURBED THOUGHT PROCESSES

Related Factors: Physiologic changes

Defining Characteristics: Confusion; memory deficit; disorientation; lethargy

OUTCOMES

Short Term

Improvement in neurologic function and mentation, as evidenced by stability in orientation and mental functioning (expected in 1 week)

Long Term

Appropriate level of mental function within limitations imposed by disease status (expected in 2 to 4 weeks)

NURSING INTERVENTIONS/INSTRUCTIONS

1. Assess mentation, including confusion, lethargy, irritability, depression, personality and behavioral changes, slurred speech, and psychotic ideations, and instruct client to report any of these conditions to physician (each visit).
2. Encourage client to participate in interactions with others and to use clock, calendar, newspaper, radio, and other stimulation that may be preferred (first visit).
3. Inform client of reason for mental changes if they occur (first visit).
4. Refer client to psychologic counseling if appropriate (any visit).
5. Refer HHA to assist with ADL (first visit).

CLIENT AND FAMILY/CAREGIVER INTERVENTIONS

1. Client identifies and reports mental and emotional changes.
2. Client provides stimulation and reality reinforcement.
3. Client administers medications if prescribed.

NURSING DIAGNOSIS DISTURBED BODY IMAGE

▎**Related Factors:** Biophysical factors caused by disease process

▎**Defining Characteristics:** Jaundice; pruritus; skin irritation from scratching; chronic fatigue; estrogen-androgen imbalance; ascites; edema

OUTCOMES

▎**Short Term**
Improvement in self-image, as evidenced by participation in care and interest in appearance and by some resumption of outside activities or interactions (expected in 3 to 7 days)

▎**Long Term**
Adaptation to temporary and permanent changes in body image, as evidenced by resumption of self-care activities and social and work activities to achieve optimal level of function within disease limitations (expected in 1 to 3 months)

NURSING INTERVENTIONS/INSTRUCTIONS

1. Assess client's and family's ability to cope and adapt (first visit).
2. Allow time for and acceptance of expressions of concern and negative comments about appearance (each visit).
3. Assess behavioral and emotional trends and changes, and integrate them into clinical profile for disease progression and encephalopathy (each visit).
4. Assess and discuss appearance and measures to minimize the effects of edema, jaundice, weight changes, loss of hair, menstrual irregularities, impotence, and changes in sex characteristics (first visit; reinforce as needed).
5. Initiate referral to social services, counseling, or support group (any visit).

CLIENT AND FAMILY/CAREGIVER INTERVENTIONS

1. Client expresses concerns and feelings about changes.
2. Client supports and adapts to physical changes.
3. Client participates in daily care and uses measures to conceal body changes and appearance.
4. Client reports signs and symptoms of hormonal imbalance or central nervous system dysfunction.
5. Client seeks counseling if needed, occupational retraining if appropriate.

NURSING DIAGNOSIS | DEFICIENT KNOWLEDGE

▌**Related Factors:** Lack of information about disease and care

▌**Defining Characteristics:** Request for information about disease process, causes, treatments, preventive measures, and medical regimen; denial as result of absence of symptoms or alcohol abuse

OUTCOMES

▌Short Term
Adequate knowledge, as evidenced by client's statement of status of disease and symptoms of worsening condition and of need for compliance in medication and activity regimens and alcoholism rehabilitation (expected in 1 week)

▌*Long Term*

Functional knowledge, as evidenced by compliance with requirements to maintain liver function and obtain optimal level of health (expected in 2 to 3 months)

NURSING INTERVENTIONS/INSTRUCTIONS

1. Assess lifestyle, abilities to learn and adapt to treatments, interests and diversional activities, family participation and support, and presence of alcoholism (first visit).

2. Perform abdominal assessment, including measurement for changes in abdominal girth indicating ascites palpation for splenomegaly, hepatic level and hardness, and abdominal discomfort, and instruct client in performing this assessment (first visit and ongoing).

3. Assess complaints of nausea, vomiting, anorexia, weight loss or gain, constipation or diarrhea, fatigue, or pruritus, and instruct client to report these conditions to physician if they occur (each visit).

4. Assess for history of alcohol abuse, use of hepatotoxic drugs, exposure to chemicals, or gastrointestinal (GI) surgery (first visit).

5. Discuss and reinforce importance of alcohol abstinence (first visit; reinforce when needed).

6. Instruct client to schedule 6 to 8 hours of sleep per 24 hours and to schedule rest hours around meals and activities (first visit).

7. Instruct client to report any signs or symptoms of complications or worsening condition, including fever, bleeding, shortness of breath, increase in abdominal girth, weight or urinary output changes, edema, confusion or personality changes, abdominal pain, or jaundice (first week).

8. Instruct client to avoid exposure to toxic agents, medications, or environments and to possible infection (first visit).

9. Instruct client in medication administration, including vitamins, antipruritic agents, stool softeners, diuretics, electrolyte replacement products, aldosterone-blocking agents, digestive enzymes, lactulose, and others as ordered; inform client of dose; frequency; route; side effects; and food, drug, and alcohol interactions (first visit; reinforce on second visit).

10. Advise client of importance of keeping appointments with physician and laboratory (first visit).

11. Provide information about community agencies and groups, such as Alcoholics Anonymous (AA), for support, counseling, or educational materials (first visit).

CLIENT AND FAMILY/CAREGIVER INTERVENTIONS

1. Client complies with medical regimen and changes lifestyle if needed.
2. Client reports signs and symptoms of complications.
3. Client avoids intake of alcohol and other substances toxic to liver.
4. Client administers medications correctly and safely.
5. Client avoids stressful situations; seeks counseling if needed.
6. Client schedules adequate rest and sleep and promotes as part of daily routine.
7. Client maintains physician and laboratory appointments.
8. Client contacts AA or other support groups for assistance.
9. Client returns to work and activities within limitations.

✳ *Hepatitis*

Hepatitis is the inflammation of the liver as the result of alcohol, drugs, or viruses. Viral hepatitis may be classified as hepatitis A, hepatitis B, or hepatitis C, depending on the viral strain. Hepatitis A is transmitted by the oral-fecal route; hepatitis B and C are transmitted by the parenteral route. The disease varies in severity, which determines the degree of liver cell injury and scarring and resolution or chronicity of the condition.

Home care is primarily concerned with proper testing and treatment necessary to prevent transmission and increased incidence of the disease in the community and with the teaching involved in the care and treatment of the acute stage of the disease and the prevention of permanent liver damage.

Primary Diagnoses:
Hepatitis—ICD code: 573.3
Hepatitis, Viral—ICD code: 070.9
Hepatitis B—ICD code: 070.30
Hepatitis C—ICD code: 070.51
Hepatitis C, Chronic—ICD code: 070.54

NURSING DIAGNOSIS	IMBALANCED NUTRITION: LESS THAN BODY REQUIREMENTS

Related Factors: Inability to ingest food; inability to digest foods because of biologic factors

Defining Characteristics: Nausea; vomiting; anorexia; abdominal diarrhea; inability to store nutrients; inability to metabolize fats, proteins, and carbohydrates; excessive fluid losses; tenderness; weight loss

OUTCOMES

Short Term
Adequate nutrition, as evidenced by consumption of increased carbohydrates and increased calories and by prescribed protein intake (expected in 3 days)

Long Term
Nutritional status optimal, as evidenced by intake of prescribed diet and by weight maintenance for health and functioning during course of disease (expected in 1 to 2 months)

NURSING INTERVENTIONS/INSTRUCTIONS

1. Assess nutritional and GI status, taking into consideration dietary preferences and restrictions or inclusions (see Gastrointestinal System Assessment, p. 22, for guidelines) (first visit).
2. Measure height and weight and calculate weight requirements (first visit).
3. Measure abdominal girth, and determine weight on same scale, at same time of day, with client wearing similar clothing (each visit).
4. Instruct client to keep food diary that includes types, portions, and preparation method of foods consumed (first visit).
5. Using these data as a basis for diet teaching, assist client in food selection for a high-carbohydrate, high-calorie diet, which also should be high in protein in the absence of edema; provide sample menu/meal plan (first visit; reinforce on second visit).
6. Instruct client to eat smaller, more frequent meals rather than three large meals per day; advise client to eat larger amounts during the day rather than in the evening (first visit).

7. Instruct client to drink 3000 ml of fluids per day (in absence of edema) and to estimate adequacy of output (first visit).
8. Suggest hard candy, sips of carbonated beverages, or dry food for nausea (first visit).
9. Instruct client in administration of prescribed antiemetic 30 minutes before meals (first visit).

CLIENT AND FAMILY/CAREGIVER INTERVENTIONS

1. Client maintains a food and fluid intake diary.
2. Client measures and records weight daily or as needed.
3. Client maintains prescribed carbohydrate and caloric intake.
4. Client spreads meals over entire day, with most eaten early in the day, and intersperses meals with fluid intake.
5. Client administers antiemetic before meals.
6. Client performs oral care as needed.
7. Client uses hard candy and other dietary aids to control nausea.
8. Client limits protein and fluid intake if edema is present.

NURSING DIAGNOSIS RISK FOR IMPAIRED SKIN INTEGRITY

■ *Related Factors:* Internal factor of altered pigmentation

■ *Defining Characteristics:* Jaundice; pruritus; dry skin; scratches or disruptions on skin

OUTCOMES

■ *Short Term*
Skin intact and free from irritation, as evidenced by absence of rash, abrasions, excoriations, or disruptions (expected in 1 week)

■ *Long Term*
Skin integrity maintained, with optimal comfort and health achieved (expected in 1 month)

NURSING INTERVENTIONS/INSTRUCTIONS

1. Assess skin for color, temperature, integrity, and sensation; assess for presence of jaundice or pruritus and for evidence of scratching (see Integumentary System Assessment, p. 39, for guidelines) (each visit).
2. Instruct client in relief measures, such as cool or warm shower or cool compresses to area, mild soap for bathing, patting

instead of rubbing dry, diversional methods, and use of emollients in water and topically (first visit).

3. Instruct client to maintain clean, short nails and to apply pressure to itchy areas instead of scratching (first visit).

4. Instruct client in use of antipruritic medications and antihistamines, including dose, time, frequency, and side effects; inform client of drug or alcohol interactions (first visit).

5. Inform client to wear loose clothing and to avoid tight, restrictive types of clothing, which might increase itching (first visit).

CLIENT AND FAMILY/CAREGIVER INTERVENTIONS

1. Client administers medications for relief of itching.
2. Client uses other relief measures to control pruritus.
3. Client avoids scratching.
4. Client notifies physician if symptoms are not relieved or if breaks appear on skin.

NURSING DIAGNOSIS IMPAIRED SOCIAL INTERACTION

Related Factors: Therapeutic isolation; body image disturbance

Defining Characteristics: Verbalized discomfort in social participation; jaundiced appearance; fear of transmitting disease to others; stated lack of diversional activity and interactions

OUTCOMES

Short Term

Minimal boredom, loneliness, and impaired body image, as evidenced by client's statement that body image is improving as condition resolves and by participation in activities to provide stimulation (expected in 1 week)

Long Term

Adaptation to temporary restrictions in social relationships to prevent transmission of disease and adaptation to sensory deficits by maintenance of optimal level of health and functioning (expected in 1 month)

NURSING INTERVENTIONS/INSTRUCTIONS

1. Instruct client in reasons for isolation precautions and that length of time restrictions must be observed (first visit).

2. Instruct family to provide separate room and bathroom for client if possible (first visit).
3. Instruct family to spend time with client at intervals during day (first visit).
4. Inform client and family of precautions to take to prevent transmission, including handwashing and care of utensils and articles used for meals and for bowel elimination (first visit).
5. Encourage family to provide for diversional activities, such as books, cards, television, radio, newspaper, and telephone (first visit).
6. Inform client that jaundice is not permanent and that it disappears as disease is resolved (first visit).
7. Remove mirrors and cover body parts to preserve body image if jaundice is present (first visit).
8. Note negative attitudes and comments regarding skin color and pruritus, and provide support (each visit).
9. Refer to social services as indicated (any visit).

CLIENT AND FAMILY/CAREGIVER INTERVENTIONS

1. Client encourages visits from friends.
2. Client maintains precautions to prevent transmission of disease.
3. Family provides diversional activities when client is confined to room.
4. Family promotes and supports positive attitude about temporary jaundice.

NURSING DIAGNOSIS DEFICIENT KNOWLEDGE

▌**Related Factors:** Lack of information about disease

▌**Defining Characteristics:** Request for information about disease and its transmission and about prevention of complications or relapse or recurrence

OUTCOMES

▌**Short Term**

Adequate knowledge, as evidenced by client's stating methods of disease transmission, treatment, and prevention of complications and by client's compliance with diet, activity, and hygiene and sanitation regimens (expected in 3 days)

▌*Long Term*

Optimal knowledge, as evidenced by client's meeting requirements to achieve optimal level of liver function and absence of symptoms and complications or transmittal of disease to others (expected in 1 to 2 months)

NURSING INTERVENTIONS/INSTRUCTIONS

1. Assess lifestyle, ability and interest to learn, ability to adapt, and family participation and support (first visit).
2. Review history of flulike symptoms such as nausea, vomiting, anorexia, weight loss, fatigue, malaise, headache, myalgia, or constipation or diarrhea; also note recent travel, transfusions, injections or sharing of needles, or exposure to toxins or to carriers (first visit).
3. Perform abdominal assessment (see Gastrointestinal System Assessment, p. 22, for guidelines) and note liver size and tenderness; enlarged nodes; and presence of dark urine, clay-colored stools, scleral icterus, or jaundice (each visit).
4. Instruct client in causes, transmission, signs and symptoms, and treatment of disease (first visit).
5. Instruct client in handwashing and isolation protocols, and emphasize washing hands, especially after toileting (first visit).
6. Instruct client to avoid tiring self and to participate only in activity that is tolerated (first visit).
7. Instruct client to report edema in extremities or abdomen, unexplained weight gain, changes in personality or behavior, or evidence of bleeding (first visit).
8. Instruct client to avoid intake of alcohol or toxins; review drug profile for hepatotoxic drugs (first visit).
9. Instruct client not to donate blood (first visit).
10. Instruct client to temporarily avoid sexual contact (first visit).
11. Instruct client with hepatitis C (HCV) in administration of prescribed interferon-based regimens (first, second, and third visits).
12. Instruct client to keep appointments with physician and for laboratory testing, and monitor laboratory results as available (each visit).
13. Initiate referral to appropriate health care facility for possible prophylactic care of household contacts and regular sexual partners (first visit).

14. Provide information on community agencies and groups, such as drug rehabilitation or counseling groups, for educational literature and support (first visit).

CLIENT AND FAMILY/CAREGIVER INTERVENTIONS

1. Client avoids transmission of disease by taking the following precautions:

   - Properly washing hands
   - Properly disinfecting food utensils, clothing, and linens
   - Avoiding sharing food, utensils, personal grooming items, toilet, clothing, or linens
   - Properly disposing tissues

2. Client states cause, transmission, signs and symptoms, and treatment of disease.
3. Client avoids intake of alcohol or hepatotoxic drugs and exposure to toxins.
4. Client avoids sexual contact.
5. Client refrains from donating blood.
6. Client avoids stressful situations; sets aside rest periods during day.
7. Client with HCV demonstrates safe administration of prescribed interferon-based medications.
8. Client reports signs and symptoms to physician as instructed.
9. Client reports for physician and laboratory appointments.
10. Client has contacts report for prophylactic therapy.
11. Client reports pregnancy status to all health workers.
12. Client contacts support groups or counselor for assistance if appropriate.

✳ *Peptic Ulcer*

A peptic ulcer is a sharp, circumscribed ulceration of the mucous membrane of the stomach (i.e., gastric ulcer, which is usually at the lesser curvature) or of the duodenum (i.e., duodenal ulcer, which is usually at the point where the stomach contents enter the small intestine). The condition may be acute or chronic and may be caused by the effect on the mucosal barrier of drug ingestion, high

levels of hydrochloric acid and enzyme secretions, prolonged illness, trauma or stress, or autoimmune disorders.

Home care is primarily concerned with the teaching involved in
the healing of the ulcer and with preventing factors that are associated with chronicity or recurrence.

Primary Diagnosis:
Peptic Ulcer—ICD code: 555.90

NURSING DIAGNOSIS — ACUTE PAIN

Related Factors: Biologic, chemical, or psychologic injuring
agents

Defining Characteristics: Communication of pain descriptors
(e.g., epigastric pain, burning, gnawing, aching, soreness that
occurs before or during eating); heartburn; indigestion; weight loss
or gain; high level of stress; ingestion of drugs (e.g., steroids, antiinflammatory drugs, antihypertensive agents)

OUTCOMES

Short Term
Increased comfort, as evidenced by client stating that he or she
feels better and that pain is decreased or absent (expected in 2 to 3
days)

Long Term
Absence of or minimal pain with decreased incidence of recurrence or relapse and achievement of optimal health and functioning (expected in 2 to 3 months)

NURSING INTERVENTIONS/INSTRUCTIONS

1. Assess abdomen (see Gastrointestinal System Assessment, p. 22,
   for guidelines); note vital signs, including temperature; type,
   intensity, and location of pain; radiation; bowel sounds; and
   precipitating and alleviating factors (each visit).
2. Instruct client in administration of medications that will assist
   in relieving pain, such as antacids, sedatives, and histamine
   (H_2) blockers, if ordered (first visit).
3. When pain is minimal or relieved, review health regimen to
   include diet, rest and activity, and avoidance of stressors (each
   visit).

CLIENT AND FAMILY/CAREGIVER INTERVENTIONS

1. Client correctly administers medications for pain as instructed.
2. Client avoids stressors and stressful situations.
3. Client reports new, increased, or uncontrolled pain to physician.

NURSING DIAGNOSIS DEFICIENT KNOWLEDGE

▌*Related Factors:* Lack of information about disorder

▌*Defining Characteristics:* Request for information about disease, causes, treatment (diet and medications), and importance of compliance

OUTCOMES

▌*Short Term*
Adequate knowledge, as evidenced by client stating signs and symptoms of deteriorating condition or complication; diet, activity, and medication regimens; and lifestyle adaptations (expected in 3 days)

▌*Long Term*
Optimal knowledge, as evidenced by client meeting requirements to achieve optimal level of health and functioning (expected in 2 weeks)

NURSING INTERVENTIONS/INSTRUCTIONS

1. Assess nutritional status, food preferences, and cultural or religious restrictions (first visit).
2. Assess height and weight and calculate desired weight; instruct client to measure and record weight weekly (first visit).
3. Instruct client on nutritionally adequate diet and prescribed modifications (first visit; reinforce on second visit):

   · Consume bland meals; eliminate food distressors such as black pepper; chili powder; raw, spicy, or fatty foods; fruit juices; and beverages containing caffeine
   · Eat smaller, more frequent meals (five or six per day), including a bedtime snack; include protein source at each meal
   · Drink skim rather than whole milk

4. Suggest that client rest before meals and that environment be quiet and pleasant during meals (first visit).
5. Instruct client to restrict alcohol intake and to refrain from smoking (first visit; reinforce on second visit).
6. Instruct client in administration of antacids (tablet or liquid), sedatives, antianxiety agents, proton-pump inhibitors, and histamine antagonists, including dose; route; frequency; side effects; and food, drug and alcohol interactions. Instruct client to avoid OTC drugs, especially aspirin or aspirin-containing drugs (first visit).
7. Assist client in identifying and exploring sources of emotional stress and in developing methods to minimize or eliminate them (first and second visits).
8. Inform client of importance of compliance with treatment regimen and expected effects (first visit).
9. Instruct client to notify physician immediately if hemorrhage occurs (signs and symptoms include weakness, apprehension, restlessness, vertigo/syncope, thirst, diaphoresis, dyspnea, tarry or bloody stools, and vomiting with frank blood or coffee ground appearance) (first visit).
10. Instruct client to notify physician immediately if obstruction occurs (signs and symptoms include bloated feeling after meals, fullness after meals, absence of bowel elimination, anorexia, weight loss, vomiting large amounts, projectile vomiting, and dehydration) (first visit).
11. Instruct client to call ambulance and go to emergency department if perforation occurs (signs and symptoms include sudden sharp epigastric or abdominal pain, pain radiation to shoulders, abdominal rigidity, diaphoresis, fever, rapid and shallow respirations, and increased pulse rate) (first visit).
12. Encourage modification rather than complete lifestyle changes to increase compliance (first visit).
13. Suggest community resources and groups for smoking cessation, stress reduction, and dietary counseling and support (first visit).
14. Encourage client to keep appointments with physician and for laboratory tests (first visit).
15. Instruct client to avoid aspirin and aspirin-containing products (first visit).

CLIENT AND FAMILY/CAREGIVER INTERVENTIONS

1. Client eats a well-balanced, bland diet in small and frequent meals; avoids dietary stressors.
2. Client avoids alcohol, tobacco, and caffeine intake.
3. Client avoids stress in environment and avoids relationships and situations that may create stress.
4. Client administers medications correctly and as instructed; avoids aspirin and nonsteroidal antiinflammatory drugs.
5. Client notifies physician of signs and symptoms of complications if they occur.
6. Client asks questions and clarifies information when needed.
7. Client seeks reinforcement and support from community groups that might be helpful.
8. Client keeps appointments with physician for follow-up care.

NURSING DIAGNOSIS ANXIETY

Related Factors: Threat to or change in health status

Defining Characteristics: Increased tension and apprehension about change in health and lifestyle; client's verbalization of inability to manage stress and symptoms of the disease

OUTCOMES

Short Term
Decreased anxiety, as evidenced by more relaxed posture and facial expression, statements that anxiety has decreased and has been controlled, and decrease in symptoms as a result of compliance with health regimen (expected in 3 to 7 days)

Long Term
Anxiety minimal or controlled, as evidenced by client's acceptance of changes in lifestyle to achieve optimal health and functioning (expected in 4 weeks)

NURSING INTERVENTIONS/INSTRUCTIONS

1. Assess mental and emotional status (see Psychosocial Assessment, p. 52, for guidelines) (first visit).

2. Explore with client historical coping patterns and problem-solving ability; relate them to condition and pain episodes (first visit).
3. Assist client in developing effective coping and stress-reducing mechanisms (first visit; reinforce on second visit).
4. Include client in all aspects of planning care at home (each visit).
5. Provide continuing information about condition and progress (each visit).
6. Suggest counseling and/or relaxation techniques to reduce anxiety if chronic (first visit).
7. Refer to social services for counseling as indicated (any visit).

CLIENT AND FAMILY/CAREGIVER INTERVENTIONS

1. Client identifies current coping mechanisms and explores options for improved coping and stress control.
2. Client participates in planning of care, including adherence to dietary, activity, and medication regimens.
3. Client performs relaxation exercises when feeling anxious.
4. Client consults physician if unable to control anxiety.

✳ *Ulcerative Colitis and Crohn's Disease*

Inflammatory bowel diseases include ulcerative colitis, involving the large intestine, and Crohn's disease, involving any part of the intestinal tract but most commonly the terminal ileum. Ulcerative colitis affects the mucous membranes, causing purulent exudate and bleeding. Segments of the colon or the entire colon may be affected, with periods of remission and exacerbation of inflammation. Ulcerative colitis may be confused with Crohn's disease. Crohn's disease affects all layers of the mucous membranes, and segments separated by normal bowel may be inflamed. Both diseases exhibit extracolonic manifestations and affect absorption of nutrients. Complications include intestinal obstruction, anemia, and nutritional and fluid and electrolyte imbalances.

Home care is primarily concerned with the teaching aspects of care and treatment for the disease and preventive measures to maintain health and avoid exacerbation.

Primary Diagnosis:
Ulcerative Colitis—ICD code: 556.9

NURSING DIAGNOSIS CHRONIC PAIN

▮ *Related Factors:* Biologic injuring agents of inflammatory disease

▮ *Defining Characteristics:* Verbalization of pain descriptors; groaning; abdominal guarding; restlessness; abdominal cramping

OUTCOMES

▮ Short Term

Pain controlled, as evidenced by client's statement that pain has subsided, relaxed posture and facial expressions, and participation in ADL and other activities (expected in 3 to 4 days)

▮ Long Term

Pain controlled, as evidenced by return to normal GI function achieved as a result of compliance with medical regimen (expected in 2 to 4 weeks)

NURSING INTERVENTIONS/INSTRUCTIONS

1. Assess pain type; location; characteristics; duration; intensity; and relationship to diet, activity, and elimination (first visit).
2. Instruct client in medication administration, including analgesics and antiinflammatory medications that have been prescribed (first visit).
3. Instruct client in relaxation exercises and guided imagery and to practice these techniques between episodes (first visit).
4. Instruct client to notify physician if pain is not relieved or if it increases in severity and if bloating, distension, vomiting, or abdominal rigidity is associated with increasing pain (first visit).

CLIENT AND FAMILY/CAREGIVER INTERVENTIONS

1. Client administers medication for optimal effects.

2. Client practices diversional activities for relaxation and pain reduction.
3. Client notifies physician if pain persists or escalates or if new symptoms develop.

NURSING DIAGNOSIS	IMBALANCED NUTRITION: LESS THAN BODY REQUIREMENTS

▌*Related Factors:* Inability to ingest or absorb nutrients because of biologic factors

▌*Defining Characteristics:* Weight loss; inadequate intake of nutrients; anorexia; diarrhea; nausea

OUTCOMES

▌*Short Term*
Adequate nutrition, as evidenced by client's statement of compliance with dietary requirements and regimen and by stabilization of weight (expected in 1 week)

▌*Long Term*
Optimal nutritional status, as evidenced by intake of required nutrients for optimal health and functioning (expected in 1 month and ongoing)

NURSING INTERVENTIONS/INSTRUCTIONS

1. Assess nutritional status, including food preferences, cultural and religious restrictions, and effect of different foods on illness (first visit).
2. Calculate ideal weight for size, sex, frame, and height (first visit).
3. Assess for nausea, vomiting, anorexia, weight loss, fatigue, malaise, and reactions to meals (each visit).
4. Instruct client to schedule rest periods after meals and to get 6 to 8 hours of sleep per night (first visit).
5. Inform client of measures that facilitate eating, including eliminating odors; providing a relaxed atmosphere and a quiet environment; eating smaller, more frequent meals; and taking antiemetics 30 minutes before meals (first visit).
6. Include client in planning a bland, high-protein, reduced-fiber, low-residue, possibly high-calorie diet. Avoid highly seasoned

foods; raw fruits and vegetables; foods containing coarse cereals, bran, seeds, or nuts; milk; and fatty or fried foods. Provide sample menus/meal plans (first visit).

7. Instruct client about administration of total parenteral nutrition when indicated (first and second visits).
8. Initiate referral to nutritionist if indicated (first visit).

CLIENT AND FAMILY/CAREGIVER INTERVENTIONS

1. Client maintains or gains weight as determined.
2. Client participates in planning and ingestion of a well-balanced diet with restrictions as determined.
3. Client promotes pleasant environment and dietary pattern that enhances intake.
4. Client maintains rest and sleep schedule.
5. Client avoids stress and irritants during meals.
6. Client includes increased calories and protein in diet plans.

NURSING DIAGNOSIS DIARRHEA

■**Related Factors:** Inflammation, irritation, or malabsorption of bowel

■**Defining Characteristics:** Abdominal pain; cramping; increased frequency; loose, liquid stools; urgency; mucus in stool; increased frequency of bowel sounds

OUTCOMES

■Short Term

Return of baseline bowel pattern, as evidenced by decrease in the frequency of bowel eliminations and by stool characteristics within baseline parameters (expected in 1 week)

■Long Term

Minimal or absence of diarrheal bowel eliminations, as evidenced by soft, formed stools eliminated according to baseline pattern (expected in 2 weeks)

NURSING INTERVENTIONS/INSTRUCTIONS

1. Assess bowel elimination patterns and stool characteristics (see Gastrointestinal System Assessment, p. 22, for guidelines) (first visit).

2. Instruct client to maintain a record of bowel movements, including number and when they occur and characteristics such as color; amount; consistency; odor; and presence of mucus, blood, or pus (first visit).
3. Monitor and instruct client in administration of antidiarrheal, anticholinergic, and antiinfective medications and corticosteroids (each visit).
4. Instruct client to notify physician if diarrhea becomes more severe or frequent or if bleeding, fatigue, or weakness is noted (first visit).

CLIENT AND FAMILY/CAREGIVER INTERVENTIONS

1. Client monitors and records bowel elimination.
2. Client administers medications correctly and as instructed.
3. Client notifies physician if diarrhea worsens and condition deteriorates or if complications occur.

NURSING DIAGNOSIS RISK FOR IMPAIRED SKIN INTEGRITY

■ *Related Factors:* Excretions and secretions

■ *Defining Characteristics:* Diarrhea; irritation, redness, or disruption of perianal area; perianal pain

OUTCOMES

■ Short Term
Minimized risk for skin breakdown, as evidenced by appropriate care of perianal area, which should be free of maceration or excoriation caused by excretions (expected in 3 to 4 days)

■ Long Term
Skin integrity maintained, as evidenced by perianal area free of any irritation or breaks (expected in 1 week and ongoing)

NURSING INTERVENTIONS/INSTRUCTIONS

1. Assess perianal area for tissue integrity, color, and odor; note presence of drainage, excoriation, maceration, abscess, fistula, or fissure formation (each visit).
2. Instruct client in perianal care to be performed every morning and possibly after every bowel elimination, including sitz bath,

cleansing with agent dispensed in a peri-bottle (perineal squirt bottle), and application of protective ointment; advise client to continue care during periods of remission (first visit; reinforce on second visit).

3. Instruct client to notify physician if irritation is unrelieved and bleeding or if drainage is noted (first visit).

CLIENT AND FAMILY/CAREGIVER INTERVENTIONS

1. Client provides perianal care daily or as needed.
2. Client protects perianal area from irritation.
3. Client maintains intact perianal tissue integrity.
4. Client notifies physician of severe excoriation or breakdown of perianal area.

NURSING DIAGNOSIS **RISK FOR IMBALANCED FLUID VOLUME**

▌*Related Factors:* Active fluid loss

▌*Defining Characteristics:* Diarrhea; vomiting; diaphoresis; decreased urine output in relation to intake; dry skin and mucous membranes; weight loss; electrolyte (i.e., sodium, potassium) imbalance

OUTCOMES

▌*Short Term*
Adequate fluid and electrolyte balance, as evidenced by absence of signs and symptoms of dehydration, balanced intake and output, and electrolyte levels within normal ranges (expected in 1 week)

▌*Long Term*
Fluid and electrolytes within balance, with optimal health and functioning achieved whether during remission or during exacerbation of disease (expected in 2 weeks and ongoing)

NURSING INTERVENTIONS/INSTRUCTIONS

1. Assess fluid needs according to age, weight, and estimated fluid losses (each visit).
2. Monitor for dehydration, including thirst, decreased urinary output, poor skin turgor, dry mucous membranes, and furrowed tongue (each visit).

3. Instruct client to take and record daily weight and estimated intake and output (first visit).
4. Instruct client to drink 8 to 10 glasses of fluid per day in small, spaced servings and to avoid fluids that are too hot or cold (first visit).
5. Instruct client in administration of potassium supplements and intake of foods containing potassium, including bananas, citrus juices, and dried fruits (first visit).
6. Monitor for electrolyte imbalance, and instruct client in recognition of signs and symptoms, including muscle weakness, cramping, twitching, confusion, paresthesias, and pulse irregularities (first visit).
7. Monitor laboratory values for potassium, sodium, calcium, chloride, magnesium, hemoglobin, and hematocrit if available (any visit).

CLIENT AND FAMILY/CAREGIVER INTERVENTIONS

1. Client maintains fluid intake according to calculated needs and fluid losses.
2. Client administers or increases intake of potassium replacement.
3. Client measures weight daily; compares intake and output of fluids in relation to diarrhea.
4. Client reports any signs and symptoms of dehydration or electrolyte decreases.

NURSING DIAGNOSIS INEFFECTIVE COPING

Related Factors: Multiple life changes; chronic illness

Defining Characteristics: Verbalization of inability to cope or ask for or seek out help; inability to solve problems and use defense mechanisms effectively; exacerbation of symptoms; chronic anxiety; depression

OUTCOMES

Short Term
Improved coping ability, as evidenced by client's statement that recognizing need for and adapting to changes in lifestyle are necessary (expected in 1 week)

▌*Long Term*

Effective coping, as evidenced by compliance with treatment regimen and by changes in lifestyle to adapt to illness and to requirements for optimal health achievement (expected in 1 to 2 months and ongoing)

NURSING INTERVENTIONS/INSTRUCTIONS

1. Assess for developmental level and dependency needs, behavioral and emotional changes, use of defense mechanisms and their effectiveness, and ability to solve problems (first visit).
2. Establish a trusting relationship, and facilitate an open discussion to explore options and develop skills in coping and problem solving (each visit).
3. Identify coping skills that work, and encourage positive feeling about success of any adaptation or changes (each visit).
4. Include client in all planning and formulating of realistic goals; assist if requested to do so (each visit).
5. Encourage expression of fears about possible surgery and threat to life (each visit).
6. Refer to social services for assistance with coping strategies as indicated (any visit).

CLIENT AND FAMILY/CAREGIVER INTERVENTIONS

1. Client shares feelings, fears, and concerns with caregiver or family.
2. Client plans and participates in own care and health promotion.
3. Client sets goals and strategies for remissions and exacerbations.
4. Client participates in support group with persons who have similar condition.

NURSING DIAGNOSIS DEFICIENT KNOWLEDGE

▌*Related Factors:* Lack of information about disease and treatments

▌*Defining Characteristics:* Request for information about disease, causes, signs and symptoms, medications, and need for compliance and for prevention of exacerbations

OUTCOMES

▌*Short Term*

Adequate knowledge, as evidenced by client's statement of precipitating, aggravating, and alleviating factors in symptomatology and
signs and symptoms of exacerbation or worsening condition (expected in 3 days)

▌*Long Term*

Optimal knowledge, as evidenced by client's meeting requirements
to achieve optimal health and GI functioning with reduction in
exacerbations (expected in 1 to 2 months and ongoing)

NURSING INTERVENTIONS/INSTRUCTIONS

1. Assess client's lifestyle, learning and coping abilities, interest
   level, and family participation and support (first visit).
2. Instruct client to maintain log of ADL that includes food diary,
   fluid intake, and descriptions of GI episodes (first visit).
3. Assist client in identifying characteristic trends and influencing
   factors that precipitate or alleviate symptoms; use data as a
   physiologic and psychologic baseline and a basis for teaching
   (first visit).
4. Instruct client to notify physician of any change in condition
   that indicates complications or exacerbation (first visit).
5. Instruct client in correct medication administration, including
   sulfasalazine, vitamins, electrolyte replacement products,
   antiemetic agents, antidiarrheal medications, steroids, immunosuppressants, antibiotics, and others prescribed; emphasize
   dosage, frequency, side effects, expected results, and food and
   drug interactions; and instruct client to avoid OTC drugs without physician recommendation (first visit).
6. Instruct client about care of ileostomy, as indicated, including
   skin and appliance care and diet requirements; initiate referral
   to wound specialist (each visit).
7. Instruct client to maintain scheduled physician appointments
   (first visit).
8. Provide information about agencies or groups for educational
   material, support or counseling, or new trends (first visit).

CLIENT AND FAMILY/CAREGIVER INTERVENTIONS

1. Client maintains log of progress and changes.

2. Client monitors for influences of diet, fluids, activity, and stress.
3. Client administers medications safely and correctly.
4. Client notifies physician of unremitting or escalating symptoms.
5. Client participates in educational and support programs.
6. Client carries out measures to prevent exacerbation.
7. Client safely cares for ileostomy as indicated.

✳ *Diabetes Mellitus*

Diabetes mellitus is characterized by absence of or inadequate production of insulin by the pancreas to meet body needs for carbohydrate, fat, and protein metabolism. Long-term effects include vascular changes, retinopathy, and neuropathy. The most common type found in adults is non–insulin-dependent diabetes mellitus (NIDDM), or type 2. A second type is insulin-dependent diabetes mellitus (IDDM), or type 1.

Home care is primarily concerned with the teaching aspects of nutrition, medication regimens, monitoring of glucose levels, and measures to take for control of the disease to prevent complications.

Primary Diagnoses:
Diabetes Mellitus, Insulin-dependent—ICD code : 250.01
Diabetes Mellitus, Non–insulin-dependent—ICD code: 250.00
Diabetes Mellitus, Neuropathy—ICD code: 250.60
Diabetic Retinopathy—ICD codes: 250.50, 250.51
Diabetes Mellitus, Circulatory Manifestations—ICD code: 250.70
Diabetes Mellitus, Renal Manifestations—ICD code: 250.42

NURSING DIAGNOSIS INEFFECTIVE COPING

Related Factors: Multiple life changes; chronic illness and its consequences

Defining Characteristics: Chronic worry, anxiety, and complaints; tension; inability to cope with necessary lifestyle changes

OUTCOMES
Short Term
Improvement in use of coping skills, as evidenced by effective use of coping mechanisms and by verbalization of need to change

lifestyle and to request assistance when needed to meet needs (expected in 1 week)

▌*Long Term*

Effective coping with chronic illness, as evidenced by acceptable level of anxiety and concern and by adaptation to lifestyle changes (expected in 2 to 3 months)

NURSING INTERVENTIONS/INSTRUCTIONS

1. Assess for appropriate use of coping mechanisms, ability to solve problems, inner resources to manage anxiety and stress, and support system (each visit).
2. Provide accepting, nonjudgmental attitude and environment when teaching and discussing needs and changes to be made in lifestyle (each visit).
3. Instruct client to avoid events that produce stress or prevent use of constructive coping mechanisms or behavior (first visit).
4. Instruct client in coping, communication, and problem-solving skills (first and second visits).
5. Instruct client in relaxation and diversional techniques, such as music, muscle relaxation, and reading (first visit).
6. Encourage expression of concerns and mutual goal setting (each visit).
7. Initiate referral to social services to assist with coping strategies as indicated (any visit).

CLIENT AND FAMILY/CAREGIVER INTERVENTIONS

1. Client develops effective use of coping mechanisms.
2. Client avoids stress-provoking events.
3. Client engages in relaxation and diversional activities.
4. Client requests assistance when needed.
5. Client reduces and/or controls anxiety level.
6. Client adapts to change in lifestyle to comply with medical regimen.

NURSING DIAGNOSIS	IMBALANCED NUTRITION: LESS THAN BODY REQUIREMENTS

▌*Related Factors:* Inability to metabolize nutrients

■*Defining Characteristics:* Hyperglycemia; hypoglycemia; noncompliance with dietary, activity, and insulin regimens in controlling condition

OUTCOMES

■*Short Term*
Adequate nutrition, as evidenced by compliance with recommended American Diabetic Association (ADA) diet and absence of hyperglycemic or hypoglycemic states (expected in 1 week)

■*Long Term*
Adequate nutritional intake and metabolic process, as evidenced by appropriate dietary planning and intake in relation to insulin production or administration and by blood and urinary glucose levels that are within normal ranges (expected in 1 month and ongoing)

NURSING INTERVENTIONS/INSTRUCTIONS

1. Assess nutritional status, including food preferences, religious and cultural restrictions, emotional factors related to food and eating, and actual and desired weight levels (first visit).
2. Instruct client to keep a diary of total carbohydrates consumed, amounts and methods of food preparation, and weekly weights (first visit).
3. Instruct client about and review total carbohydrate count and prescribed diet; use diary as a guide and make changes as needed; provide written instructions and information about diet (first visit; reinforce on second visit).
4. Instruct in diabetic diet as prescribed, with reduced calories, sodium, and fat and cholesterol content if necessary; include avoidance of simple sugars (use sugar substitutes) and concentrated sweets and the importance of evenly spaced, regular meals and scheduled snacks; instruct client to eat all of meals and to avoid skipping or delaying a meal or bunching required foods in one meal (first visit; reinforce each visit).
5. Inform client of early signs and symptoms of hypoglycemia, including hunger, shakiness, palpitations, headache, weakness, irritability, nervousness, and visual disturbances (first visit).
6. Instruct client to carry candy or sugar at all times. Instruct client that, at first sign of hypoglycemic attack, he or she must take milk (preferred) or fruit juice, nondiet soft drink, 4 teaspoons of sugar, 4 to 5 pieces of hard candy, or cake frosting from a tube

or rub sugar preparation from a tube onto gums (first visit; reinforce after any hypoglycemic episodes).

7. Inform client of signs and symptoms of hyperglycemia and possible ketoacidosis, including fatigue, malaise, flushed face, nausea and vomiting, marked thirst, fruity (acetone) breath, hyperpnea, or changes in mentation (first visit).

8. Instruct client to notify physician (first visit) in the following circumstances:

   · If diet is not tolerated
   · If foods cannot be retained
   · At first onset of any sign or symptom of high or low glucose levels
   · If ketones are present in urine

9. Refer client to diabetic educator for assistance in ADA diet and exchanges if needed (first visit).

10. Review activity and exercise in relation to prescribed diet (first visit).

CLIENT AND FAMILY/CAREGIVER INTERVENTIONS

1. Client maintains record of food intake, weekly weight, and incidence of dietary changes to accommodate test results of blood and urine.

2. Client formulates meal menus and plans for dietary inclusions and restrictions.

3. Client eats regularly scheduled meals following prescribed ADA diet and exchange lists.

4. Client carries emergency sugar supply at all times.

5. Client identifies signs and symptoms of hypoglycemia and hyperglycemia.

6. Client takes extra nutrition before engaging in strenuous activities.

NURSING DIAGNOSIS DEFICIENT KNOWLEDGE

▌*Related Factors:* Lack of knowledge about disease and procedures to control disease and prevent complications

▌*Defining Characteristics:* Request for information and instruction about disease and procedures to control disease and prevent complications; verbalization of unfamiliarity with medication administration; dietary and exercise inclusions and restrictions; blood and urine testing for glucose; care of feet, skin, teeth, and eyes; signs and symptoms of hyperglycemia and hypoglycemia; and measures to take to treat these conditions

OUTCOMES

▌*Short Term*
Adequate knowledge, as evidenced by client's ability to describe medication administration; blood and urine testing; activity regimen; care of feet, skin, and eyes; signs and symptoms of altered glycemic states; and treatment (expected in 4 to 7 days)

▌*Long Term*
Optimal knowledge, as evidenced by absence of complications following daily compliance with treatment regimen (expected in 1 month and ongoing)

NURSING INTERVENTIONS/INSTRUCTIONS

1. Assess all body systems for baselines; assess history of drug, hormone, and alcohol use (first visit).
2. Instruct client in and demonstrate self-administration of insulin, noting technique; rotation of sites; onset, peak, and duration of action; and expected results of the insulin(s). Instruct in possibility of local reaction to injection and use and care of pump if applicable. Refer to diabetic educator for assistance with pump usage (first and second visits and ongoing as needed).
3. Instruct client in administration of oral hypoglycemic agents, noting dose; frequency; side effects; food, drug, and alcohol interactions; and expected action and results (first visit).
4. Instruct client in and demonstrate blood collection and testing for glucose and use of glucometer; relate to insulin administration and diet; and instruct client in urinary glucose and ketone testing to be done if blood glucose reaches a predetermined level (first visit; reinforce on second visit).
5. Assess activities of daily living and exercise pattern; instruct client to exercise daily, implementing a consistent routine; and instruct client in actions to take if exercise is increased (first visit).
6. Encourage client to stop smoking; suggest support groups (first visit).

7. Inform client of importance of complying with medication, exercise, and diet regimens to maintain glucose level within normal range; instruct client to notify physician of continuous signs and symptoms of hypoglycemia or hyperglycemia (first visit).

8. Impress on client the importance of notifying physician if stress, trauma, or infection is present (first visit).

9. Instruct client in meticulous care of feet, including daily bathing in tepid water and rinsing well and patting dry, especially between toes. Instruct client to see podiatrist for foot care; to apply cream to lower extremities (avoid cream between toes); to wear well-fitting shoes and cotton socks; and to check feet for cuts, scratches or blisters, ulcers, delayed healing, and reduced sensation (first visit; reinforce on second visit).

10. Discuss sexual concerns (e.g., impotence, family planning) as appropriate (first visit).

11. Instruct client to inform all health care personnel (e.g., dentist, surgeon) of diagnosis (first visit).

12. Instruct client to wear and/or carry identification indicating condition and medications (first visit).

CLIENT AND FAMILY/CAREGIVER INTERVENTIONS

1. Client administers insulin or hypoglycemic correctly and in timely manner.

2. Client uses insulin pump effectively if prescribed.

3. Client tests blood and urine at appropriate times and analyzes results for proper actions to take.

4. Client checks blood glucose before driving vehicle. If level is below 120 mg, client eats or drinks a carbohydrate; rechecks blood glucose in 20 minutes.

5. Client exercises daily and maintains constant day-to-day program.

6. Client ceases smoking or joins support group for assistance.

7. Client states signs and symptoms of hypoglycemia and hyperglycemia and appropriate actions to take.

8. Client states signs and symptoms of infection to report to physician.

9. Client reports any visual disturbances; participates in periodic eye examinations.

10. Client notes neuropathies and reports any trauma to physician.

11. Client performs consistent, meticulous foot care; caregiver examines feet daily if visual or neurologic disturbances are present.
12. Client follows up on sexual concerns to make informed decisions as indicated.
13. Client wears or carries identification information.
14. Client consults podiatrist, ophthalmologist, and dentist for specific care.

NURSING DIAGNOSIS NONCOMPLIANCE

Related Factors: Health beliefs and practices

Defining Characteristics: Failure to adhere to medical regimen, with resulting development of complications or exacerbation of symptoms; failure to keep appointments or report to physician

OUTCOMES

Short Term
Compliance with medical regimen, as evidenced by client identifying and performing dietary and activity modifications, medication regimen, blood and urine testing, and foot and skin care (expected in 1 week)

Long Term
Optimal and effective compliance, as evidenced by participation in all aspects of care, absence of complications, and functioning at optimal level (expected in 2 to 3 months)

NURSING INTERVENTIONS/INSTRUCTIONS

1. Establish rapport and provide a nonthreatening, accepting environment for care and teaching (each visit).
2. Assess coping and learning abilities, developmental level and achieved tasks, economic level, and support system; note perceived implications of disorder for lifestyle (each visit).
3. Evaluate knowledge and performance of dietary, activity, medication, and testing procedures and modifications (first visit).
4. Include client and family/caregiver in planning and teaching of health care (each visit).

5. Help client modify lifestyle with as few changes as possible; explore options and praise efforts and successes (each visit).
6. Suggest counseling or support groups such as the ADA for information, supplies, and support (first visit).
7. Encourage expression of perception of disease (each visit).

CLIENT AND FAMILY/CAREGIVER INTERVENTIONS

1. Client participates in all aspects of health care; complies with requirements.
2. Client accepts support from family, friends, and agencies.
3. Client demonstrates facility in performance of all procedures and planning of care for optimal health and functioning.

HEMATOLOGIC SYSTEM

✳ Acquired Immunodeficiency Syndrome

Acquired immunodeficiency syndrome (AIDS) is characterized by extreme immunosuppression, allowing for the development of malignancies and opportunistic infections caused by viruses, bacteria, fungi, and protozoa. It is a life-threatening illness whose cause is unknown. The disease demonstrates suppression of T-helper cells and an increase in T-suppressor cells, both of which decrease the body's ability to respond to an acute inflammatory reaction and depress a defensive response. AIDS is transmitted by administration of contaminated blood or blood products; sexual contact; use of contaminated needles, syringes, or instruments; or accidental exposure to contaminated blood through breaks in the skin or mucous membranes; perinatal transmission also occurs.

Home care is primarily concerned with the care and teaching aspects of infection prevention, activities of daily living (ADL), the medication regimen, and transmission prevention.

Primary Diagnosis:
AIDS—ICD code: 042.0

NURSING DIAGNOSIS ANXIETY

■ **Related Factors:** Threat of death; change in health status

■ **Defining Characteristics:** Presence of human immunodeficiency virus (HIV); presence of AIDS-related complex (ARC); apprehension and increased helplessness; absence of any effective treatment; fear of transmission to others

OUTCOMES

▌*Short Term*

Decreased anxiety, as evidenced by client's statement of reduced fear and apprehension about change in health status and possible early death (expected in 1 week)

▌*Long Term*

Management or control of anxiety level, as evidenced by compliance with and acceptance of treatment regimen and change in lifestyle to prevent transmission of the disease to others (expected in 1 to 2 months and ongoing)

NURSING INTERVENTIONS/INSTRUCTIONS

1. Assess client's mental and emotional status in relation to life-threatening illness and associated stigma (see Psychosocial Assessment, p. 52, for guidelines) (first visit).
2. Encourage expression of fears and concerns in a supportive and nonjudgmental environment; instruct client in relaxation techniques (each visit).
3. Assist client in identifying needed changes in lifestyle and methods to make necessary changes (first visit and as needed).
4. Inform client about activities allowed, treatments and tests to expect, and testing of contacts (first visit).
5. Initiate referral to social services, counseling, support groups, or agencies that may assist with legal, economic, and health care needs (first visit).
6. Encourage expression of concerns and mutual goal setting (each visit).

CLIENT AND FAMILY/CAREGIVER INTERVENTIONS

1. Client develops coping skills for long-term treatment and possible outcome.
2. Client maintains manageable level of anxiety.
3. Client seeks information that will help reduce anxiety.
4. Client expresses fears and concerns about necessary changes in lifestyle.
5. Client contacts and consults with available support services.

NURSING DIAGNOSIS RISK FOR INFECTION

█ **Related Factors:** Inadequate secondary defenses

█ **Defining Characteristics:** Immunodeficiency; potential for opportunistic infection, hyperthermia, prostration, change in breathing pattern (with *Pneumocystis pneumonia*), change in thought process (with cytomegalovirus) with dementia

OUTCOMES

█ **Short Term**

Absence of infection, as evidenced by temperature and blood tests within normal ranges and by freedom from signs and symptoms of any opportunistic infection (expectation depends on immune system status)

█ **Long Term**

Absence of infection with optimal functioning of all systems (expected to be ongoing)

NURSING INTERVENTIONS/INSTRUCTIONS

1. Perform complete physical assessment to establish baseline data and note any signs and symptoms associated with the disease (first visit).
2. Instruct client to monitor for and report presence of fever, malaise, night sweats, cough, dyspnea, headache, enlarged glands, epigastric or abdominal pain, vomiting or diarrhea, skin lesions, rashes, weakness, joint pain, or sensory or intellectual deficits (first visit).
3. Instruct client in preventive measures regarding infections, including handwashing, personal hygiene, and avoiding crowds and persons with infection or who are ill (first visit).
4. Instruct client in administration of antiinfective agents and specific preventive drugs for disease and to avoid any immunosuppressive drugs (first visit).
5. Encourage health promotion, including rest, nutritious diet, and stress management (each visit).

CLIENT AND FAMILY/CAREGIVER INTERVENTIONS

1. Client bathes daily; inspects for and reports rashes, skin lesions, vesicles, or skin disruptions.

2. Client washes hands after toileting, before meals, and before any procedures.
3. Client takes temperature if any symptoms appear and reports elevation.
4. Client monitors for and reports signs and symptoms of infection in any system.
5. Client administers medications as instructed.
6. Client avoids exposure to persons with infections.
7. Client maintains healthy lifestyle that includes nutritious meals, 6 to 8 hours of sleep per night, and social and diversional activities.

NURSING DIAGNOSIS   ACTIVITY INTOLERANCE

▌*Related Factors:* Generalized weakness

▌*Defining Characteristics:* Verbalization of fatigue and weakness; inability to perform ADL and to ambulate; repeated infections; malnutrition; wasting; lack of sleep

OUTCOMES

▌*Short Term*

Increased activity and energy, as evidenced by performance of ADL and use of energy-conservation techniques (expected in 1 week)

▌*Long Term*

Adequate activity within disease limitations, as evidenced by achievement of optimal level of self-care and general functioning (expected in 2 to 3 months as realistic)

NURSING INTERVENTIONS/INSTRUCTIONS

1. Assess client's ability to carry out ADL and energy and endurance levels; note strength, gait, posture, balance, presence of fatigue, general weakness, and sensory deficits (each visit).
2. Encourage rest after activity and at least 6 to 8 hours of sleep per night (first visit).
3. Assist client in identifying activities that need pacing and in setting limits (first visit; reinforce on second visit).
4. Inform client of available energy-conserving aids to assist in dressing, bathing, grooming, toileting, and eating (first visit).

5. Assess support system; include support system in care planning and administration (first visit).
6. Coordinate social services and community resources for assistance and support (first visit).
7. Refer home health aide (HHA) to assist with ADL (first visit).

CLIENT AND FAMILY/CAREGIVER INTERVENTIONS

1. Client bases rest and sleep on individual needs and condition.
2. Client participates in activities within set limits.
3. Client uses energy-saving devices in ADL.
4. Caregiver assists with any activity requiring support.
5. Client uses private and public resources for assistance.

NURSING DIAGNOSIS | **IMBALANCED NUTRITION: LESS THAN BODY REQUIREMENTS**

▌*Related Factors:* Inability to ingest food and absorb nutrients

▌*Defining Characteristics:* Anorexia; infection of oroesophageal tract; gastroenteritis; diarrhea; weight loss; wasting

OUTCOMES

▌*Short Term*

Adequate nutrition, as evidenced by intake of nutritious and high-calorie foods and by maintenance of stable weight pattern (expected in 1 week)

▌*Long Term*

Optimal nutritional status, as evidenced by weight stability and by absence of disease manifestations that affect food intake necessary to maintain health and functioning (expected in 1 month and ongoing)

NURSING INTERVENTIONS/INSTRUCTIONS

1. Assess nutritional status, including height, actual and ideal weight, food preferences, and cultural and religious restrictions (first visit).
2. Perform gastrointestinal assessment (see Gastrointestinal System Assessment, p. 22, for guidelines); note presence of anorexia, nausea, vomiting, weight loss, persistent diarrhea,

oroesophageal inflammation or lesions, and temperature elevation; cross-reference signs and symptoms with drug profile (each visit).

3. Instruct client in regular, scrupulous oral hygiene and in use of soft toothbrush, topical antifungal agents, mouthwashes, and topical anesthetics as prescribed in the presence of oral inflammation or lesions (first visit).

4. Instruct client to eat high-calorie, well-balanced diet and to include foods that will prevent or minimize distressing manifestations (first visit).

5. Instruct client to eat smaller, more frequent meals that include commercially prepared supplements (first visit).

6. If nausea is present, suggest that client eat toast or dry crackers, choose foods that are less aromatic and less strong in taste, and drink beverages 30 minutes before meals rather than with meals (first visit).

7. Instruct client to eat when rested and to rest with head elevated for 30 minutes after meals (first visit).

8. Instruct client to administer vitamin and mineral supplements daily (first visit).

9. Instruct client in administration of antidiarrheal and antiemetic medications if prescribed (first visit).

10. Inform client of alternative feeding methods such as tube feedings or total parenteral nutrition (TPN), and instruct client in procedures if implemented (applicable visit; reinforcement as needed).

11. Initiate referral to nutritionist for consultation and to community resources for food preparation and delivery if needed (first visit).

CLIENT AND FAMILY/CAREGIVER INTERVENTIONS

1. Client measures and records daily weight and reports any significant, progressive losses.

2. Client eats small, frequent, high-calorie meals that include preferences and nutritional requirements.

3. Client performs mouth care after meals and if oral mucous membrane is impaired and protects oral cavity from further trauma.

4. Client treats nausea with dry foods and timely intake of fluids.

5. Client supplements meals with foods and beverages of high nutritional value.

6 Client administers vitamin and mineral supplements, antidiarrheals, antifungals, antibiotics, and topical anesthetics as instructed.
7. Client monitors tube feedings or TPN if present and performs procedures for administration and care of these methods of feeding if capable of managing them.
8. Client consults with nutritionist.
9. Client uses community resources for food service.

NURSING DIAGNOSIS IMPAIRED SOCIAL INTERACTION

Related Factors: Therapeutic isolation; inability to engage in satisfying personal relationship

Defining Characteristics: Stigma associated with AIDS and unaccepted social behavior (drug abuse, sexual behavior); fear of transmission of disease; fear of loss of confidentiality and loss of or rejection by significant others and community as result of diagnosis

OUTCOMES

Short Term
Involvement in social interaction, as evidenced by verbalization of behaviors resulting from isolation and of options to reverse these and to adapt to requirements for meaningful relationships (expected in 1 week)

Long Term
Optimal social relationships, as evidenced by participation in social activities with significant others and support group (expected in 1 month)

NURSING INTERVENTIONS/INSTRUCTIONS

1. Provide continuity of care by providing same professional caregiver for treatment and care (each visit).
2. Use therapeutic communication, including touch (each visit).
3. Identify type and amount of support available in home and community (first visit).
4. Provide an understanding, nonjudgmental environment (each visit).

5. Facilitate individual and group interaction; note that behavior or personality changes may be the result of neurologic dysfunction (each visit).
6. Provide a range of diversional options, including books, games, collecting, and visits from friends (first visit).
7. Refer to AIDS support group, social services, or counseling as needed (any visit).

CLIENT AND FAMILY/CAREGIVER INTERVENTIONS

1. Client occupies time with diversional activities.
2. Client accepts visits from friends.
3. Client verbalizes understanding of social fears and lack of knowledge regarding disease.
4. Client interacts with support groups and services.
5. Client consults counseling or other agencies for assistance.

NURSING DIAGNOSIS ANTICIPATORY GRIEVING

Related Factors: Perceived potential loss of physiopsychosocial well-being

Defining Characteristics: Expression of distress at potential loss; anger; guilt; denial of potential loss; sorrow; choked feelings; changes in sleep, eating, and activity patterns

OUTCOMES

Short Term
Progress in grieving, as evidenced by attitude and behavior changes manifested by stage in process (expected in days)

Long Term
Grief process resolving, as evidenced by resumption of lifestyle with or without changes as needed and by integration of grieving stage into lifestyle and activities (expected in 2 to 3 months and ongoing)

NURSING INTERVENTIONS/INSTRUCTIONS

1. Assess degree and stage of grief (each visit).
2. Inform client of stages of grieving process and that behavior is acceptable for specific stage and that acceptance will be final stage (first visit).

3. Allow expression of feelings and perceptions about disabilities and potential loss and death in a nonjudgmental environment (each visit).
4. Initiate referral for social services, psychologic and spiritual counseling, and hospice care as appropriate (any visit).

CLIENT AND FAMILY/CAREGIVER INTERVENTIONS

1. Client progresses through grief process to acceptance.
2. Client seeks counseling as needed.
3. Client verbalizes stages and behaviors during grief process.

NURSING DIAGNOSIS DEFICIENT KNOWLEDGE

Related Factors: Lack of exposure to information

Defining Characteristics: Request for information about changes in sexual patterns and social behavior necessary to prevent transmission of disease, legal and medical rights and assistance, and community resources available

OUTCOMES

Short Term
Adequate knowledge, as evidenced by client's statements regarding disease progression and transmission and treatments (expected in 3 days)

Long Term
Optimal knowledge, as evidenced by compliance in meeting requirements of changed lifestyle, within limitations imposed by condition, to achieve optimal level of functioning (expected in 1 month)

NURSING INTERVENTIONS/INSTRUCTIONS

1. Instruct caregivers to use standard (universal) precautions in all aspects of client care (first visit).
2. Include significant others in instruction; allow for active participation in care planning (each visit).
3. Assess for and instruct client in recognition of opportunistic infection, recurrence, reinfections, neoplasms, and neurologic manifestations and in treatment available for these conditions (each visit).

4. Instruct client in transmission modes, and stress that disease is not transmitted by casual contact or living with others but by sexual contact, exchange of needles in drug use, administration of blood or blood products, or sharing of razors or other items that might contain the virus (first visit).

5. Instruct client in general cleaning and disinfection methods; bleach solution (1 part bleach to 10 parts water) may be used to clean contaminated materials but must be reconstituted every 24 hours (first visit).

6. Advise client of need for testing sexual contacts or high-risk contacts in addition to concurrent counseling about transmission (first visit).

7. Instruct client in options for sexual activity, including abstinence, use of latex condoms lubricated with nonoxynol 9, and birth control planning (first visit; reinforce second visit).

8. Encourage rehabilitation of intravenous drug users; instruct them not to share needles or paraphernalia and to wash syringes with soap and water and then cleanse with bleach and rinse thoroughly after each use (each visit).

9. Instruct client in administration of antiretroviral, antibiotic and antiinfective, psychotropic, anticonvulsant, and immunomodulating medications; analgesics; antipyretic agents; and chemotherapy as prescribed, including dose, route, frequency, side effects, and interactions; inform client of possible resources for medications (first visit; reinforce as needed).

10. Instruct client not to donate blood or organs (first visit).

11. Instruct client to inform all nursing, medical, dental, and laboratory personnel of condition (first visit).

12. Assist client in organizing health care information; provide written instructions and reminders for care, medications and schedules, and resource and emergency telephone numbers (first visit).

13. Inform client of importance of follow-up with physician and laboratory visits (first visit).

14. Refer client to community groups; resources; and organizations, including hospice, for support, information, and financial and legal needs (first visit and ongoing).

CLIENT AND FAMILY/CAREGIVER INTERVENTIONS

1. Client monitors and reports any signs and symptoms of opportunistic infections.

2. Client prevents transmission to others.
3. Client reports contacts to be tested.
4. Client administers medications as prescribed and instructed; uses a written plan and schedule.
5. Client avoids activities that will spread disease and verbalizes how disease is transmitted and measures to take to protect others from disease.
6. Client informs those who need to know diagnosis, with assurance of confidentiality.
7. Client seeks out support services available for persons with AIDS.

NURSING DIAGNOSIS   RISK FOR CAREGIVER ROLE STRAIN

Related Factors: Severity of illness of the care receiver; complexity and number of caregiving tasks

Defining Characteristics: Caregiver's report of not having enough resources (e.g., emotional and physical strength; help from others) to provide care and of difficulty in performing specific caregiving activities (e.g., bathing, cleaning up after incontinence, managing client's weakened condition and discomforts)

OUTCOMES

Short Term
Potential for caregiver role strain identified, as evidenced by caregiver's verbalization of difficulties encountered in performing care and concern about ability and conflicts in giving care (expected in 1 week)

Long Term
Prevention of caregiver role strain, as evidenced by continued safe and appropriate care provided without compromise to own physical and emotional needs (expected in 1 month and ongoing)

NURSING INTERVENTIONS/INSTRUCTIONS

1. Assess severity of illness; needs of the receiver of care; and caregiver's ability to perform role (first visit).
2. Assess relationship between care receiver and caregiver before illness and stressors placed on the relationship by the illness (first visit).

3. Assist caregiver in monitoring continued ability to perform care and treatments, changes in day-to-day needs, changes in stressors and strains, maintenance of routines, and need for additional resources (e.g., aides, homemaker, respite care, friends, family) (first visit).
4. Discuss role performance and whether expectations are realistic, flexibility of role, and decision-making process (first visit).
5. Initiate referral to HHA, social worker, or psychologic counseling to assist with economic and mental or physical health needs (any visit).

CLIENT AND FAMILY/CAREGIVER INTERVENTIONS

1. Caregiver develops ability to cope with caregiver role and flexibility in day-to-day functioning.
2. Caregiver explores financial, legal, and physical assistance resources and considers a referral to these services.
3. Caregiver maintains own health and well-being in caregiver role.
4. Caregiver maintains ongoing care and treatment regimen.

✳ *Anemia*

Anemia is a condition characterized by decreases in red blood cell (RBC), hemoglobin, and hematocrit levels. It may be caused by excessive blood loss (i.e., hypovolemic), decreased production of RBCs by bone marrow (i.e., aplastic), decreased production of RBCs from inadequate intake of iron and folic acid (i.e., iron deficiency), decreased development of RBCs because of the lack of the intrinsic factor needed for vitamin B_{12} absorption (i.e., pernicious), or the destruction of RBCs (i.e., hemolytic). Whatever the type, the decrease in RBCs affects the transport of oxygen in the body, with severity dependent on the degree of decrease.

Home care is primarily concerned with iron-deficiency and pernicious anemias and the teaching aspects for compliance with the medical regimen to control the disorder and prevent relapses.

Primary Diagnoses:
Anemia, Unspecified—ICD code: 285.9
Anemia, Vitamin B_{12} Deficiency—ICD code: 281.1

Anemia, Pernicious—ICD code: 281.0
Anemia, Aplastic—ICD code: 284.9

NURSING DIAGNOSIS	IMBALANCED NUTRITION: LESS THAN BODY REQUIREMENTS

▍*Related Factors:* Inadequate intake of iron and folic acid

▍*Defining Characteristics:* Reduced intake of food containing iron and folic acid; weight loss; weakness; anorexia; nausea; vomiting; glossy red tongue; lesions on oral mucosa; shortness of breath; pallor; headaches; irritability; dysphagia; fissures at angles of tongue

OUTCOMES

▍*Short Term*

Adequate nutrition, as evidenced by consumption of a well-balanced diet with necessary supplementation, and maintenance of appropriate weight for height, frame, and age (expected in 4 days)

▍*Long Term*

Optimal nutritional status achieved, as evidenced by maintenance of daily requirements and supplemental therapy, with optimal level of health and physiologic functioning (expected in 1 month)

NURSING INTERVENTIONS/INSTRUCTIONS

1. Review history and focus on source and remediation of deficiency, including increased iron requirements, inadequate intake, decreased or inadequate absorption, or chronic blood loss (first visit).

2. Assess hematologic, cardiovascular, neurologic, integumentary, gastrointestinal, and endocrine systems for status and effect of anemic condition on them (see specific system assessments for guidelines) (first visit).

3. Assess nutritional status, including food preferences and cultural or religious and medical restrictions (first visit).

4. Instruct client to measure and record weights weekly (first visit).

5. Instruct client to maintain a food diary for 1 week that includes all foods consumed and amounts and methods of preparation; use data as a basis for dietary teaching (first visit).

6. Instruct client in a well-balanced diet that includes snacks and foods that will supply nutrients to lessen the deficiency; inform client that more frequent, smaller meals are recommended if nausea, vomiting, or fatigue interferes with intake (first visit; reinforce on second visit).

7. Instruct client in (and supply list of) sources of dietary iron and/or vitamin B_{12}, including red meat, organ meats, fish, milk, egg yolks, green leafy vegetables, dried legumes, enriched breads and cereals, and dried fruits (first visit).

8. Instruct client in good oral hygiene, especially after meals and if mouth is sore (first visit).

9. Instruct client in administration of iron preparation and vitamin C, and inform client that stools may turn dark green or black and that milk and antacids will decrease absorption of iron (first visit).

10. Suggest that client eat a bland diet and avoids irritating, hot, spicy foods if tongue is sore or in presence of gingival or mouth irritation or lesions (first visit).

11. Refer client to nutritionist or counselor if needed (any visit, based on evaluation).

CLIENT AND FAMILY/CAREGIVER INTERVENTIONS

1. Client measures and records weekly weight using same scale, wearing same type of clothing, and at same time of day.

2. Client maintains daily log of intake and reviews each week for possible changes.

3. Client eats a well-balanced diet that includes sources of iron and folic acid.

4. Client maintains oral hygiene; applies lubricant to lips if needed.

5. Client administers medications safely and as instructed.

6. Client modifies diet if oral discomfort occurs.

7. Client consults with nutritionist if needed.

NURSING DIAGNOSIS ACTIVITY INTOLERANCE

▍*Related Factors:* Generalized weakness; imbalance between oxygen supply and demand

▍*Defining Characteristics:* Decreased RBCs and hemoglobin; hypoxia; fatigue; inability to carry out ADL; decreased stamina;

weakness; loss of positional and vibratory senses; numbness and tingling of extremities

OUTCOMES

▌*Short Term*
Tolerance and endurance improved, as evidenced by modification of ADL and increased participation in activities (expected in 1 week)

▌*Long Term*
Optimal activity tolerance, as evidenced by increased energy and endurance and independence in ADL and mobility for optimal or higher level of health and functioning (expected in 1 month)

NURSING INTERVENTIONS/INSTRUCTIONS

1. Assess client's ability to perform ADL by having client demonstrate several typical activities and noting vital signs afterward for increases in pulse or dyspnea (first visit).
2. Instruct client to personalize and pace activities and to schedule rest periods between these activities; include work and home schedules (first visit).
3. Instruct client to change position slowly and to sit down if dizzy (first visit).
4. Instruct client to request assistance in ADL and ambulation if needed, especially if there are sensory changes in extremities (first visit).
5. Encourage self-care with use of aids if they promote independence (first visit).
6. Instruct client to elevate head of bed to facilitate respirations and to administer supplemental oxygen if needed, with instructions about hazards associated with oxygen therapy (first visit).
7. Refer HHA to assist with ADL as needed (first visit).

CLIENT AND FAMILY/CAREGIVER INTERVENTIONS

1. Client follows plan for rest and activity.
2. Client performs ADL independently with increasing endurance.
3. Client obtains assistance or aids as needed.
4. Client administers supplemental oxygen as instructed.
5. Client sleeps with head elevated; takes steps to eliminate dyspnea associated with activity by resting.

NURSING DIAGNOSIS ▐ DEFICIENT KNOWLEDGE

▌*Related Factors:* Lack of exposure to information

▌*Defining Characteristics:* Request for information about medical regimen, maintenance therapy, and prevention of recurrence of signs and symptoms of anemia

OUTCOMES

▌*Short Term*

Adequate knowledge, as evidenced by client stating precautions needed for specific anemia being treated, medication regimen and implications, course of disease and treatment, and complications if not treated (expected in 3 days)

▌*Long Term*

Optimal knowledge, as evidenced by compliance with medication, dietary, and activity regimens and other treatment to prevent recurrence of anemia and complications (expected in 1 month)

NURSING INTERVENTIONS/INSTRUCTIONS

1. Instruct client to inform all physicians and dentists of disorder (first visit).
2. Inform client that, for pernicious anemia, parenteral vitamin B_{12} must be administered monthly for life, and instruct client in administration (first and second visits).
3. Instruct client to avoid infections by handwashing, good personal hygiene, and avoiding exposure to persons with upper respiratory tract infections; encourage client to update immunizations (first visit).
4. Instruct client to report any presence of infection with fever to physician; any recurrence of skin color changes (pallor), changes in motor or sensory responses in extremities, presence of dizziness, or dyspnea should also be reported (first visit).
5. Instruct client to keep warm with extra clothing and blankets if needed and to avoid using heating pads and hot water bottles (first visit).
6. Instruct client in skin care, including use of mild soap, gentle massage, and emollients; note pressure points for erythema and reduced sensation (first visit).

7. Inform client of measures to avoid trauma to skin if vasomotor disturbance or peripheral neuropathies exist (first visit).
8. Inform client that diet inclusions and several medications may be used for anemia, including iron, pyridoxine, vitamin B_{12}, and folic acid, and to avoid all over-the-counter medications unless approved by physician (first visit).
9. Instruct client to keep physician and laboratory appointments and emphasize need for compliance as symptoms decrease (first visit).

CLIENT AND FAMILY/CAREGIVER INTERVENTIONS

1. Client maintains dietary and medication regimens for specific anemia.
2. Client follows personal hygiene practice; avoids contact with possible infection; maintains immunizations.
3. Client maintains warmth and avoids injury to skin and dry, irritated skin.
4. Client notifies physician of signs and symptoms of infection or recurrence of condition.
5. Client complies with physician and laboratory visits for injection of vitamin B_{12} and assessment of condition.
6. Client wears clothes and shoes that maintain warmth and prevent trauma to extremities.
7. Client states cause of disorder and reason for treatment regimen.

MUSCULOSKELETAL SYSTEM

❋ *Amputation*

An amputation is the surgical removal of all or part of an extremity. The procedure may be performed at a joint or in the middle of a limb to treat a malignancy, severe infectious process, circulatory impairment, traumatic event or injury, or congenital defect. Care management includes the use of a prosthesis as part of the rehabilitative program and treatment for the underlying condition that is associated with the amputation.

Home care is primarily concerned with the teaching aspects of stump care, prosthesis care, and compliance with the rehabilitative phase of the medical regimen.

> Primary Diagnoses:
> Amputation, Surgical—ICD code: 997.6
> Amputation, Infected—ICD code: 997.62

NURSING DIAGNOSIS   IMPAIRED PHYSICAL MOBILITY

▌**Related Factors:** Intolerance to activity; musculoskeletal impairment (lower extremity amputation)

▌**Defining Characteristics:** Inability to purposefully move in physical environment; reluctance to attempt movement and ambulation; improper prosthesis fit; inadequate healing and conditioning of stump

OUTCOMES

▌**Short Term**
Adequate mobility, as evidenced by progressive independence in ambulation with prosthesis without falls or trauma (expected in 1 week)

▊*Long Term*

Maximum mobility achieved, as evidenced by effective use of prosthesis for ambulation and activities of daily living (ADL) with independence and optimal functioning (expected in 2 to 3 months)

NURSING INTERVENTIONS/INSTRUCTIONS

1. Assess client's mobility and activity status, effectiveness of use of prosthesis for ambulation, balancing difficulties, and use of assistive aids for walking (see Musculoskeletal System Assessment, p. 31, for guidelines) (first visit and each visit as needed).
2. Assess prosthesis fit, healing and conditioning of stump, and presence of pain when client is using prosthesis (each visit).
3. Instruct client in use of crutches, cane, or walker with or without prosthesis as appropriate (first visit).
4. Instruct client to balance on one leg without support and to ambulate with extension of stump (first visit).
5. Instruct client to ambulate with proper gait, using prosthesis as taught (first visit).
6. Provide and instruct in range-of-motion (ROM) exercises for unaffected joints (first visit).
7. Instruct client in exercises to tighten gluteal and abdominal muscles and to transfer from bed to sitting or standing position and back to bed (first and second visits).
8. Instruct client in prescribed exercises to legs, use of weights, push-ups and knee bends, and standing or walking with one foot (each visit).
9. Instruct client to progress in ambulation from 5-minute periods to daily increases as tolerated and within restrictions; advise client to have assistance until stability and coordination are achieved (first visit).
10. Instruct client in arranging pathways and in furniture arrangement that promotes support in ambulation and prevents accidents from bumping or falling and injuring operative or other site (first visit).
11. Inform client of resources for purchasing or renting supplies and equipment (first visit).
12. Initiate referral to or reinforce instructions of physical therapist (any visit).
13. Refer home health aide (HHA) for assistance in mobility and ADL (first visit).

CLIENT AND FAMILY/CAREGIVER INTERVENTIONS

1. Client performs daily progressive muscle and joint exercises.
2. Client ambulates safely with or without use of prosthesis.
3. Client provides safe environment for ambulation without trauma.
4. Client uses aids such as crutches, cane, and walker as needed.
5. Client performs prescribed physical rehabilitation as instructed by therapist.
6. Client avoids strain, fatigue, and falls while using prosthesis.
7. Client achieves independence in mobility with use of prosthesis, including transfer and position changes.
8. Client complies with appointments for physical therapy.

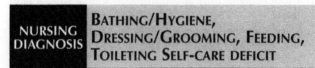

NURSING DIAGNOSIS **BATHING/HYGIENE, DRESSING/GROOMING, FEEDING, TOILETING SELF-CARE DEFICIT**

▌*Related Factors:* Impaired mobility and activity ability (upper or lower extremity amputation)

▌*Defining Characteristics:* Inability to wash body parts, put on or take off clothing, maintain appearance, bring food to mouth for ingestion, use toilet or commode, and carry out toilet hygiene

OUTCOMES

▌*Short Term*
Adequate participation in ADL, as evidenced by progressive independence in daily activities with use of prosthesis (expected in 1 week)

▌*Long Term*
Optimal participation in ADL achieved, as evidenced by effective use of prosthesis for all personal care, with optimal functioning and independence (expected in 2 to 3 months)

NURSING INTERVENTIONS/INSTRUCTIONS

1. Assess client's activity status; ability to perform ADL with or without prosthesis; and ability to use assistive aids for bathing, grooming, dressing, toileting, and eating (see Functional Assessment, p. 55, for guidelines) (first visit).

2. Assess prosthesis (e.g., artificial arm, hook, or cosmetic hand) fit and healing and condition of stump (any visit).
3. Instruct client in use of one arm or hand and aids for cooking, personal care, and other activity needs (each visit).
4. Instruct client in ROM exercises for unaffected joints and prescribed exercises for arm and shoulder, including frequency, length of time, and progressive increases (first and second visits).
5. Initiate referral to or reinforce instructions of physical and/or occupational therapists (any visit).
6. Refer HHA to assist with ADL as needed (first visit).

CLIENT AND FAMILY/CAREGIVER INTERVENTIONS

1. Client performs daily progressive ADL with or without prosthesis.
2. Client uses aids to assist with toileting, eating, bathing, dressing, grooming, cooking, working in home, and returning to occupation.
3. Client avoids accidents and fatigue during use of prosthesis for ADL.
4. Client performs prescribed physical and occupational rehabilitation as instructed by therapists.
5. Client achieves independence in ADL with use of prosthesis.
6. Client complies with appointments for therapy.

NURSING DIAGNOSIS RISK FOR IMPAIRED SKIN INTEGRITY

▌*Related Factors:* External mechanical factor of pressure

▌*Defining Characteristics:* Weight bearing on stump; improper fit of prosthesis; improper care of stump; improper conditioning; redness, pain, edema, and irritation at stump site

OUTCOMES

▌*Short Term*

Preservation of skin integrity, as evidenced by intactness at stump surgical site and by absence of irritation, pain, or edema (expected in 1 week and after prosthesis use)

▌*Long Term*

Absence of skin damage or breakdown, as evidenced by maintenance of optimal skin integrity for health and prosthesis use (expected to be ongoing)

NURSING INTERVENTIONS/INSTRUCTIONS

1. Assess stump site for redness, tenderness, irritation, edema, flabbiness, fit of prosthesis, and pressure against stump (see Integumentary System Assessment, p. 39, for guidelines) (every visit).
2. Instruct client to assess stump and to report changes to physician or prosthetist (first visit).
3. Instruct client in cleansing and gentle drying of stump and in massaging and exposing to air for 20 minutes each day (first visit).
4. Instruct client in removal and reapplication of dressing or bandage, with proper wrapping to avoid tightness and to promote shaping (first and second visits).
5. Instruct client to avoid use of powders or lotions on stump; instruct client in application of stump sock after cleansing and drying and to change daily (first visit).
6. Instruct client to pad pressure areas on skin and stump (first visit).
7. Instruct client to discontinue use of prosthesis if skin is red or irritated and to have prosthesis checked for fit if this occurs (first visit).
8. Advise client to seek assistance from prosthetist for problems with fit or use of prosthesis, whether for arm or leg (first visit).

CLIENT AND FAMILY/CAREGIVER INTERVENTIONS

1. Client maintains integrity and cleanliness of stump skin.
2. Client protects stump from pressure of prosthesis.
3. Client avoids skin damage from improper fit of prosthesis.
4. Client uses proper stump sock, mild soap and warm water, and thorough drying in stump care.
5. Client bandages or wraps stump properly.
6. Client secures services of prosthetist when needed.

NURSING DIAGNOSIS DISTURBED BODY IMAGE

■ *Related Factors:* Biophysical factor of amputation procedure

■ *Defining Characteristics:* Verbal response to change in structure and function of body part or to loss of body part; negative feelings about body; feelings of helplessness or powerlessness; change in social involvement

OUTCOMES

■ *Short Term*
Improved body image adaptation, as evidenced by statement of feelings and concerns about changes in appearance and limitations imposed by loss of body part and need to change lifestyle (expected in 1 week)

■ *Long Term*
Optimal adaptation to body image, as evidenced by improvement in role performance and interpersonal relationships and by willingness to change functional patterns and integrate them into lifestyle (expected in 2 to 3 months)

NURSING INTERVENTIONS/INSTRUCTIONS

1. Assess client's lifestyle, roles, and ability to adapt to changes (first visit).
2. Allow client to express fears and concerns about ability to resume normal life (each visit).
3. Allow time for questions and clarifications; provide accepting, nonjudgmental environment (each visit).
4. Instruct client to encourage visits from friends, clergy, and other amputees (any visit).
5. Encourage client to express strengths, and inform client of options for lifestyle changes, including sexual activity, ADL, social and occupational interactions, and recreational and leisure activities (any visit).
6. Inform client of and refer to sex therapist, occupational rehabilitation, social or counseling services, and driving instruction (first visit).
7. Inform client of clothing that deemphasizes lost limb (first visit).

CLIENT AND FAMILY/CAREGIVER INTERVENTIONS

1. Client verbalizes concerns and feelings about loss.
2. Client allows for grieving over loss.
3. Client participates in all aspects of care independently.
4. Client returns to work or enters vocational rehabilitation.
5. Client adapts to limitations imposed by loss of limb.
6. Client resumes close relationships with others and activities, interests, and social interactions with others.

NURSING DIAGNOSIS DEFICIENT KNOWLEDGE

■ *Related Factors:* Lack of information about condition and care

■ *Defining Characteristics:* Request for information about prosthesis care, medical regimen for progressive rehabilitation, and signs and symptoms of complications

OUTCOMES

■ *Short Term*
Adequate knowledge, as evidenced by client's statement of treatment regimen, care of prosthesis, and signs and symptoms to report (expected in 4 days)

■ *Long Term*
Optimal knowledge, as evidenced by compliance with medical regimen and prevention of complications to achieve optimal level of health and functioning (expected in 2 to 3 months)

NURSING INTERVENTIONS/INSTRUCTIONS

1. Assess lifestyle changes, ability to adapt, ability and interest to learn, and family participation and support (first visit).
2. Instruct client to assess for complications, including swelling, color change, pain, purulent drainage from stump site, temperature elevation, and pulse and respiration changes, and to report these signs and symptoms to physician (first visit).
3. Inform client that pain in the amputated limb (i.e., phantom pain) is a normal response and instruct about measures to overcome, including exercise, diversional activities, and pharmacologic agents (first visit).

4. Instruct client in washing and drying socket of prosthesis, application of prosthesis, wearing of proper shoes with prosthesis for proper gait, and having prosthesis checked for fit or adjustment as needed (first visit; each visit thereafter as needed).
5. If medication is prescribed, instruct client in administration, including dose, frequency, time, food and drug interactions, and side effects (first visit).
6. Instruct client to keep all appointments with physician, laboratory, prosthetist, and therapists (first visit).
7. Inform client of community agencies and support groups for information and securing equipment and supplies (any visit).

CLIENT AND FAMILY/CAREGIVER INTERVENTIONS

1. Client assesses and monitors stump and remaining limbs for signs and symptoms of complications, and reports to physician.
2. Client cleans stump and prosthesis and applies prosthesis correctly.
3. Client administers medications correctly and safely, achieving desired results.
4. Client adapts to change in lifestyle.
5. Client complies with medical regimen and keeps appointments with interdisciplinary professionals.
6. Client contacts agencies, clubs, and groups for assistance, equipment, information, and support.

✳ *Osteoarthritis and Rheumatoid Arthritis*

Arthritis includes conditions that affect and cause damage to joints, cartilage, and connective tissue and result in activity and mobility limitations. Osteoarthritis is a chronic degenerative disease that is localized and progressive; it results in cartilage erosion and most commonly affects weight-bearing joints. Rheumatoid arthritis is a chronic inflammatory disease; it is systemic and progressive and affects the synovial joints and related structures.

Home care is primarily concerned with the care of the involved joints and with teaching aspects of the medical regimen, prevention of injury to the joints, and progression of the disease.

Primary Diagnoses:
Osteoarthritis, Acute Exacerbation—ICD code: 715.90
Osteoarthritis, Hip—ICD code: 715.95
Osteoarthritis, Leg, Knee—ICD code: 715.96
Osteoarthritis, Spine—ICD code: 715.90
Rheumatoid Arthritis—ICD code: 714.0

NURSING DIAGNOSIS CHRONIC PAIN

Related Factors: Chronic physical disability

Defining Characteristics: Verbal report of pain experienced for more than 6 months; fear of reinjury; altered ability to continue previous activities; guarded movement; physical and social withdrawal; depression

OUTCOMES

Short Term
Minimal pain or reduction in pain, as evidenced by client's statements that pain medication and measures to increase comfort are effective in controlling pain (expected in 3 days)

Long Term
Absence or control of pain, as evidenced by optimal mobility and activity necessary for functioning, socializing, and independently performing ADL (expected in 2 to 3 weeks)

NURSING INTERVENTIONS/INSTRUCTIONS

1. Assess pain and characteristics, including remissions and exacerbations or, if the pain is continuous, factors that relieve or precipitate pain (each visit).
2. Instruct client in administration of analgesics, antirheumatics, and steroidal and nonsteroidal antiinflammatory drugs, including dose, action of drug, times, frequency, side effects (especially steroids); instruct client to take drugs continuously regardless of improvement and to avoid abrupt discontinuation of steroid therapy (first visit).

3. Instruct client to coordinate medication for pain with activities and to avoid overworking or activities that cause stress to joints (first visit).
4. Instruct client to avoid stressful situations; damp, moist environments; and extremes in environmental temperatures (first visit).
5. Instruct client to avoid sudden movements and prolonged activities, including walking, standing, and sitting (first visit).
6. Instruct client in use of bed cradle, footboard, and bed board (first visit).
7. Instruct client in application of heat treatments, including warm baths and showers; electric blanket; and warm, wet compresses. Inform client of possible paraffin application during physical therapy session (first visit; reinforce on second visit).
8. Instruct client in application of splints to reduce pain by immobilizing the joints, including when to remove and reapply them (first visit).
9. Suggest relaxation techniques and methods of distraction (first visit).

CLIENT AND FAMILY/CAREGIVER INTERVENTIONS

1. Client assesses and administers analgesics for pain.
2. Client places affected joints in position of comfort.
3. Client applies heat treatments as instructed.
4. Client administers medications as instructed; observes and reports side effects.
5. Client applies splints, footboard, soft linens, pillows, bed cradle, or other devices as appropriate to control pain and support joints.
6. Client uses relaxation and diversional activities during painful episodes.
7. Client avoids overactivity, stress, and environmental changes that affect joints.
8. Client reports time, intensity, duration, and site(s) of pain.

NURSING DIAGNOSIS   IMPAIRED PHYSICAL MOBILITY

▌***Related Factors:*** Pain and discomfort; musculoskeletal impairment

■*Defining Characteristics:* Reluctance to attempt movement; inability to purposefully move in physical environment; limited ROM; imposed restrictions of movement

■OUTCOMES

Short Term
Adequate activity and mobility, as evidenced by progressive ambulation and movement within restrictions or limitations imposed by the disease process and by participation in ADL (expected in 1 week)

■*Long Term*
Optimal achievement of physical mobility, as evidenced by ability to maintain health and functioning and by performance of ADL within restrictions without complications (expected in 1 to 2 months)

NURSING INTERVENTIONS/INSTRUCTIONS

1. Assess ability to ambulate and to participate in ADL, limitations of joint movement, presence of pain on movement, and need for assistive aids (see Musculoskeletal System Assessment, p. 31, for guidelines) (first visit).
2. Instruct client in prescribed limitations in use of joints, 1-hour rest periods throughout day to rest affected parts, and scheduling of activities to avoid fatigue and joint injury (first and second visits).
3. Instruct client to allow plenty of time to perform all activities and to take pain medication before exercising if drug is not too potent (first visit).
4. Instruct client in correct body alignment and in body mechanics in a resting position and for transferring, lifting, reaching, stooping, bending, pushing, and ambulating (first visit; reinforce on second visit).
5. Instruct client in use of assistive aids and supportive devices, such as crutches, braces, corrective shoes, cane, walker, and wheelchair, and in use of aids to perform ADL, such as long-handled pickups, Velcro closures, holders for mirrors and books, and zippered clothing (first visit).

6. Instruct client in exercises for involved and uninvolved joints, including type and frequency of ROM and muscle-setting exercises (each visit as needed).

7. Instruct client in joint protection during activities and in the use of immobilization aids to rest joints when needed (first visit).

8. Encourage client to participate in ADL and diversional activities within restrictions (first visit and as needed).

9. Instruct client in skin protection for areas under splints and at enlarged joint areas because these are susceptible to breakdown (each visit).

10. Initiate referral to physical therapist for exercise regimen and occupational therapist for ADL and fine-motor exercises (any visit).

11. Refer HHA to assist with ADL as needed (first visit).

CLIENT AND FAMILY/CAREGIVER INTERVENTIONS

1. Client performs planned exercises and activities, with progressive increases daily or weekly.

2. Client ambulates, transfers, reaches, and changes position using proper body mechanics and maintaining body alignment.

3. Client participates in ADL as able, with progress until independence is achieved.

4. Client provides rest periods throughout day as needed to avoid overactivity.

5. Client uses assistive and supportive aids for joint protection.

6. Client adjusts work hours according to activity tolerance.

7. Client uses assistive aids for ADL, eating, reaching, and dressing and grooming, and a raised toilet seat, as needed.

8. Client reports to physician any prolonged pain that is not controlled and that limits activity and exercise.

9. Client maintains physical and occupational therapy regimens with changes as indicated.

10. Client administers analgesic before activity or ambulation, as appropriate.

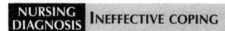

NURSING DIAGNOSIS | **INEFFECTIVE COPING**

▌*Related Factors:* Personal vulnerability; multiple life changes

∎Defining Characteristics: Verbalization of inability to cope with chronic illness or to ask for help; inability to meet basic needs and role expectations; chronic worry and anxiety; chronic fatigue; inability to solve problems; immobility; chronic pain; social isolation

OUTCOMES

∎Short Term

Improved coping skills, as evidenced by client's statement of chronic nature of the disease and knowledge of need to develop new coping and problem-solving skills for compliance with long-term treatments (expected in 1 week)

∎Long term

Positive coping with chronic illness, as evidenced by optimal participation in care and willingness to adapt to lifestyle changes to achieve maximum health and functioning status (expected in 2 months)

NURSING INTERVENTIONS/INSTRUCTIONS

1. Assess mental and emotional status, ability to adapt, level of anxiety, and coping mechanisms used and their effect (first visit).
2. Provide an accepting environment, and allow expressions of fears, concerns, and feelings regarding deformity and effect on body image (each visit).
3. Allow client to control planning of care and to make decisions for goal setting (each visit).
4. Assist client in identifying desires and ways to change lifestyle, which coping mechanisms work, and which are destructive (each visit).
5. Instruct client in methods to develop new coping skills and to try changes without fear of failing (first visit).
6. Initiate referral for psychotherapy, support group assistance, or counseling as indicated (any visit).
7. Refer to social worker if social services and mental health assistance are needed (any visit).

CLIENT AND FAMILY/CAREGIVER INTERVENTIONS

1. Client develops effective coping and problem-solving skills.

2. Client verbalizes feelings and concerns about body image and long-term disability with family members and requests assistance when needed.
3. Client identifies negative and positive behaviors and maintains productive coping methods.
4. Client uses significant others, groups, and agencies for help and support.
5. Client joins and participates in the Arthritis Foundation.
6. Client manages own care effectively and maintains a positive attitude.

NURSING DIAGNOSIS DEFICIENT KNOWLEDGE

Related Factors: Lack of information about care and preventive measures

Defining Characteristics: Request for information about disease process, cause, and treatment; risk of falls or injury in an unsafe environment; signs and symptoms of complications; need to modify lifestyle

OUTCOMES

Short Term
Adequate knowledge, as evidenced by client's statement of cause, treatment, measures to prevent injury or trauma, signs and symptoms to report, and medication regimen (expected in 1 week)

Long Term
Optimal knowledge, as evidenced by client's complying with medical regimen and meeting requirements of modified lifestyle necessary to achieve optimal health and musculoskeletal functioning (expected in 1 to 2 months)

NURSING INTERVENTIONS/INSTRUCTIONS

1. Assess lifestyle, ability to adapt to change and disabilities, learning ability and interest, and family participation and support (first visit).
2. Inform client of cause and chronicity of disease, remissions and exacerbations, need for long-term consistent therapy, and progressive joint weakness and instability (first visit).

3. Instruct client in fluid, nutrition, and rest plan and in need to avoid weight gain (first and second visits).

4. Instruct client in signs and symptoms of complications to report, including uncontrolled pain, redness, swelling, and inability to move joint (first visit).

5. Inform client of prevalence of advertised quack cures and misinformation (first visit).

6. Inform client of alternative timing and positioning for sexual closeness (any visit).

7. Instruct client to provide safe environment to reduce injury from falls, including removing small rugs; using night lights and hand rails; using cane or walker; wearing well-fitting, sturdy shoes; and clearing all pathways (first visit).

8. Instruct client in medication administration, including analgesics, steroids, salicylates, and gold injections, with action, dose, frequency, side effects, expected results, and food and drug interactions (first visit; reinforce each visit thereafter).

9. Inform client of need for and importance of all physical and occupational therapy recommendations and of need to keep appointments for laboratory work and with physician (first visit).

10. Instruct client to adjust daily schedules, to change activities that are not tolerated well, and to take 1-hour rest periods frequently during the day (first visit; reinforce as needed).

11. Initiate referral to community agencies and support groups, such as the Arthritis Foundation, for literature and for information about where to acquire supplies and equipment (any visit).

CLIENT AND FAMILY/CAREGIVER INTERVENTIONS

1. Client states cause, prescribed treatments, fluid and dietary requirements, rest needs, and signs and symptoms to report to physician.

2. Client assesses daily for changes that are positive and negative in terms of progress.

3. Client administers medications correctly and reports any untoward responses.

4. Client avoids stressful situations when possible.

5. Client adjusts sexual activities as needed.

6. Client avoids unrecognized treatments that may cause disappointment or injury.

7. Client maintains therapy regimens, laboratory testing schedule, and appointments with physician or other referrals.
8. Client participates in and accepts assistance from agencies and support groups as needed.
9. Client adapts to lifestyle changes in a realistic manner.

✳ *Fractured Hip and Hip or Knee Prosthesis Replacement*

Hip fractures include fractures of the head, neck, and trochanter parts of the femur. They usually result from osteoporosis or falls. The surgical procedure for hip/knee replacement includes the removal of the ball and socket of the hip joint and insertion of a prosthesis or includes the replacement of the surfaces of the tibia and femur with a prosthesis. Either procedure is performed to correct damage caused by fracture, deformity, or rheumatoid or degenerative arthritis.

Home care is primarily concerned with the teaching of the medical and rehabilitative regimen to ensure optimal mobility.

Primary Diagnoses:
Hip Fracture—ICD code: 820.80
Knee, Degenerative Arthritis—ICD code: 715.96
Osteoarthritis, Hip—ICD code: 715.95
Hip Replacement, Total—ICD code: 81.51
Knee Replacement—ICD code: 81.54

NURSING DIAGNOSIS IMPAIRED PHYSICAL MOBILITY

▮ *Related Factors:* Musculoskeletal impairment

▮ *Defining Characteristics:* Inability to purposefully move in environment; reluctance to attempt movement; limited ROM; fear of dislocating prosthesis

OUTCOMES

▌*Short Term*

Adequate activity and mobility, as evidenced by progressive ambulation and movement in imposed limitations (expected in 1 week)

▌*Long Term*

Optimal physical mobility and independence in ADL achieved within restrictions to maintain health and functioning without complications (expected in 1 month)

NURSING INTERVENTIONS/INSTRUCTIONS

1. Assess client's ability to participate in ADL, mobility status, and need for assistive aids for ambulation and self-care (see Musculoskeletal System Assessment, p. 31, for guidelines) (first visit and as needed).
2. Instruct client in transferring and pivoting techniques to get on toilet and to get into car, bed, wheelchair, shower, or other places (first and second visits).
3. Instruct client in muscle-strengthening exercises to prepare for use of devices for ambulation and ADL; instruct client in use of walker, cane, or crutches as appropriate (each visit).
4. Instruct client in ROM exercises as permitted and instruct client to perform them on all functioning joints, including number of times and frequency (first visit; reinforce on second visit).
5. Instruct client in and encourage him or her to perform all personal care; instruct client to increase ambulation daily (each visit).
6. Instruct client in weight-bearing limitation on operative side (first visit).
7. Initiate referral to physical, occupational, and vocational therapists (any visit).
8. Refer HHA to assist in ADL as needed (first visit).
9. Arrange for equipment in home, including hospital bed, wheelchair, walker, or other aids (first visit).

CLIENT AND FAMILY/CAREGIVER INTERVENTIONS

1. Client performs daily planned exercise regimen, including ROM exercises and ambulation using appropriate assistive aids.
2. Client progresses in independence in walking and in transfer techniques.

3. Client uses assistive aids for ADL, including raised toilet seat, long-handled tongs for reaching or picking up articles, and other aids, depending on needs associated with dressing, meal preparation, and bathing.
4. Client participates in therapy programs.
5. Client carries out prescribed rehabilitation as instructed by therapists.

NURSING DIAGNOSIS RISK FOR TRAUMA

Related Factors: Internal factors of surgical procedure affecting movement; external factors of unsafe environment

Defining Characteristics: Weakness; reduced weight-bearing ability; reduced movement of limb; lack of safety precautions; inability or refusal to use assistive aids

OUTCOMES

Short Term
Absence of falls or injury, as evidenced by ability to move without pain and weakness and by increased weight-bearing ability using assistive aids (expected in 1 week)

Long Term
Ongoing absence of trauma, as evidenced by maintenance of optimal health and functioning, and increased mobility without injury (expected in 1 month and ongoing)

NURSING INTERVENTIONS/INSTRUCTIONS

1. Assess for signs of prosthesis dislocation, such as shortening of or inability to move or bear weight on operative extremity and severe pain and spasms during movement; instruct client to observe for these signs and symptoms (each visit).
2. Instruct client to maintain weight-bearing restrictions and to avoid hip flexion, elevating knees, stooping, crossing legs, twisting of the limb, and positions during intercourse that cause hip to turn inward or rotation of the knee (first visit).
3. Instruct client to use assistive aids for ambulation and holding bars to assist with movement and to provide stability (first visit).

4. Instruct client to turn on side when in bed only as instructed and to avoid lifting heavy objects (first visit).
5. Instruct client to provide clear pathways; to remove rugs, cords, furniture, or other objects that may interfere with ambulation; to avoid stairways; and to take plenty of time for all activities (first visit).
6. Instruct client to take rest periods and to avoid activities when fatigued (first visit).

CLIENT AND FAMILY/CAREGIVER INTERVENTIONS

1. Client provides clear pathways, good lighting, and assistive aids to prevent falls.
2. Client avoids positions, turning, weight bearing, sitting, lifting, and stooping as instructed to prevent dislocation.
3. Client avoids strain and fatigue as result of activity.
4. Client follows recommendations for positioning during sexual intercourse.
5. Client allows sufficient time for activities.
6. Client reports to physician any signs or symptoms indicating displacement.

NURSING DIAGNOSIS DEFICIENT KNOWLEDGE

■ *Related Factors:* Lack of information about postoperative care

■ *Defining Characteristics:* Request for information about medical regimen and rehabilitation requirements

OUTCOMES

■ Short Term
Adequate knowledge, as evidenced by client's statement of signs and symptoms of complications to report and client's ability to perform postoperative wound care and to correctly administer medications (expected in 1 week)

■ Long Term
Optimal knowledge, as evidenced by achievement of optimal health and return of functioning within prescribed limitations (expected in 2 to 3 months)

NURSING INTERVENTIONS/INSTRUCTIONS

1. Assess lifestyle and ability to adapt, learning abilities, and family assistance and support (first visit).
2. Inform client of signs and symptoms of complications, including persistent or increased pain in extremity; numbness in extremity; bleeding, edema, redness, or pain at incision site; and continued difficulty in bearing weight on extremity. Instruct client to report any complications to physician (first visit).
3. Instruct client in administration of analgesics and antibiotics, including action, dose, frequency, route, and side effects (first visit).
4. Instruct client in sterile dressing changes and allow for return demonstration; instruct client to note and report drainage characteristics (first visit; reinforce on second visit).
5. Encourage client to participate in diversional activities according to interests (first visit).
6. Instruct client to report any changes in elimination pattern (e.g., constipation) for advice in taking stool softener or for changing fluid and nutritional intake (first visit).
7. Inform client of importance of complying with physical and occupational rehabilitation program (any visit).

CLIENT AND FAMILY/CAREGIVER INTERVENTIONS

1. Client correctly administers medications as prescribed.
2. Client provides care to surgical site as needed, using sterile technique.
3. Client establishes and maintains bowel elimination pattern.
4. Client monitors for complications and reports them to physician if present.
5. Client satisfactorily complies with rehabilitation program.
6. Client participates in diversional and stress-reducing activities.

❈ *Fractures and Cast Application*

A fracture is a break in a bone caused by trauma (e.g., falls or accidents) or disease (e.g., osteoporosis with pathologic fracture). It is usually accompanied by contusion of the surrounding soft tissue. Fractures may be complete or incomplete and simple or compound, and they may affect any bone in the body. A fracture is corrected by closed reduction or open reduction and immobilization of the part by casting, splinting, or traction.

Home care is primarily concerned with the teaching of care for the affected body part, ensuring immobilization and healing of the fracture, and preventing complications of the fracture.

> Primary Diagnoses:
> Fracture, Ankle—ICD code: 824.8
> Fracture, Humerus—ICD code: 812.20
> Fracture, Tibia—ICD code: 823.80
> Fracture, Ulna and Radius—ICD code: 813.83
> Fracture, Wrist—ICD code: 813.41

NURSING DIAGNOSIS   ACUTE PAIN

▌**Related Factors:** Physical injuring agents of bone fracture

▌**Defining Characteristics:** Verbal descriptors of pain; guarding and protective behavior; altered muscle tone

OUTCOMES

▌Short Term

Minimal pain or absence of pain, as evidenced by client's statement that pain has been reduced or controlled and that measures to promote comfort are effective (expected in 3 days)

▌Long Term

Absence of pain, as evidenced by achievement of optimal comfort level and mobility for health and functioning in presence of casted body part (expected in 1 week or when cast removed)

NURSING INTERVENTIONS/INSTRUCTIONS

1. Assess, and instruct client and family to assess, type of fracture and associated pain, tight cast (insert finger between cast and skin), swelling, pallor or cyanosis, coolness of skin, loss of sensation, and decreased peripheral pulse in casted extremity; assess every 30 minutes for 24 hours and then every 3 to 4 hours (first visit).
2. Instruct client to handle involved extremity gently, with smooth movement, especially first 24 hours, and to elevate on pillow for comfort (first visit).
3. Instruct client in administration of analgesic, including dose, frequency, and relief to expect (first visit).
4. Instruct client to participate in diversional activities and relaxation exercises to reduce pain (e.g., music, reading, watching television, or using imagery) (first visit).
5. Instruct client to change position every 2 hours to prevent pressure of cast to one area (first visit).

CLIENT AND FAMILY/CAREGIVER INTERVENTIONS

1. Client assesses pain and administers analgesic accordingly.
2. Client provides comfort measure to reduce pain.
3. Client uses diversional methods and interactions to relieve pain.

NURSING DIAGNOSIS RISK FOR IMPAIRED SKIN INTEGRITY

▎**Related Factors:** External factors of pressure of cast and physical immobilization

▎**Defining Characteristics:** Redness, swelling, irritation of skin at cast edges or bony prominences; immobility of injured part

OUTCOMES

▎**Short Term**

Skin integrity preserved, as evidenced by intactness at pressure areas (expected in 2 to 3 days)

▎**Long Term**

Absence of skin damage, as evidenced by maintenance of optimal skin integrity and by return to normal functioning (expected to be ongoing)

NURSING INTERVENTIONS/INSTRUCTIONS

1. Assess skin at edges of cast, splint, or other device used to immobilize fractured bone; note redness, irritation, breaks, or pain; and instruct client to assess and report these signs and symptoms if they are present (first visit).
2. Petal (i.e., cover) the edges of cast or device with soft adhesive, and inform client of rationale and of procedure to replace petaling (first visit).
3. Instruct client to avoid sticking things into cast to scratch itchy areas (first visit).
4. Encourage client to frequently change positions (first visit).

CLIENT AND FAMILY/CAREGIVER INTERVENTIONS

1. Client maintains skin integrity at areas prone to irritation.
2. Client protects skin from rough edges of cast or rubbing from device.
3. Client avoids skin damage caused by foreign objects in cast and prolonged pressure.

NURSING DIAGNOSIS IMPAIRED PHYSICAL MOBILITY

▌*Related Factors:* Pain and discomfort; musculoskeletal impairment

▌*Defining Characteristics:* Inability to purposefully move in physical environment; imposed restriction of movement by cast or splint; inability to use assistive aids and provide self-care

OUTCOMES

▌*Short Term*
Adequate activity and mobility within limitations of cast or splint, as evidenced by movement with use of assistive aids (expected in 2 to 3 days)

▌*Long Term*
Optimal physical mobility and independence in ADL achieved within restrictions to maintain health and functioning without complications (expected in 1 week or at time of cast removal)

NURSING INTERVENTIONS/INSTRUCTIONS

1. Assess client's mobility status with cast and ability to progress daily with or without assistive aids; assess for mobility with leg cast or for ADL with arm cast (see Musculoskeletal System Assessment, p. 31, for guidelines) (first and second visits).
2. Instruct client in use of walking cast, crutches, or arm sling as appropriate (first visit or when weight bearing is allowed).
3. Instruct client in transferring to bed, chair, car, and toilet and in use of aids for bathing, dressing, grooming, and personal hygiene as needed (first visit).
4. Instruct client to arrange furniture and clear pathways for ambulation and to place articles in easy reach and for convenience (first visit).
5. Instruct client in ROM exercises for uncasted parts and to move unaffected body parts frequently while progressing in ADL and other activities; include digits on casted extremity (first visit).
6. Initiate referral to physical therapist if needed (any visit).
7. Refer HHA to assist in ADL as appropriate (first visit).

CLIENT AND FAMILY/CAREGIVER INTERVENTIONS

1. Client ambulates and participates in ADL at earliest possible time using assistive aids.
2. Client ambulates when weight bearing is allowed; applies sling properly; avoids activities that might damage cast.
3. Client provides and promotes activities that require use of all muscles and independence in ADL.
4. Client performs ROM and other strength-maintaining muscle exercises.
5. Client maintains clear, safe pathways and safe environment to prevent falls and injury and bumping or damage to cast.

NURSING DIAGNOSIS **RISK FOR PERIPHERAL NEUROVASCULAR DYSFUNCTION**

▌*Related Factors:* Fracture; mechanical compression (e.g., cast)

▌*Defining Characteristics:* Pallor; cyanotic color and coolness of skin at cast edges; decreased peripheral pulses; change in sensation or feeling proximal to cast edges; numbness or loss of sensation at cast site

OUTCOMES

▌*Short Term*

Neurovascular function preserved, as evidenced by digits or areas proximal to cast warm and pink and perception to touch present (expected in 2 to 3 days)

▌*Long Term*

Absence of neurovascular dysfunction in presence of cast, as evidenced by optimal color, temperature, sensation, and peripheral pulses until cast is removed and fracture is healed (expected for period of cast application[s])

NURSING INTERVENTIONS/INSTRUCTIONS

1. Assess skin at cast edges and on digits for color, presence of pain or numbness, peripheral pulses and capillary refill, and warmth or coolness; instruct client to assess and report any changes to physician (first visit).
2. Instruct client in monitoring neurovascular status of casted part by noting swelling; taking peripheral pulses bilaterally and comparing them; placing pressure on digits to note capillary refill when pressure is released; and noting color of skin, which may be pink, red, pallid, or cyanotic, and temperature of skin, which may be cool or warm to touch. Inform client of frequency (possibly twice daily) of assessment (first visit).
3. Position casted part for comfort, usually elevated; instruct client to avoid trauma or pressure to casted areas to prevent injury (each visit).

CLIENT AND FAMILY/CAREGIVER INTERVENTIONS

1. Client assesses neurovascular status of casted area at least once a day.
2. Client provides positioning and comfort to casted area.
3. Client reports signs and symptoms of neurovascular complications of fracture and/or cast application.

NURSING DIAGNOSIS · DEFICIENT KNOWLEDGE

▌*Related Factors:* Lack of information

▌*Defining Characteristics:* Request for information about cast care and safety precautions to prevent falls or complications

OUTCOMES

█ *Short Term*

Adequate knowledge, as evidenced by client's statement of measures to care for cast and to prevent complications of cast application (expected in 1 week)

█ *Long Term*

Optimal knowledge, as evidenced by client's meeting requirements of modified lifestyle resulting from fracture and casted part to achieve optimal health and functioning as healing is completed (expected in 4 to 6 weeks or until cast is removed)

NURSING INTERVENTIONS/INSTRUCTIONS

1. Assess client's lifestyle, ability to adapt to change and temporary disability, learning ability and interest, and family participation and support (first visit).
2. Inform client of cause and type of fracture and type and function of cast (first visit).
3. Instruct client to handle wet cast with palms of hands for at least 24 hours until cast is completely dry; use fan to dry cast by placing fan 18 to 24 inches from the cast; expose all parts to air for drying, and avoid covering cast until dry (first visit).
4. Instruct client to wear comfortable, loose clothing to fit over cast (first visit).
5. Instruct client to maintain skin integrity (clean, dry, and free of irritants) and to assess for complications to report, including foul, musty odor from cast; evidence of staining that comes from wound under cast; elevated temperature; pallor or cyanotic color and cool skin; decreased peripheral pulse; change in sensation or feeling; and increasing pain (first visit).
6. Instruct client to decrease itching by using alcohol swabs or blowing cool air into cast with fan and to avoid use of powders or lotion under cast (first visit).
7. Instruct client to petal cast edges with soft tape or to pad edges to prevent irritation of skin (first visit).
8. Instruct client to cover cast with a plastic bag while bathing or taking a shower (first visit).
9. Instruct client to clean cast with a damp cloth if soiled (first visit).

10. Instruct client to protect cast from damage or breakage by avoiding weight bearing or activities until cast is completely dry (first visit).

11. If medications are prescribed, instruct client in administration, including dose, frequency, time, side effects, and food and drug interactions (first visit).

CLIENT AND FAMILY/CAREGIVER INTERVENTIONS

1. Client assesses for and reports signs and symptoms of complications of fracture and cast application, including circulatory, neurologic, or skin symptoms or presence of infectious process.

2. Client states purpose and importance of cast and immobilization of body part.

3. Client maintains dry, intact cast and cleans it with damp cloth or shoe polish.

4. Client protects skin at edges of cast with petaling.

5. Client avoids inserting anything into cast or allowing cast to get wet.

6. Client administers medications correctly and safely.

7. Client secures rental or purchase of equipment and supplies.

✳ *Laminectomy and Spinal Fusion, Lumbar or Cervical*

A laminectomy is the surgical removal of the posterior arch of a vertebra to treat a herniated nucleus pulposus, tumor, or bone fragment that creates pressure on the spinal nerve roots and causes chronic pain. The procedure is usually performed on a cervical or lumbar vertebra. The fusion of bone fragments from the iliac crest may be performed to provide stability for the spine if degenerative disease is present.

Home care is primarily concerned with the teaching aspects of postoperative care to promote healing and function, prevent complications, and achieve successful outcome of the surgery.

Primary Diagnoses:
Lumbar Stenosis—ICD code: 724.02
Spinal Stenosis—ICD code: 724.00

NURSING DIAGNOSIS **IMPAIRED PHYSICAL MOBILITY**

■ *Related Factors:* Pain and discomfort; neuromuscular and musculoskeletal impairment

■ *Defining Characteristics:* Reluctance to attempt movement of legs or arms; limited ROM; decreased muscle strength and control; difficulty in performing ADL

OUTCOMES

■ *Short Term*
Adequate activity and mobility within prescribed limits, as evidenced by progressive ambulation within imposed limitations and movement within proposed restrictions (expected in 3 days)

■ *Long Term*
Return to optimal physical mobility and self-care activities within restrictions to maintain health and functioning without complications (expected in 2 to 3 weeks)

NURSING INTERVENTIONS/INSTRUCTIONS

1. Assess ability to participate in ADL, body alignment, ambulation limitations, and knowledge of prescribed restrictions (see Musculoskeletal System Assessment, p. 31, for guidelines) (first visit and as needed).
2. Instruct client to apply brace and collar before ambulation to stabilize surgical site (first visit).
3. Instruct client in logrolling, ambulating, sitting, bending, and stooping using proper body mechanics (first visit; reinforce on second visit).
4. Instruct client to sit in straight-backed chair and seat for driving and to splint back when sitting or rising from chair (first visit).
5. Instruct client in ROM and other exercises as permitted (first visit; reinforce on second visit).
6. Advise client to sleep on firm mattress with hips and knees flexed or in proper body alignment (first visit).

7. Instruct client in use of assistive aids for ADL within recommended restrictions (each visit).
8. Initiate referral to physical therapist (first visit).
9. Refer to HHA to assist with ADL as needed (first visit).

CLIENT AND FAMILY/CAREGIVER INTERVENTIONS

1. Client performs progressive ambulation, ADL, and other activities allowed, using proper body mechanics.
2. Client participates in exercise regimen as instructed.
3. Client correctly applies cervical collar, corset, and brace and wears as prescribed.
4. Client limits or avoids sexual activity, driving, and lifting as instructed.
5. Client takes rest periods as needed and stops activity if weak or tired or if painful response occurs.
6. Client changes mattress if necessary and uses aids in turning in bed or getting up.
7. Client participates in physical therapy program.
8. Client resumes work on a part-time basis or considers the need for a change in occupation.

NURSING DIAGNOSIS DEFICIENT KNOWLEDGE

▌*Related Factors:* Lack of information about postoperative care

▌*Defining Characteristics:* Request for information about postoperative activity restrictions, wound care, urinary and bowel elimination, and medication regimen

OUTCOMES

▌Short Term
Adequate knowledge, as evidenced by client's statement of postoperative care requirements and performance of postoperative procedures (expected in 1 week)

▌Long Term
Optimal knowledge, as evidenced by compliance with postoperative medical regimen and meeting requirements to return to optimal health and functioning (expected in 4 to 6 weeks)

NURSING INTERVENTIONS/INSTRUCTIONS

1. Assess lifestyle, ability to adapt, learning ability and interest, and family participation and support (first visit).
2. Inform client of cause of vertebral abnormality and surgical procedure performed to correct it (first visit).
3. Instruct client in administration of analgesics and muscle relaxants as ordered, including times, dose, frequency, side effects, and food and drug interactions (first and second visits).
4. Instruct client in wound care, including dressing change using sterile technique, and to report pain, redness, or swelling at site; allow for return demonstration of dressing change (first and second visits).
5. Instruct client to report leg or arm pain, numbness, or weakness (first visit).
6. Inform client of bowel and bladder elimination changes and their causes and of use of stool softener, fluid intake, and exercises to assist in return to normal pattern (first visit).
7. Inform client of importance of compliance with proposed activity and exercise regimen and of avoiding activities that place stress on operative area (e.g., changing position, lifting, pushing, pulling, or stooping) (first visit).
8. Instruct client in padding brace, cast, neck collar, or any other device to protect skin from rough edges or excessive tightness; check skin for changes caused by pressure when removing device (first visit).
9. Instruct client to comply with follow-up appointments with physician (first visit).

CLIENT AND FAMILY/CAREGIVER INTERVENTIONS

1. Client correctly administers medications as prescribed.
2. Client provides care to surgical site as needed, using sterile technique.
3. Client assesses skin under collar, brace, or other immobilizing device and provides skin care to prevent irritation and breakdown.
4. Client participates in prescribed activities safely and within restrictions imposed by surgery.
5. Client establishes and maintains bowel and urinary elimination pattern.
6. Client reports adverse effects of medications, treatments, and surgical intervention if appropriate.

❊ *Osteomyelitis*

Osteomyelitis is an infection of the bone, which may be acute or chronic. It may occur as a result of surgery or compound fractures, in which case the infectious agent is introduced directly into the bone, or the bloodstream may carry an infectious agent to the bone from infected soft tissue or joints. The infection may spread through the marrow, cortex, and periosteum. Causative agents include *Staphylococcus aureus* (most common), group A streptococcus, *Escherichia coli,* and *Pseudomonas* and *Klebsiella* organisms.

Home care is primarily concerned with treating symptoms and with teaching of the medication regimen and prevention of secondary infection or transmission of infection to others.

Primary Diagnoses:
Osteomyelitis, Acute or Subacute—ICD code: 730.00
Osteomyelitis, Chronic—ICD code: 730.10

NURSING DIAGNOSIS ACUTE PAIN

▐ *Related Factors:* Biologic injuring agents (infection)

▐ *Defining Characteristics:* Communication of pain descriptors; guarded or protective behavior toward painful part

OUTCOMES

▐ *Short Term*
Pain minimized or controlled, as evidenced by client's statement that pain is relieved by initiation of measures to prevent discomfort; relaxed posture and expressions (expected in 3 days)

▐ *Long Term*
Absence of pain and achievement of optimal functioning without pain (expected in 2 weeks)

NURSING INTERVENTIONS/INSTRUCTIONS

1. Assess and instruct client to assess pain and characteristics and precipitating and alleviating factors, with an emphasis on early recognition of onset (first visit).
2. Assess pain for type, location over long bones with redness and edema, sudden onset, intensity, and duration (first visit).
3. Instruct client in administration of analgesics and antibiotics as ordered to control pain and to reduce infectious process causing pain (first visit; reinforce on second visit).
4. Immobilize part with pillows and splints to prevent increased pain, and instruct client in need for bed rest and in methods to immobilize limb (first visit).
5. Instruct client to prevent pressure or further injury to limb by using a bed cradle and supporting limb and handling gently when moving in bed (first visit).
6. Maintain body alignment and correct positioning of limb (each visit).

CLIENT AND FAMILY/CAREGIVER INTERVENTIONS

1. Client maintains bed rest and position of comfort.
2. Client administers analgesic and monitors response in controlling pain.
3. Client performs measures to prevent pain and injury to limb.
4. Client maintains immobilization of part during acute phase.

NURSING DIAGNOSIS IMPAIRED PHYSICAL MOBILITY

▮*Related Factors:* Pain and discomfort; intolerance to activity

▮*Defining Characteristics:* Limited ROM; imposed restrictions of movement by splint or traction; reluctance to attempt movement; decreased muscle strength

OUTCOMES

▮*Short Term*

Increasing tolerance to activity, as evidenced by increased endurance and participation in ADL within imposed restrictions (expected in 1 week)

▌*Long Term*

Optimal mobility, energy, endurance, and participation in activities, as evidenced by performance of ADL and progressive ambulation (expected in 1 month)

NURSING INTERVENTIONS/INSTRUCTIONS

1. Assess discomfort, weakness, muscle strength or atrophy, ROM in all joints, and presence of traction or splints (see Musculoskeletal System Assessment, p. 31, for guidelines) (first visit).
2. Perform ROM exercises within limitations set by physicians as healing allows, and instruct client to perform ROM and muscle exercises (first and second visits).
3. Progressively allow ambulation with use of assistive aids as needed when healing allows, and encourage client to comply daily as instructed while limiting activity (each visit).
4. Refer HHA to assist in ADL until healing allows self-care (first visit).

CLIENT AND FAMILY/CAREGIVER INTERVENTIONS

1. Client performs ROM exercises, ADL, and ambulation daily, with increases as endurance and healing allow.
2. Client performs ADL with assistance and eventual independence.
3. Client applies and uses splint for ambulation.
4. Client prevents muscle wasting and contractures by practicing exercise regimen.
5. Client plans activities around rest periods.
6. Client uses assistive aids or devices for ambulation if needed.

NURSING DIAGNOSIS RISK FOR INFECTION

▌*Related Factors:* Inadequate primary defenses (traumatized tissue)

▌*Defining Characteristics:* Altered bone integrity with fracture or risk of fracture; spread of infectious agent; redness, swelling, drainage at entry site of catheter used for medication administration (right atrium); septicemia; meningitis

OUTCOMES

▌*Short Term*

Prevention of infection spread, as evidenced by normal range of temperature and vital signs and by absence of purulent drainage (expected in 1 week)

▌*Long Term*

Maintenance of infection-free state, as evidenced by the absence of septicemia, meningitis, or pathologic fracture (expected in 1 to 2 months)

NURSING INTERVENTIONS/INSTRUCTIONS

1. Assess temperature for elevation; note amount and characteristics of drainage if present (each visit).
2. Instruct client to avoid heat application to the area or exercises that would increase circulation to the part and stimulate the spread of infection (first visit).
3. Instruct client in administration of antiinfective medication, including dose, frequency, method, route, food and drug interactions, and side effects, for oral administration and topical administration via dressing if applicable (first visit).
4. Instruct client in sterile dressing change (dry, wet) and in disposal of soiled dressings using standard precautions; allow for return demonstration (first visit).
5. Instruct client to avoid exposure to persons with infections or illnesses that might be transmitted to client (first visit).

CLIENT AND FAMILY/CAREGIVER INTERVENTIONS

1. Client administers antiinfective medication for 6 to 8 weeks as prescribed.
2. Client performs handwashing and sterile dressing changes.
3. Client takes temperature daily and reports to physician if chilled or if drainage becomes purulent.
4. Client provides light clothing and linens in a comfortable, cool environment.
5. Client avoids exposure to persons with infections; prevents transmission of pathogens to client.
6. Client uses proper precautions in disposal of contaminated articles and supplies.

NURSING DIAGNOSIS | DEFICIENT KNOWLEDGE

▌*Related Factors:* Lack of information about treatment measures

▌*Defining Characteristics:* Request for information about medication regimen, nutrition, fluids, and activity requirements

OUTCOMES

▌*Short Term*
Adequate knowledge, as evidenced by client's statement of medical regimen requirements and adaptive lifestyle behaviors necessary to achieve optimal health (expected in 1 week)

▌*Long Term*
Functional knowledge, as evidenced by compliance with medical regimen and meeting the requirements to achieve return to health and optimal functioning with absence of recurrent infection (expected in 1 to 2 months)

NURSING INTERVENTIONS/INSTRUCTIONS

1. Assess lifestyle; adapting abilities; learning interest, abilities, and readiness; and family participation and support (first visit).
2. Instruct client in high-protein and vitamin C diet inclusions to facilitate healing, and inform client of more-than-normal nutritional requirements; offer a list and sample menus that include preferences and meet the recommended standards for height and weight; and instruct client to weigh weekly on same scale, at same time, and with similar clothing (first visit and second visit if needed).
3. Instruct client in administration of antiinfective, analgesic, and antipyretic medications, following guidelines and a schedule that are mutually planned (first visit).
4. Inform client of activity restriction and rationale (first visit).
5. Instruct client in daily requirements of fluid intake, especially if temperature is elevated (first visit).
6. Instruct client in skin protection and care if splints or traction are used and prolonged rest and immobilization are advised; instruct client in massage of bony prominences and in position changes and to report any reddened areas (first and second visits).

7. Discuss effect of disease process on self-concept and body image when long-term care is necessary and possible deformity occurs; allow client to express feelings and explore coping strategies (first visit).

CLIENT AND FAMILY/CAREGIVER INTERVENTIONS

1. Client administers medications correctly and records any side effects.
2. Client complies with dietary and fluid requirements and increases protein and vitamin C intake.
3. Client adapts to long-term immobilization and restriction in activity.
4. Client maintains intact skin, with protection of pressure points.
5. Client displays optimistic attitude for a recovery without deformity.

❋ *Osteoporosis*

Osteoporosis is a condition characterized by reduced bone mass or density resulting from increased bone resorption. It is associated with liver or renal diseases, menopause, hyperthyroidism, hyperparathyroidism, and Cushing's syndrome. Reduced mobility and inadequate dietary calcium intake contribute to the disorder. Bone fracture and deformity are common results of long-term osteoporosis.

Home care is primarily concerned with the teaching of the medical regimen to prevent or control the progression of bone mass loss and subsequent fractures.

Primary Diagnosis:
Osteoporosis—ICD code: 733.00

NURSING DIAGNOSIS RISK FOR TRAUMA

▌*Related Factors:* Bone weakness from reduced bone mass

▌*Defining Characteristics:* Falls; spontaneous fractures

OUTCOMES

Short Term

Minimal risk for trauma, as evidenced by client's compliance with safety measures to prevent falls and with treatment regimen (expected in 4 to 7 days)

Long Term

Absence of bone fracture, as evidenced by intact skeletal system and achievement of mobility and ADL for optimal health and functioning (expected in 1 month and ongoing)

NURSING INTERVENTIONS/INSTRUCTIONS

1. Assess environment for safety hazards; assess client for weakness, past falls and fractures, and presence of back pain (first visit).
2. Instruct client to remove small rugs, objects that obstruct pathways, and water on floors; to install hand grips, holding bars, and antislip equipment; to have adequate lighting and sturdy chairs; and to use low bed or footstool (first visit).
3. Instruct client to use cane, walker, or other method of support (first visit).
4. Instruct client in activity needs, daily walking and exercises, and other activities to maintain bone density (first visit; reinforce on second visit).
5. Inform client of and recommend therapist for weight-bearing exercises (first visit).

CLIENT AND FAMILY/CAREGIVER INTERVENTIONS

1. Client performs daily exercise regimen, including recommended frequency and number of times for each exercise.
2. Client joins activity group for exercises if appropriate.
3. Client wears corset to prevent vertebral collapse.
4. Client maintains mobility and ADL without falls.
5. Client maintains a hazard-free environment to prevent trauma.
6. Client provides aids to maintain safe mobility and self-care.

NURSING DIAGNOSIS DEFICIENT KNOWLEDGE

Related Factors: Lack of information

Defining Characteristics: Request for information about causes, treatment, and measures to prevent condition

OUTCOMES

▌*Short Term*
Adequate knowledge, as evidenced by client's verbalization of cause, medication regimen, and complications of the disease (expected in 3 days)

▌*Long Term*
Optimal knowledge, as evidenced by client's compliance with requirements for health and functioning and prevention of complications (expected in 2 weeks and ongoing)

NURSING INTERVENTIONS/INSTRUCTIONS

1. Assess client's lifestyle, ability to adapt, learning abilities and interest in health maintenance, and family participation and support (first visit).
2. Assess client's history to determine underlying cause of condition, including diabetes mellitus, cirrhosis of liver, kidney disease, hyperthyroidism, or hyperparathyroidism (first visit).
3. Instruct client in cause of disease, effects of bone loss, and risk for deformity or pathologic fracture (first visit).
4. Instruct client in prescribed medication regimen, including estrogen therapy and calcium and vitamin D supplements, with action, dose, frequency, time, side effects, and food, drug, and alcohol interactions. Instruct client in administration of calcium injection if prescribed (first visit; reinforce on second visit).
5. Inform client of foods containing calcium and vitamin D to include in diet if supplements are not prescribed (first visit).
6. Inform client of importance of follow-up x-ray studies and bone density procedures if ordered (first visit).
7. Instruct client to report to physician bone pain or inability to move any part of the body (first visit).

CLIENT AND FAMILY/CAREGIVER INTERVENTIONS

1. Client verbalizes cause, treatment, and complications of the disease.
2. Client accurately administers prescribed medications as instructed.

3. Client includes foods high in calcium and vitamin D in dietary intake.
4. Client complies with requirement of 1000 mg/day of calcium and estrogen therapy if postmenopausal.
5. Client maintains appropriate follow-up appointments with physician and diagnostic laboratory.

✳ *Kidney Transplantation*

Kidney transplantation is the surgical placement of a donor kidney (from a cadaver or from a live donor) into a recipient with end-stage renal disease who has a matching tissue type. Recipients of kidney transplants require immunosuppression to prevent rejection. The advisability of transplantation is dictated by the client's age and health problems, the availability of a donor kidney, and the client's preference for the procedure rather than relying on dialysis. Graft rejection may be acute or chronic, with the least acute response resulting from the most adequately matched donor and recipient.

Home care is primarily concerned with teaching the client about immunosuppressive therapy and monitoring for signs and symptoms of rejection.

Primary Diagnosis:
Renal Failure, Chronic—ICD code: 585.00

NURSING DIAGNOSIS — ANXIETY

▍**Related Factors:** Threat to or change in health status

▍**Defining Characteristics:** Verbalization of fear of organ rejection and consequences; apprehension; uncertainty; focus on self

OUTCOMES

▍Short Term
Decreased anxiety, as evidenced by client's statement of increased interest in care, increased participation by client in care, and relaxed posture and facial expression (expected in 3 days)

▍Long Term
Optimal level of anxiety or control of anxiety, as evidenced by client's compliance with and acceptance of treatment and by positive treatment response (expected in 1 month)

NURSING INTERVENTIONS/INSTRUCTIONS

1. Assess client's mental and emotional status (see Psychosocial Assessment, p. 52, for guidelines) (first visit).
2. Provide an accepting environment and allow for expression of fears and concerns about organ rejection (each visit).
3. Provide continuing information about progression to wellness; explain that one or more rejection episodes may occur in several months of transplant but they do not mean that kidney will be lost (each visit).
4. Initiate referral to social services, counseling, and/or support group if indicated (last visit).

CLIENT AND FAMILY/CAREGIVER INTERVENTIONS

1. Client seeks information that will reduce anxiety.
2. Client develops coping strategies for possibility of rejection.
3. Client maintains manageable level of anxiety.
4. Client consults with social worker, counselor, or support group for control of anxiety.

NURSING DIAGNOSIS INTERRUPTED FAMILY PROCESSES

■ *Related Factors:* Situational crisis from transplant surgery

■ *Defining Characteristics:* Family system unable to meet needs of donor and recipient, both physical and emotional; inappropriate level and direction of energy; inability to accept or receive help; inability of family to adapt to situation

OUTCOMES

■ Short Term
Beginning progress toward family's acceptance of and adaptation to organ transplant, as evidenced by open communication, mutual support, and participation in care (expected in 1 week)

■ Long Term
Return of family to former positive interactions and support as client returns to wellness (expected in 1 to 2 months)

NURSING INTERVENTIONS/INSTRUCTIONS

1. Assess family interaction, dynamics, and supportive behaviors (see Family Assessment, p. 59 for guidelines) (first visit).
2. Include family members in teaching in a nonjudgmental environment; allow family members to ask questions (each visit).
3. Encourage openness among family members; inform them of importance of maintaining own health and social activities (first visit).
4. Suggest family counseling, social services or support groups, rehabilitative services, or financial resources as needed (first visit).

CLIENT AND FAMILY/CAREGIVER INTERVENTIONS

1. Family verbalizes feelings and concerns.
2. Family identifies problems in family and ways to solve them together.
3. Family resolves lifestyle changes together.
4. Family seeks out and participates in support group activity.
5. Family participates in rehabilitation.
6. Client participates in family activities and contributes to family cohesiveness.

NURSING DIAGNOSIS DEFICIENT KNOWLEDGE

■ **Related Factors:** Lack of exposure to information about medical regimen

■ **Defining Characteristics:** Request for information about immunosuppressive therapy, signs and symptoms of rejection to report, and health-promotion behaviors

OUTCOMES

■ **Short Term**
Adequate knowledge, as evidenced by client's statement of treatment protocols, compliance with intensive medication regimen, and active participation in preventive health care (expected in 7 to 10 days)

▌*Long Term*

Optimal knowledge, as evidenced by client's meeting requirements for changed lifestyle and achievement of optimal level of health and functioning (expected in 4 to 6 weeks)

NURSING INTERVENTIONS/INSTRUCTIONS

1. Instruct client in progressive resumption of activity; emphasize avoidance of contact sports or any activity that might be traumatic to operative site (first visit).

2. Assess operative area for size, color, temperature, approximation of edges, and presence of drainage, and instruct client to notify physician of any changes in site (first visit).

3. Instruct client in administration of immunosuppressive agents and steroids, including dose, frequency, multiple side effects, and possible interactions with over-the-counter (OTC) drugs, foods, and alcohol (first visit).

4. Assess client for side effects of drug therapy, including gastrointestinal irritation and bleeding, hepatotoxicity, cushingoid body changes, decreased wound healing, visual changes, and personality changes (each visit).

5. Instruct client in monitoring of weight, intake and output, and vital signs; demonstrate and have client return demonstration; instruct client to keep log on results (first visit; reinforce on second visit).

6. Inform client of possible signs and symptoms of organ rejection, including flulike symptoms, urination difficultly, oliguria, weight gain, edema, increased blood pressure, and pain or tenderness over operative site; instruct client to report any of these signs to physician (first visit; reinforce each visit).

7. Instruct client to avoid active, live virus immunizations and children who have recently been immunized (e.g., oral polio vaccination) (first visit).

8. Instruct client in proper collection of random, midstream, or 24-hour urine specimens (whichever is ordered), and stress importance of delivery to laboratory (first visit).

9. Inform client of importance of keeping physician appointments and laboratory testing for complete blood count, drug levels, electrolytes, renal function tests, urinalysis, and culture and sensitivities (first visit).

10. Instruct client to wear or carry identification and medical information, including surgery and date, medications, and physician's name and telephone number (first visit).
11. Initiate referral to nutritionist, dentist, and specialist physician as appropriate (first visit).

CLIENT AND FAMILY/CAREGIVER INTERVENTIONS

1. Client resumes activities within limitations and avoids trauma to site.
2. Client correctly and consistently administers prescribed medications and monitors for side effects to report.
3. Client monitors and records daily or weekly weight, vital signs, and intake and output.
4. Client lists signs and symptoms of graft rejection and reports to physician if they occur.
5. Client engages in multisystem regimen to avoid infection and reports any signs and symptoms of renal/urinary or respiratory tract infection.
6. Client maintains clean wound with progressive healing stages.
7. Client maintains appointments with physicians and laboratory.
8. Client wears identifying medical information at all times.
9. Client consults with health professionals for regular health maintenance and advice.

✳ *Prostatic Hypertrophy and Prostatectomy*

Benign prostatic hypertrophy is the enlargement of the prostate gland, which is thought to be caused by an imbalance between the male and female sex hormones that occurs in men older than 50 years. The condition results in partial or complete obstruction of the urethra or incomplete emptying of the bladder. Prostatectomy, the partial or complete surgical removal of the prostate gland, can be performed to relieve obstruction caused by compression on the urethra (i.e., suprapubic or transurethral) or to remove a malignant mass (i.e., perineal or retropubic). The surgical approach depends on age, size and location of the obstruction or mass, and severity of symptoms.

Home care is primarily concerned with the maintenance of urinary elimination before and after surgery, wound care after surgery, and the teaching of medical or surgical regimens and prevention of complications as applicable.

Primary Diagnoses:
Prostate Cancer—ICD code: 185.00
Benign Prostatic Hypertrophy—ICD code: 600.0
Urinary Retention—ICD code: 788.20

NURSING DIAGNOSIS URINARY RETENTION

Related Factors: Blockage

Defining Characteristics: Bladder distension; frequent voiding of small amounts; absence of urinary output; dribbling; dysuria; residual urine; overflow incontinence; pain with bladder fullness and overdistension; small urinary stream; hesitancy in urinating

OUTCOMES

Short Term
Distress associated with urination minimized, as evidenced by client's statement of relief of retention with use of palliative measures (evidenced in 2 days)

Long Term
Urinary bladder distension and symptoms controlled, with optimal urinary elimination (expected in 1 to 2 weeks and ongoing)

NURSING INTERVENTIONS/INSTRUCTIONS

1. Assess renal/urinary and reproductive systems (see Renal/Urinary System Assessment, p. 35, and Reproductive System Assessment, p. 42, for guidelines), and note decreased size and force of urinary stream, difficulty in starting to urinate, urgency, frequency, dribbling, nocturia, hematuria, inability to completely empty bladder, and presence of overflow incontinence (first visit).

2. Assess for suprapubic distension by palpation and for possible complete retention with anuria and suprapubic pain (each visit).

3. Instruct client to note times and amounts of urinary elimination and to compare with times and amounts of fluid intake (first visit).

4. Instruct client to maintain hydration with intake of 8 to 10 glasses of water per day and to avoid alcoholic and caffeine-containing beverages (first visit).

5. Instruct client to notify physician if he or she is unable to void or if signs and symptoms of urinary elimination problems escalate (first visit).

6. Instruct client to avoid straining at bowel elimination; instruct client in administration of stool softener if needed (each visit).

7. Instruct client to take warm sitz baths to facilitate voiding and decrease distress (first visit).

8. Instruct client to empty bladder every 2 to 3 hours and not to delay voiding when urge is present (first visit).

9. Instruct client in administration of urinary antispasmodic and urinary analgesic medications as ordered, including dose; frequency; side effects; and food, drug and alcohol interactions (first visit).

10. Catheterize client using aseptic technique when ordered or when voiding has been absent for 6 to 8 hours (any visit).

CLIENT AND FAMILY/CAREGIVER INTERVENTIONS

1. Client keeps a record of changes in urinary elimination patterns and signs and symptoms of distress.

2. Client notifies physician of failure of relief measures to control signs and symptoms.

3. Client avoids constipation and straining by administration of stool softener.

4. Client maintains fluid intake of 2 to 3 L/day; avoids fluids that increase diuresis.

5. Client empties bladder at designated times and when urge is present.

6. Client takes medications prescribed for specific complaints.

NURSING DIAGNOSIS RISK FOR INFECTION

▮ *Related Factors:* Inadequate primary defenses (e.g., stasis of urine, broken skin)

▮ *Defining Characteristics:* Invasive procedure (e.g., surgery or catheterization); surgical wound with redness, edema, pain, purulent drainage; urinary retention; wound or urine culture positive for infectious organism; cloudy, foul-smelling urine

OUTCOMES

▮ *Short Term*

Absence of infection, as evidenced by decreased urinary retention and by proper care of surgical site (expected in 3 to 4 days)

▮ *Long Term*

Absence of infection, as evidenced by temperature and white blood count in normal ranges, surgical site clean and healing, clear urine, and urination without symptoms (expected in 4 to 6 weeks)

NURSING INTERVENTIONS/INSTRUCTIONS

1. Assess temperature, pulse and respiratory rates, and blood pressure, and instruct client to report chills and fever higher than 100° F to physician (each visit).
2. Assess incisional drains and operative wounds as applicable for pain, color, temperature, swelling, drainage, and approximation of edges (each visit).
3. Perform sterile wound care and catheter or meatal care (each visit).
4. Instruct client in care of catheter, placement and emptying of drainage bag, and use of leg bag (first visit).
5. Instruct client to inform physician of changes in urine characteristics, including cloudiness and foul odor (first visit).
6. Monitor for hematuria, and assess client's ability to empty bladder after catheter is removed (each visit).
7. Instruct client to administer antibiotic and urinary antiseptic medications as ordered for treatment or prophylaxis (first visit).

CLIENT AND FAMILY/CAREGIVER INTERVENTIONS

1. Client monitors vital signs and temperature and reports changes.

2. Client reports changes in urine characteristics, hematuria, or changes in appearance of wound.
3. Client maintains closed drainage system for indwelling catheter.
4. Client performs wound and catheter care using sterile technique.
5. Client maintains adequate hydration.
6. Client administers antibiotic agents for full course and other medications for urinary bladder treatment.

NURSING DIAGNOSIS SEXUAL DYSFUNCTION

Related Factors: Altered body function

Defining Characteristics: Impotence; decreased libido; erectile dysfunction following surgery; sterility

OUTCOMES

Short Term
Temporary dysfunction progressing to normal function, as evidenced by client's statement of understanding of surgical outcome and changes that can be expected in sexual functioning (expected in 1 week)

Long Term
Optimal sexual functioning within physiologic limitations resulting from surgical procedure (expected in 1 month)

NURSING INTERVENTIONS/INSTRUCTIONS

1. Provide a nonjudgmental, nonthreatening environment for client to have time and opportunity to ask questions or discuss sexual function according to comfort level (each visit).
2. Inform client of sexual implications of surgery and possibility of sterility or impotence (first visit).
3. Inform client of change in urine clarity after intercourse if transurethral procedure is performed (first visit).
4. Inform client that sexual intercourse may resume 6 to 8 weeks after surgery, and provide information about alternative methods of gratification for partner (first visit).

5. Inform client about possible aids available to assist with penile erection if applicable (first visit).
6. Initiate referral for sexual counseling if indicated or requested (any visit).

CLIENT AND FAMILY/CAREGIVER INTERVENTIONS

1. Client expresses feelings and concerns about sexuality for resolution.
2. Client communicates needs and abilities to perform sexual intercourse and response of partner.
3. Client consults sex therapist with or without partner.
4. Client explores use of aids for impotence.

NURSING DIAGNOSIS ANXIETY

▌**Related Factors:** Threat to health status; threat to change in role functioning

▌**Defining Characteristics:** Urinary incontinence; blood in urine; change in role and relationships; altered body image if dribbling or incontinence is chronic or with use of retention catheter; urgency and inability to reach bathroom in time

OUTCOMES

▌Short Term
Decreased and manageable anxiety level, as evidenced by client's statements of knowledge of postoperative course and improved bladder control (expected in 3 days)

▌Long Term
Anxiety controlled, as evidenced by maintenance of improved urinary elimination pattern and by improved body image (expected in 1 month)

NURSING INTERVENTIONS/INSTRUCTIONS

1. Assess client's coping abilities and ability to adapt to changes in health status; assist in identification and use of positive and effective coping mechanisms and problem-solving skills (each visit).

2. Instruct client to avoid heavy lifting, carrying heavy objects, or prolonged sitting or driving for 3 to 6 weeks (first visit).
3. Inform client that some blood may remain in urine for several weeks (first visit).
4. Instruct client to become acquainted with locations of bathrooms when away from home and to refrain from fluid intake before going out and at bedtime (first visit).
5. Inform client that postoperative dribbling and some incontinence are common and may be minimized by exercising; instruct client in perineal exercises (first visit).
6. Assist client in formulating an exercise schedule that is progressive in frequency and number of times (first visit).

CLIENT AND FAMILY/CAREGIVER INTERVENTIONS

1. Client uses positive coping strategies that reduce anxiety and improve body image.
2. Client avoids postoperative activities that cause complications.
3. Client verbalizes normal postoperative course and expectations.
4. Client performs perineal exercises daily to strengthen sphincter tone.
5. Client reduces embarrassment of dribbling and incontinence by limiting fluids and wearing waterproof undergarment.
6. Client uses bathroom as frequently as needed, at least every 2 hours.

�֍ *Renal Failure, Chronic*

Chronic renal failure (CRF) is the progressive, gradual deterioration of kidney function, resulting in decreased glomerular filtration rate, renal blood flow, resorption ability, and function of the tubules. The condition is irreversible as it progresses toward uremia but may be controlled by dietary and fluid restrictions. As the kidneys lose the ability to maintain fluid and electrolyte balance, the client is provided with renal dialysis. Diseases that predispose a person to the development of CRF are immunologic (e.g., glomerulonephritis), infectious (e.g., pyelonephritis and tuberculosis), urinary obstructive (e.g., prostatic hypertrophy and renal calculi), metabolic (e.g., diabetes mellitus), congenital (e.g., poly-cystic disease), vascular (e.g., hypertension), or nephrotoxic (i.e., from drugs). All organs of the body are affected by CRF.

Home care is primarily concerned with providing for activities of daily living (ADL) as needed; administration of peritoneal dialysis if appropriate; and teaching the client about dietary and fluid restrictions, compliance with hemodialysis, and prevention of complications of the disease.

Primary Diagnosis:
Renal Failure, Chronic—ICD code: 585.0

NURSING DIAGNOSIS ANXIETY

■ *Related Factors:* Threat of death; threat to or change in health status

■ *Defining Characteristics:* Apprehension; uncertain outcome; increased helplessness and tension; possible future need for kidney dialysis or transplant; changes in lifestyle

OUTCOMES

■ Short Term
Decreased anxiety, as evidenced by client's statement of reduced fear and apprehension about change in health status and possible dialysis and transplant availability (expected in 3 days)

■ Long Term
Management or control of anxiety level, as evidenced by compliance with and acceptance of treatment regimen and change in lifestyle (expected in 1 to 2 months)

NURSING INTERVENTIONS/INSTRUCTIONS

1. Assess client's mental and emotional status regarding life-threatening illness (see Psychosocial Assessment, p. 52, for guidelines) (first visit).
2. Encourage expressions of fears, concerns, and questions regarding therapy and its effects in an accepting environment (each visit).

3. Assist client in identifying needed changes in lifestyle and methods for making necessary changes (first visit; reinforce each visit).
4. Inform client of all activities, treatments, and tests and effects to expect (first visit).
5. Initiate referral to social services, counseling, or support group (any visit).

CLIENT AND FAMILY/CAREGIVER INTERVENTIONS

1. Client develops coping mechanisms for long-term treatment and possible outcome.
2. Client maintains manageable level of anxiety.
3. Client seeks information that will reduce anxiety.
4. Client expresses fears and concerns about necessary changes in lifestyle.
5. Client consults with social worker, counselor, clergy, or support group.

NURSING DIAGNOSIS EXCESS FLUID VOLUME

■ *Related Factors:* Compromised regulatory mechanism

■ *Defining Characteristics:* Edema; weight gain; decreased urinary output; electrolyte (e.g., potassium, sodium, calcium, magnesium, and phosphorus) imbalance; increased blood pressure and pulse rate; decreased specific gravity; increased blood urea nitrogen and creatinine

OUTCOMES

■ Short Term
Balanced intake and output, as evidenced by decreasing edema, compliance with fluid and electrolyte restrictions, and stable weight and blood pressure (expected in 1 week)

■ Long Term
Adequate renal function, as evidenced by optimal intake and output ratio and by maintenance of renal status within limitations imposed by disease (expected in 1 to 2 months)

NURSING INTERVENTIONS/INSTRUCTIONS

1. Assess client's renal status (see Renal/Urinary System Assessment, p. 35, for guidelines); evaluate baseline weight, hydration, peripheral edema, vital signs, output trends, and urine characteristics (each visit).
2. Instruct client in techniques for taking blood pressure and weight and for monitoring edema and intake and output, and allow for return demonstration (first visit).
3. Instruct client in formula for fluid restriction as prescribed, which is generally the previous day's urinary output plus 500 to 600 ml; include allotment and measurement of fluids, rationale for therapy, and how to distribute fluids over 24-hour period (first visit; reinforce on second and third visits).
4. Instruct client to restrict sodium intake by avoiding adding table salt and eating cold cuts; processed, canned, or convenience foods; and other foods high in sodium (first visit).
5. Instruct client to restrict potassium intake by avoiding citrus products, dried fruits, and bananas (first visit).
6. Instruct client to notify physician of increasing weight gain and edema, decreased urinary output, or increased blood pressure (first visit).
7. Instruct client and reinforce instruction in need for continual kidney dialysis, procedure for peritoneal dialysis in the home, and performance of procedure by client or family member if realistic and possible (first visit and ongoing).
8. Instruct client in administration of diuretic and antihypertensive agents, including dose, frequency, route, side effects, possible interferences with OTC drugs, and possible reactions with foods (first visit).

CLIENT AND FAMILY/CAREGIVER INTERVENTIONS

1. Client monitors and records blood pressure, weight, intake and output, and edema daily.
2. Client restricts fluid intake; uses ice chips; spreads limited fluids over 24-hour period; and measures fluids at mealtime, snack time, and medication time.
3. Client restricts foods containing large amounts of sodium or potassium.
4. Client administers medications correctly and as instructed.

5. Client reports signs and symptoms of increasing failure or increased sodium or potassium levels.
6. Client participates in hemodialysis or performs peritoneal dialysis as appropriate in home.

NURSING DIAGNOSIS	IMBALANCED NUTRITION: LESS THAN BODY REQUIREMENTS

■ *Related Factors:* Inability to ingest foods

■ *Defining Characteristics:* Anorexia; dietary protein restriction; nausea; vomiting; hiccups

OUTCOMES

■ *Short Term*
Adequate nutrition, as evidenced by absence of anorexia and by ingestion of protein-restricted diet (expected in 1 week)

■ *Long Term*
Optimal nutrition, as evidenced by compliance with special dietary restrictions throughout illness, including achievement of caloric, electrolyte, and protein requirements (expected in 1 month)

NURSING INTERVENTIONS/INSTRUCTIONS

1. Assess nutritional status and eating patterns, including food preferences and cultural and religious adaptations; note presence of anorexia, nausea, vomiting, stomatitis, bad taste in mouth, or tissue wasting (each visit).
2. Instruct client in protein-restricted diet if client is not on dialysis; emphasize proteins with high biologic value (each visit).
3. Instruct client in adequate foods to increase caloric intake, derived primarily from carbohydrates and unsaturated fats; integrate information about fluid and electrolyte requirements or restrictions into instruction (each visit).
4. Instruct client in administration of vitamin supplements, phosphorus-binding agents, and calcium supplements (first visit).
5. Instruct client in oral hygiene, especially after meals; encourage client to brush teeth and use mouthwash, hard candy, or sour candy for breath control (first visit).

6. Instruct client to eat smaller, more frequent meals and to take antiemetic agents 30 minutes before eating if nauseated (first visit).
7. Provide written instructions, sample menus, and recipes, and emphasize that compliance with dietary regimen will ease distressing symptoms of anorexia, nausea, vomiting, fatigue, and edema (each visit).
8. Initiate referral for dietary consultation as appropriate (first visit).

CLIENT AND FAMILY/CAREGIVER INTERVENTIONS

1. Client adjusts eating schedule to rest periods and to antiemetic administration.
2. Client frequently performs mouth care during day.
3. Client follows restrictions (e.g., protein, sodium, and/or potassium) in diet using planned menus.
4. Client eats smaller, more frequent meals.
5. Client administers vitamin and mineral supplements and other medications as instructed.
6. Client maintains ideal weight as closely as possible.
7. Client reads labels on foods and avoids foods containing large amounts of sodium or potassium; notes caloric value of purchased foods.

NURSING DIAGNOSIS RISK FOR IMPAIRED SKIN INTEGRITY

■ *Related Factors:* External factors of immobility; internal factors of urea deposits and peripheral neuropathy

■ *Defining Characteristics:* Pruritus; yellow pigmentation; scratching with breaks in skin; redness at pressure points; buildup of uremic frost on skin; dryness of skin; numbness in feet and legs

OUTCOMES

Short Term

Skin integrity intact, as evidenced by decreased pruritus and by compliance with skin care regimen (expected in 4 days)

▌*Long Term*

Skin integrity maintained, as evidenced by absence of skin disruption with skin in optimal condition (expected in 1 month and ongoing)

NURSING INTERVENTIONS/INSTRUCTIONS

1. Assess skin (see Integumentary System Assessment, p. 39, for guidelines) and note color, turgor, integrity, temperature, presence of scratch marks, and presence of uremic frost or pruritus (each visit).
2. Instruct client to bathe daily and to use superfatted soap and emollients if itching is present (first visit).
3. Instruct client to maintain short, clipped nails and to cut them straight across when trimming (first visit).
4. Instruct client to avoid scratching or rubbing skin (first visit).
5. Instruct client in perineal care after toileting (first visit).
6. Instruct client in use of oral and topical antipruritic agents (first visit).
7. Instruct client in handwashing technique (first visit).

CLIENT AND FAMILY/CAREGIVER INTERVENTIONS

1. Client bathes daily; uses lotion, moisturizer, or emollients; pats and avoids rubbing skin.
2. Client performs perineal care after toileting.
3. Client avoids scratching; maintains short, clean nails.
4. Client administers medications for pruritus as instructed.
5. Client reports skin breaks, rashes, or scratches to physician.

NURSING DIAGNOSIS RISK FOR ACTIVITY INTOLERANCE

▌*Related Factors:* Deconditioned status; generalized weakness

▌*Defining Characteristics:* Verbalization of fatigue and weakness; activity restrictions; inability to produce erythropoietin, causing anemia; defect in platelet function; faulty bone metabolism

OUTCOMES

▌*Short Term*

Adequate activity, as evidenced by participation in ADL within limitations (expected in 1 week)

▌*Long Term*

Mobility and self-care in ADL achieved for optimal level of functioning within limitations imposed by illness (expected in 1 month)

NURSING INTERVENTIONS/INSTRUCTIONS

1. Assess client's level of participation in ADL, endurance, muscle strength, gait, peripheral neuropathy, and fatigue with activity (first visit).
2. Encourage independence in ADL; instruct client to prioritize and pace activities, to use aids to conserve energy, and to schedule rest periods between activities (first visit).
3. Instruct client in measures to protect feet and legs from trauma (first visit).
4. Initiate referral to physical and/or occupational therapists if indicated (any visit).
5. Refer home health aide to assist with ADL when appropriate (first visit).

CLIENT AND FAMILY/CAREGIVER INTERVENTIONS

1. Client schedules rest periods and paces activities according to endurance and energy.
2. Client participates in ADL.
3. Client wears sturdy, well-fitting shoes and clean socks.
4. Client avoids injury caused by limited energy and fatigue.
5. Client equips environment with holding bars and aids for washing, dressing, grooming, toileting, and eating.

NURSING DIAGNOSIS ▌ DISTURBED THOUGHT PROCESSES

▌*Related Factors:* Physiologic changes

▌*Defining Characteristics:* Drowsiness; inability to concentrate; memory deficit; hallucinations; seizures; high level of nitrogenous wastes

OUTCOMES

▌*Short Term*

Minimal changes in thought processes, as evidenced by appropriate attitude, behavior, and communication (expected in 1 week)

▌*Long Term*

Thought processes maintained intact, as evidenced by optimal level of mental functioning within disease limitations (expected in 1 month and ongoing)

NURSING INTERVENTIONS/INSTRUCTIONS

1. Assess client's mental and orientation status, and compare findings with previous profiles (each visit).
2. Adapt communication style and instruction to client's needs and abilities (each visit).
3. Reinforce need for compliance with dietary restrictions and medication administration and dialysis to maintain thought processes (first visit; reinforce when needed).
4. Provide stimulating and diversional experiences, including reality-based experiences (each visit).

CLIENT AND FAMILY/CAREGIVER INTERVENTIONS

1. Client complies with medical regimen.
2. Client participates in reality-based activities, using aids to reinforce orientation.
3. Client complies with dialysis protocol.
4. Client uses aids to assist with remembering medication, dietary, and fluid schedules.

NURSING DIAGNOSIS COMPROMISED FAMILY COPING

▌*Related Factors:* Prolonged, progressive disease that exhausts supportive capacity of significant people

▌*Defining Characteristics:* Less-than-satisfactory supportive behaviors and results; client's expression of concerns about others' responses to client's health needs; family's expressed need for knowledge and understanding of client's needs

OUTCOMES

▌*Short Term*

Improved coping by family, as evidenced by family's acknowledgment of disabling effects of disease and required lifestyle changes and by family's cooperation and participation in treatment regimen (expected in 1 week)

■ *Long Term*

Optimal level of participation and support of family members to facilitate client's lifestyle and improvement in health status (expected in 1 to 2 months)

NURSING INTERVENTIONS/INSTRUCTIONS

1. Assess family interactions, coping abilities, and level of participation and support; strengths of individual members; and resources available and used by family (see Family Assessment, p. 59, for guidelines) (first visit).
2. Provide accurate information to family about treatment regimen and progress; allow time for questions and clarifications (each visit).
3. Encourage family to discuss strengths and options for change and to identify coping mechanisms used (each visit).
4. Include family members in teaching and planning of care (each visit).
5. Inform client of government and community agencies available for support and assistance (first visit).
6. Initiate referral for social services as indicated (any visit).
7. Encourage family to contact counselor and to arrange for hospice care if appropriate (any visit).

CLIENT AND FAMILY/CAREGIVER INTERVENTIONS

1. Family verbalizes concerns and feelings about burden of caring for family member with long-term disorder.
2. Family seeks assistance if needed.
3. Family participates in planning and implementing care.
4. Family adapts to client's limitations and integrates them into family activity.
5. Family supports dialysis program.
6. Family continues family activities and open communication.

NURSING DIAGNOSIS — ANTICIPATORY GRIEVING

■ *Related Factors:* Perceived potential loss of physiopsychosocial well-being

■ *Defining Characteristics:* Altered sleep and communication patterns; sorrow; expression of distress at potential loss

OUTCOMES

▌*Short Term*
Progress in grieving, as evidenced by verbalization, attitude, and behavior changes manifested by stage in process (expected in days)

▌*Long Term*
Grief process resolving, as evidenced by resumption of lifestyle with or without changes as needed and by integration of grieving stage into lifestyle and activities (expected in 2 to 3 months and ongoing)

NURSING INTERVENTIONS/INSTRUCTIONS

1. Assess degree and stage of grief; include suicide potential (each visit).
2. Inform client of stages of grief and that client's behavior is acceptable for specific stage and that resolution will be final stage (first visit).
3. Allow expression of feelings about disabilities and potential loss and implications for the future (each visit).
4. Provide open communication and accepting environment for interactions (each visit).
5. Initiate referral for psychologic or spiritual counseling (any visit).

CLIENT AND FAMILY/CAREGIVER INTERVENTIONS

1. Client progresses through grieving process to resolution.
2. Client seeks counseling as needed.

NURSING DIAGNOSIS DEFICIENT KNOWLEDGE

▌*Related Factors:* Lack of exposure to information about medical regimen

▌*Defining Characteristics:* Request for information about dialysis and about care of abdominal site or arteriovenous fistula site

OUTCOMES

▌*Short Term*

Adequate knowledge, as evidenced by compliance with medication regimen, identification of signs and symptoms to report, and demonstration of shunt care or care of abdominal site for dialysis (expected in 1 week)

▌*Long Term*

Functional knowledge, as evidenced by client's meeting requirements for a modified lifestyle without complications and maintaining optimal health and functioning within disease limitations (expected in 1 to 2 months)

NURSING INTERVENTIONS/INSTRUCTIONS

1. Instruct client in administration of prescribed drugs, including diuretic agents, exchange resins, sodium bicarbonate or citrate, antibiotic medications, and clofibrate; include dose, route, frequency, side effects, and fluid allotment (first visit).
2. Instruct client in measures for preventing constipation, including high-fiber diet and exercise (first visit).
3. Instruct client in measures to prevent infection, including handwashing, caring for catheter, avoiding persons with upper respiratory tract infections, and using sterile technique in shunt or peritoneal dialysis site care (first visit; reinforce on second visit).
4. Assess for cardiovascular changes (e.g., increased blood pressure, arrhythmias, and visual changes), respiratory changes (e.g., decreased breath sounds, crackles, wheezes, chest pain, dyspnea, fever, and restlessness), neurologic changes (e.g., lassitude, apathy, decreased mental acuity, paresthesias, muscle cramps, twitching, irritability, and confusion), and hematologic changes (e.g., fatigue, pallor, easy bruising, petechiae, purpura, and bleeding from any site) (each visit).
5. Assess for signs of hypocalcemia, including confusion, emotional lability, numbness, tingling or twitching of fingers or toes, Chvostek's sign or Trousseau's phenomenon, muscle weakness, and stupor (each visit).
6. Instruct client to notify physician if symptoms increase in severity or if any complications occur (first visit).

7. Instruct client in arteriovenous shunt or fistula care (first and second visits):
   - Avoid taking blood pressure or blood samples from affected arm.
   - Avoid carrying purse or heavy item over affected arm.
   - Avoid wearing tight clothing over affected arm.
   - Avoid tugging, pulling, or lying on affected arm.
8. Instruct client in dressing change at abdominal peritoneal site, and allow for return demonstration (first visit).
9. Instruct client to monitor patency of external shunt, including presence of bright-red blood and a thrill or bruit on auscultation over site (first visit).
10. Instruct client to monitor patency of internal fistula, including checking pulsations at site (first visit).
11. Inform client of importance of compliance with total care regimen and of incorporation of regimen into daily activities (each visit).
12. Instruct client to follow up with physician and laboratory visits as scheduled; inform client of importance of dialysis schedule (each visit).
13. Instruct client to wear or carry identification information at all times, including condition and physician's name and telephone number (first visit).

CLIENT AND FAMILY/CAREGIVER INTERVENTIONS

1. Client complies with medication regimen.
2. Client manages constipation with diet and medication.
3. Client uses measures to prevent infection and other complications.
4. Client reports deteriorating condition or presence of signs and symptoms of complications associated with dialysis access site.
5. Client maintains patency of access site; takes measures to avoid injury to site.
6. Client maintains dialysis, physician, and laboratory appointments.
7. Client wears identification information for emergency care.
8. Client complies with total medical regimen and integrates into lifestyle.

❇ *Urinary Tract Infection*

Infection of the lower urinary tract (i.e., cystitis) is caused by gram-positive or gram-negative organisms that gain access to the bladder via sexual intercourse, urethral trauma, poor personal hygiene, or an indwelling catheter or by stasis of urine as a result of obstructive conditions, neurogenic bladder, or kidney disease. The condition is more common in women because of the proximity of the urethra to the vagina and anus. Cystitis may become chronic because microorganisms become resistant to therapy. Chronic cystitis is particularly common in elderly people who have indwelling catheters for long periods.

Home care is primarily concerned with the teaching of medication regimens to prevent or control recurrent bladder infections and possible spread to the kidneys.

Primary Diagnosis:
Urinary Tract Infection—ICD code: 599.0

NURSING DIAGNOSIS ACUTE PAIN

▌*Related Factors:* Biologic injuring agents (e.g., bacterial infection)

▌*Defining Characteristics:* Communication of pain descriptors; urine culture positive for infectious organism; dysuria; cloudy, foul-smelling urine

OUTCOMES

▌*Short Term*
Minimal pain or decrease in pain, as evidenced by client's statement of compliance with urinary tract analgesic and antibiotic therapy (expected in 2 days)

▌*Long Term*
Absence of pain, as evidenced by completion of antibiotic regimen and increased comfort in lower abdomen and during urination (expected in 10 days)

NURSING INTERVENTIONS/INSTRUCTIONS

1. Assess client's pain, including site, duration, and intensity; aggravating and alleviating factors; and characteristics associated with voiding (each visit).
2. Instruct client in administration of systemic antibiotic, urinary antiseptic, or urinary tract analgesic medications, including dose; frequency; side effects; and food, drug, and alcohol interactions; inform client that phenazopyridine may turn urine orange, which may stain undergarments (first visit).
3. Instruct client in use of heating pad over suprapubic area or lower back region and in use of sitz bath (first visit).

CLIENT AND FAMILY/CAREGIVER INTERVENTIONS

1. Client administers medications as instructed and for proper length of time.
2. Client applies heat for symptomatic relief.

NURSING DIAGNOSIS IMPAIRED URINARY ELIMINATION

▮*Related Factors:* Mechanical trauma of bladder infection

▮*Defining Characteristics:* Dysuria; frequency; nocturia; urgency; urinary retention and stasis; small-volume, frequent voiding

OUTCOMES

▮*Short Term*
Minimal urinary alteration, as evidenced by resumption of normal micturition pattern (expected in 2 days)

▮*Long Term*
Urinary elimination pattern within baseline and free from any abnormal changes (expected in 2 weeks)

NURSING INTERVENTIONS/INSTRUCTIONS

1. Perform renal and reproductive assessment (see Renal/Urinary System Assessment, p. 35, and Reproductive System Assessment, p. 42, for guidelines); note temperature and assess for history of urinary tract infection or renal problems, or presence of sexually transmitted diseases (first visit).

2. Instruct client to monitor pattern and frequency of urine elimination and characteristics of urine and to note pain or burning on urination, urgency, hesitancy, and force of flow (each visit).
3. Encourage client to consume up to 3000 ml of fluid per day if allowed (first visit).
4. Instruct client in acid-ash diet, including meat, fish, poultry, eggs, cheese, corn, cereals, cranberries, plums, and prunes; instruct client to avoid intake of alcohol, caffeine, and pepper because they aggravate symptoms (first visit).

CLIENT AND FAMILY/CAREGIVER INTERVENTIONS

1. Client records all output and characteristics of urine, with symptoms if present.
2. Client drinks 8 to 10 glasses of water or juice per day at regular intervals.
3. Client includes or avoids specific foods that affect condition.

NURSING DIAGNOSIS DEFICIENT KNOWLEDGE

Related Factors: Lack of exposure to information about infection

Defining Characteristics: Request for information about medication administration and measures to prevent recurrence of infection

OUTCOMES

Short Term
Adequate knowledge, as evidenced by identification of and compliance with hygienic practices and medication regimen (expected in 3 days)

Long Term
Optimal knowledge, as evidenced by completion of medical regimen and hygienic measures to prevent recurrence (expected in 10 days)

NURSING INTERVENTIONS/INSTRUCTIONS

1. Instruct client in absolute necessity of taking full course of antibiotics even if symptoms disappear (first visit).

2. Instruct client in hygienic practices (first visit):

   - Wash with soap and water daily.
   - Void when urge is felt, do not delay; void every 2 hours if possible.
   - Wipe from front to back, if female.
   - Urinate after intercourse.

3. Instruct client to notify physician if symptoms persist or escalate or if flank pain or fever is present (first visit).
4. Suggest taking showers instead of tub baths (first visit).
5. Instruct female clients to avoid use of feminine sprays and to wear cotton undergarments (first visit).
6. Advise client to have follow-up urine cultures if symptoms recur (last visit).

CLIENT AND FAMILY/CAREGIVER INTERVENTIONS

1. Client follows hygienic preventive procedures.
2. Client administers all medications as prescribed.
3. Client maintains consistency in daily care; avoids allowing irritating substances to come into contact with genital area.
4. Client collects midstream urine specimen and takes to laboratory if symptoms escalate or recur.

INTEGUMENTARY SYSTEM

❋ *Burns*

Burns are injuries that destroy layers of the skin and, in some cases, underlying tissues. Burns are classified into two categories: (1) partial-thickness burns, which may be superficial (i.e., first degree) or deep (i.e., second degree), and which involve the dermis and epidermis, with potential for epithelial regeneration, and (2) full-thickness burns (i.e., third or fourth degree), which involve all skin layers, including nerve endings, muscles, tendons, and bones, with scarring and loss of function, and which require skin grafting. With full-thickness burns, all systems are affected: cardiovascular (e.g., impaired circulation and occluded blood supply), respiratory (e.g., edema and airway obstruction), renal (e.g., reduced blood flow to kidneys with ischemia), musculoskeletal (e.g., formation of scar tissue with contractures), neurologic (e.g., disorientation and withdrawal), gastrointestinal (e.g., stress ulcer), and endocrine (e.g., stress diabetes).

Home care is primarily concerned with the rehabilitation phase of burn care and includes teaching the client about the care and treatment of the healing wounds and supporting the client's compliance with the physical and occupational therapy regimen.

Primary Diagnosis:
Burns—ICD code: 949.0
Varies with degree, percentage, and location of burn

NURSING DIAGNOSIS ACUTE PAIN

■ *Related Factors:* Biologic injuring agents

■ *Defining Characteristics:* Verbalization of pain descriptors; pain during physical therapy

OUTCOMES

▍*Short Term*
Pain minimized, as evidenced by performance of therapy with reduced pain (expected in 1 week)

▍*Long Term*
Absence of pain, as evidenced by ultimate restoration of function and by increased comfort during therapy (expected in 3 months or depending on extent of treatment)

NURSING INTERVENTIONS/INSTRUCTIONS

1. Assess pain severity during exercises and effect of pain on therapy in achieving function (first visit).
2. Assess itching of healing areas (first visit).
3. Administer and instruct client to take analgesic agent before therapy (first visit and when needed).

CLIENT AND FAMILY/CAREGIVER INTERVENTIONS

1. Client administers analgesic medication correctly.
2. Family supports client in therapy regimen.

NURSING DIAGNOSIS	IMPAIRED SKIN INTEGRITY

▍*Related Factors:* External factor of burn

▍*Defining Characteristics:* Disruption of skin surface; destruction of skin layers; sensitivity of newly healed skin to slight pressure or trauma; itching and flaking during healing

OUTCOMES

▍*Short Term*
Preservation of skin integrity, as evidenced by healing, with newly formed skin and nerve regeneration (expected in 1 week and ongoing)

▍*Long Term*
Absence of skin impairment, as evidenced by gradual return of function and new skin development (expected in 2 to 3 months, depending on extent of injury)

NURSING INTERVENTIONS/INSTRUCTIONS

1. Assess skin and grafted area for sensitivity to cold, heat, or touch; itching that occurs with healing; flaking; and formation of blisters with slight trauma (each visit).
2. Instruct client to cleanse skin with nondeodorant soap and then apply topical antihistamine cream and palliative creams to itchy, dry, flaking skin on healed areas (first visit).
3. Instruct client to apply sunscreen and to avoid direct sunlight and restrictive clothing (first visit).
4. Inform client of healing process, including discoloration and development of scar tissue with contours (first visit).
5. Instruct client in application of Jobst® pressure garments* for maintaining gentle pressure on the healed burn area and to wear 24 hours a day for possibly as long as 1 year (first visit).
6. Inform client that healing will vary based on the burn depth and that mature healing and return of suppleness and normal coloring can take 6 to 12 months (first visit).
7. Instruct client in wound care and dressing changes using sterile technique (first and second visits).

CLIENT AND FAMILY/CAREGIVER INTERVENTIONS

1. Client protects healing skin from trauma and sensitivity reactions to cold, heat, sun, and excessive pressure or constriction.
2. Client applies topical medication to allay itching.
3. Client wears pressure garment continuously, as instructed.
4. Client performs dressing changes using sterile technique; notes and reports any drainage at wound edge or fluid under the graft.

NURSING DIAGNOSIS IMPAIRED PHYSICAL MOBILITY

▌***Related Factors:*** Pain and discomfort; musculoskeletal impairment; severe anxiety

▌***Defining Characteristics:*** Reluctance to attempt movement; limited range of motion (ROM); decreased muscle strength; muscle atrophy; contractures of major joints

---

*BSN-Jobst, Inc.; 5825 Carnegie Blvd.; Charlotte, NC 28209; (704) 554-9933

OUTCOMES

▌*Short Term*

Adequate mobility, as evidenced by minimal discomfort during therapy and reduced risk for contracture formation of skin and underlying tissues (expected in 1 week)

▌*Long Term*

Optimal mobility and activity performance, as evidenced by skin healing and maturity, with absence of contractures and client's acceptance of therapy as a part of daily living (expected in 2 to 3 months and ongoing)

NURSING INTERVENTIONS/INSTRUCTIONS

1. Assess client's ability for movement of all joints and muscles and ability to ambulate and perform activities of daily living (ADL) without assistance; note especially skin at neck area, axillae, antecubital spaces, fingers, groin, popliteal area, and ankles, as appropriate, for developing skin contractures and shortening of tendons and ligaments (each visit).
2. Perform and instruct client to perform active ROM exercises, muscle-stretching exercises, and ambulation progressively and concurrently with therapy (first visit; reinforce each visit).
3. Inform client of importance of continuous long-term therapy to achieve optimal function (first visit).
4. Initiate referral to physical and occupational therapists, and encourage client to comply with the therapy programs and to correlate with ADL and social and diversional activities (first and second visits).
5. Refer home health aide to assist with ADL as needed (first visit).

CLIENT AND FAMILY/CAREGIVER INTERVENTIONS

1. Client complies with daily rehabilitation program requirements and self-care activities, using assistive aids for eating, toileting, bathing, grooming, and dressing as needed.
2. Client performs joint and muscle exercises as instructed; takes analgesic before exercising.
3. Client notes and reports pain or resistance to exercising to therapist and possibly physician.

NURSING DIAGNOSIS DISTURBED BODY IMAGE

Related Factors: Biophysical factor of effect of burns

Defining Characteristics: Verbal and nonverbal response to change in body structure and function; negative feelings about body, scarring, deformity, disfigurement, discoloration, and contour of scarring; social isolation

OUTCOMES

Short Term
Improved adaptation to body image change, as evidenced by client's statement of feelings about changed appearance and limitations imposed by condition and need to change lifestyle until restoration of function is achieved (expected in 1 to 2 weeks)

Long Term
Optimal adaptation to body image change, as evidenced by client's statement of acceptance of appearance and by client's expression of ability to cope with life changes and to meet needs for optimal health and functioning (expected in 2 to 3 months)

NURSING INTERVENTIONS/INSTRUCTIONS

1. Assess client's lifestyle, roles, and ability to adapt to long-term rehabilitation and integrate it into treatment regimen (first visit).
2. Allow client to express feelings about appearance, loss of function, presence of any deformity or disfigurement, loss of control over life situations, and inability to meet role expectations (each visit).
3. Reassure client that feelings, anxiety, and expressions of concern are a normal part of adjustment to the changes in lifestyle that occur (first visit).
4. Encourage client to ask for help when needed; to identify strengths; and to suggest options for lifestyle changes, including ADL, social and occupational interactions, and recreation and leisure activities (any visit).
5. Assist client in identifying coping mechanisms that have a positive effect on adjustment to body image changes (any visit).

6. Emphasize the positive aspects of rehabilitation and adjustment and what is achieved instead of what is not (each visit).
7. Assist client in identifying clothing that will cover scarring or deformity as appropriate (first visit or as needed).
8. Initiate referral to counseling, occupational therapist, or social services as needed (any visit).
9. Refer client to social worker for long-term planning and counseling (any visit).

CLIENT AND FAMILY/CAREGIVER INTERVENTIONS

1. Client verbalizes concern and feelings about appearance.
2. Client allows grieving over change in body image.
3. Client adapts to lifestyle changes and frustrations of long-term treatment.
4. Client uses positive coping mechanisms with success.
5. Client adapts to change in appearance and limitations imposed by disability.
6. Client resumes close interpersonal relationships.
7. Client uses counseling and/or other services as needed.

NURSING DIAGNOSIS DEFICIENT KNOWLEDGE

■ *Related Factors:* Lack of information about long-term therapy

■ *Defining Characteristics:* Request for information about risk of complications, nutritional needs, and long-term health maintenance

OUTCOMES

■ Short Term
Adequate knowledge, as evidenced by client's statement of basic needs for health promotion (expected in 1 week)

■ Long Term
Functional knowledge, as evidenced by compliance with requirements to maintain optimal health and functioning (expected to be ongoing)

NURSING INTERVENTIONS/INSTRUCTIONS

1. Assess for daily basic needs based on progression toward wellness and past patterns (first visit).

2. Instruct client in need for scheduled rest periods, especially before or after physical therapy (first visit).
3. Instruct client in high-protein, high-calorie diet as appetite improves; refer client to dietitian if appropriate (first visit; reinforce on second visit).
4. Instruct client to assess for and report any redness, swelling, pain, or drainage at burn/healing site (first visit).
5. Inform client that cosmetic or reconstructive surgery may be needed if burn is extensive and tissue destruction is major; information should reinforce physician teaching (any visit).
6. Arrange visits from other burn victims for support if appropriate (any visit).

CLIENT AND FAMILY/CAREGIVER INTERVENTIONS

1. Client assesses and monitors wound for infection and reports to physician.
2. Client provides for suggested dietary inclusions and rest and sleep opportunities.
3. Client displays optimism during therapeutic regimen.
4. Client expresses need for and fulfills daily basic requirements for health maintenance.

❈ *Herpes Zoster*

Herpes zoster is an acute, viral central nervous system infection that involves the dorsal root ganglia; it is characterized by painful skin eruptions in areas supplied by peripheral sensory nerves that arise in the affected ganglia.

Home care is primarily concerned with the relief of pain and discomfort and with teaching the client about medication administration and treatment of prolonged neuralgia.

Primary Diagnosis:
Herpes Zoster—ICD code: 053.9

NURSING DIAGNOSIS ACUTE PAIN

▌ *Related Factors:* Biologic injuring agents

■*Defining Characteristics:* Communication of pain descriptors (severity, location, duration); guarding and protective behavior toward affected area(s); self-focusing; restlessness

OUTCOMES

■*Short Term*
Increased comfort, as evidenced by client's statement that pain is decreased or absent (expected in 2 to 3 days)

■*Long Term*
Absence of or minimal pain, with decreased incidence of recurrent episodes and achievement of optimal health and functioning without pain (1 to 2 months)

NURSING INTERVENTIONS/INSTRUCTIONS

1. Assess pain, burning, or neuralgia on side of trunk or other area; assess severity of pain before and during outbreak of vesicles (first visit).
2. Instruct client in administration of oral medications to reduce pain (analgesics), inflammation (steroids), and itching (antihistamines) (first visit).
3. Instruct client in application of topical medication to reduce itching and to promote healing and comfort (first visit).
4. Instruct client to take warm tub baths with Burow's solution and to avoid rubbing skin dry, extremes in temperature or pressure against painful area, and tight clothing around area (first visit).
5. Instruct client in diversional therapy, such as music, relaxation techniques, and guided imagery (each visit).
6. Instruct client to avoid lying on affected area (first visit).

CLIENT AND FAMILY/CAREGIVER INTERVENTIONS

1. Client administers medications correctly and effectively.
2. Client reports prolonged pain to physician.
3. Client maintains calm environment including diversion from pain.
4. Client avoids actions that cause or trigger pain, including rubbing, pressure, temperature extremes, and scratching.

NURSING DIAGNOSIS DEFICIENT KNOWLEDGE

Related Factors: Lack of information about disease

Defining Characteristics: Request for information about disease causes and treatments and prevention of complications

OUTCOMES

Short Term
Adequate knowledge, as evidenced by client's statement of causes, treatments, and prognosis for the disease (expected in 1 week)

Long Term
Optimal knowledge, as evidenced by client's meeting requirements to achieve optimal level of health by compliance with the treatment regimen (expected in 1 month)

NURSING INTERVENTIONS/INSTRUCTIONS

1. Assess client's lifestyle and ability to adapt, learning abilities and interests, readiness to learn, and family participation and support (first visit).
2. Inform client of cause, course, exacerbations, and unpredictability of the disease in clear, honest language (first visit).
3. Instruct client in care of lesions and to prevent infection by avoiding scratching, touching, picking, or squeezing lesions (first visit).
4. Instruct client in handwashing and precautions to take (e.g., skin and protective isolation) if needed (first visit and ongoing).
5. Inform client of rest requirements and that inadequate rest may lengthen course of illness; instruct client to schedule rest periods and to provide a stress-free, quiet environment (each visit).
6. Inform client of importance of nutrition and fluid requirements; instruct client to note and report weight loss (first visit).
7. Instruct client in antibiotic therapy to prevent or treat infection (first visit).

CLIENT AND FAMILY/CAREGIVER INTERVENTIONS

1. Client maintains measures to prevent infection and to meet fluid, nutrition, and rest requirements for healing lesions.
2. Client correctly complies with medication regimen.

3. Client provides restful, stress-free environment.
4. Client verbalizes cause of the disease, methods of transmission, and methods for control of disease manifestations and prevention of exacerbations or sequelae.
5. Client cares for lesions and takes steps to prevent infection.

❇ *Pressure Ulcers*

Pressure ulcers (e.g., bedsores) are caused by the breakdown of the epidermal and underlying structures as a result of excessive pressure or shearing forces. Areas usually affected are the bony prominences. The risk for pressure ulcers is increased in those who are immobilized or malnourished or who have altered sensation or circulation or fecal or urinary incontinence.

Home care is primarily concerned with the care and teaching aspects of pressure ulcer prevention and control and with the healing of existing ulcers.

Primary Diagnosis:
Pressure (Decubitus) Ulcer—ICD code: 707.0

NURSING DIAGNOSIS IMPAIRED SKIN INTEGRITY

❚ *Related Factors:* External factors of pressure, shearing; internal factors of nutrition, circulation, level of consciousness, sensation

❚ *Defining Characteristics:* Redness, warmth at pressure area; disruption of skin, with pain, swelling, heat, induration, drainage, and tissue necrosis, depending on stage of pressure ulcer

OUTCOMES

❚ *Short Term*
Reduction in skin impairment, as evidenced by absence of blanching, hyperemia, or disruption in skin over stress areas (expected in 2 weeks)

▌*Long Term*

Absence of skin impairment despite immobilization, negative nitrogen balance, incontinence, or impaired innervation or circulation (expected in 1 month and ongoing)

NURSING INTERVENTIONS/INSTRUCTIONS

1. Assess skin, creases, folds, and bony prominences, including color, temperature, tone, turgor, and integrity; note presence of edema, irritation, maceration, excoriation, induration, ulceration, drainage, or necrosis (each visit).
2. Locate and measure pressure ulcers, and document degree of breakdown (each visit).
3. Instruct client in hygienic measures, including personal and skin care, bathing and cleansing after toileting, and taking sponge bath in bed; instruct client to avoid massaging reddened skin areas (first visit).
4. Instruct client in positioning in bed or sitting (first visit).
5. Instruct client in ROM exercises and in use of prophylactic and palliative measures, including appropriate cushion devices that are custom-designed for the client; instruct client to avoid using donut-type devices (each visit).
6. Apply protective topical agent and dressing as prescribed; irrigate pressure ulcer with sterile saline and apply debriding agent as prescribed; instruct client in medication and dressing changes (each visit).
7. Instruct client to reduce pressure over bony prominences; if client is on bed rest, avoid pulling or sliding client in bed (each visit).

CLIENT AND FAMILY/CAREGIVER INTERVENTIONS

1. Client maintains clean, dry skin; bathes daily with mild soap; and rinses well and pats dry.
2. Client pads and protects heels, elbows, back of head, iliac crests, and sacrococcygeal area; client applies emollient to intact skin.
3. Client maintains clean bed that is free of wrinkles and crumbs.
4. Client uses footboard and bed cradle as appropriate.
5. Client positions self hourly using overhead bar if able.
6. Family or caregiver positions client every 2 hours, provides preventive skin care, performs ROM exercises, and performs wound care as ordered.

7. Client exposes pressure ulcer to air, light, and heat for pre-scribed intervals.
8. Caregiver avoids shearing forces when moving client; lifts and rolls instead of pulling or sliding.

NURSING DIAGNOSIS DEFICIENT KNOWLEDGE

Related Factors: Lack of information about care and prevention of pressure ulcer

Defining Characteristics: Request for information about cleansing, dressing, heat application, and preventive measures to avoid new pressure ulcer formation or further breakdown of existing ulcer

OUTCOMES

Short Term
Adequate knowledge, as evidenced by client's statement about causes of skin breakdown and about care to prevent or treat pressure ulcer (expected in 1 week)

Long Term
Optimal knowledge, as evidenced by client's compliance with medical regimen and meeting requirements for adaptation of ADL to achieve optimal health and skin integrity (expected in 1 month)

NURSING INTERVENTIONS/INSTRUCTIONS

1. Assess client's nutrition and neurologic status for obesity or thinness, state of consciousness, paralysis, incontinence, immo-bility, and use of sedatives or tranquilizers (each visit).
2. Assess client's weight weekly, and compare with actual and ideal weight (any visit).
3. Encourage and instruct client in high-calorie, high-protein diet with adequate fluid intake (2 L/day) as appropriate (first visit).
4. Institute bowel and bladder training program if indicated (each visit).
5. Instruct client in prescribed treatments for skin area, such as massage, padding, heat application, cleansing and dressing area, and position changes and in recommended frequency of treatments (first visit; reinforce on second visit).

6. Inform client of use and availability of support surfaces to relieve pressure on skin (first visit).

CLIENT AND FAMILY/CAREGIVER INTERVENTIONS

1. Client maintains hydration and eats well-balanced meals that include protein and vitamin C; takes supplements as needed.
2. Client avoids medications that affect awareness and consciousness.
3. Caregiver offers toileting opportunity every 2 to 3 hours while client is awake; provides measures to prevent urine or bowel incontinence or applies device to prevent exposure to the skin.
4. Client reports progressive skin breakdown that occurs despite preventive measures.
5. Client changes position and uses aids to reduce pressure on skin.

✳ *Psoriasis*

Psoriasis is a noninflammatory, chronic dermatologic condition in which many silvery, scaly appearing red papules and plaques appear at bony prominences. The condition may affect any part of the body, including hands, feet, ears, nails, back, buttocks, and scalp. Recurrence may result from local trauma, environmental factors, withdrawal from systemic corticosteroids, emotional stress, or infection.

Home care is primarily concerned with the teaching aspects of treatments, resulting in comfort and prevention of exacerbation of the condition.

Primary Diagnosis:
Psoriasis—ICD code: 696.1

NURSING DIAGNOSIS IMPAIRED SKIN INTEGRITY

Related Factors: Alterations in skin by dermatitis

Defining Characteristics: Scales and plaques over any part of body; possible itching or scratching; disruption of skin surfaces

OUTCOMES

▌*Short Term*

Minimal skin impairment from eruptions, as evidenced by client's compliance with prescribed skin care and reduction of symptoms (expected in 1 week)

▌*Long Term*

Absence of skin impairment, as evidenced by adaptive lifestyle changes to minimize recurrences, continued compliance with prescribed skin regimen, and intact and lesion-free integument (expected in 4 to 6 weeks)

NURSING INTERVENTIONS/INSTRUCTIONS

1. Assess skin for color, integrity, and presence of papules, plaques, or pustules; include location, extent, and distribution (see Integumentary System Assessment, p. 39, for guidelines) (each visit).
2. Relate skin manifestations to implications of prescribed drug use (each visit).
3. Instruct client in skin care and application of topical petrolatum-based emollients and combinations of topical corticosteroids, keratolytics, crude coal tar, or anthralin preparations as prescribed (first visit; reinforce on second visit).
4. Instruct client in scalp care, including loosening and removal of scales, use of tar shampoo, and application of topical steroids (first visit).
5. Instruct client in medication administration (first visit).
6. Apply and instruct client in application of occlusive wraps, avoiding exposure of eye or other areas sensitive to medications (first visit).
7. Inform client of methods to minimize staining of garments (first visit).
8. Administer and instruct client in alternative therapies, such as phototherapy alone or in conjunction with medication, photochemotherapy, and protection of sensitive areas (first visit).
9. Instruct client in practices regarding teratogenic drugs and effect of systemic antimetabolites or oral retinoids on hepatic, renal, and hematopoietic systems; monitor for toxicities (each visit).
10. Provide clear written instructions for all skin care and medication protocols (first visit; review on second visit).

CLIENT AND FAMILY/CAREGIVER INTERVENTIONS

1. Client takes tub baths instead of showers for 15 to 20 minutes daily and applies topical preparations to damp skin.
2. Client uses written protocol for scheduling time, type, and method of topical medication administration; administers as directed.
3. Client loosens scales on scalp in morning, shampoos with tar preparation, and follows with topical steroid preparation.
4. Client avoids use of plastic occlusive wrap with coal tar or anthralin application.
5. Client applies topical steroid with occlusive plastic dressing; modifies vinyl jogging suit for fuller body coverage.
6. Client applies anthralin to affected area only, using gloves and a downward motion, and wears old clothes; client avoids contact with eyes or other sensitive areas.
7. Client avoids sunlight and artificial light for 24 hours following photochemotherapy and wears full protective ultraviolet filtering glasses.
8. Client follows planned schedule and family-planning practices before, during, and after therapies using retinoids and methotrexate.
9. Client consults with physician when needed for clarification and assistance in therapies.

NURSING DIAGNOSIS DEFICIENT KNOWLEDGE

▌**Related Factors:** Lack of information about disorder

▌**Defining Characteristics:** Request for information about skin disruptions, their cause, treatments, and prevention of exacerbations

OUTCOMES

▌Short Term
Adequate knowledge, as evidenced by client's identification of measures to take to minimize recurrence and to comply with skin care and medication protocols (expected in 3 days)

▌Long Term
Optimal knowledge, as evidenced by client's meeting requirements for changes in lifestyle and medical regimen to achieve optimal level of health and functioning (expected in 2 weeks)

NURSING INTERVENTIONS/INSTRUCTIONS

1. Inform family members and/or caregivers that condition is not contagious (first visit).
2. Inform client of cause of condition and that although it is chronic, it does not affect overall health, and that control of condition is possible in most cases (first visit).
3. Instruct client in general measures to reduce recurrence (first visit).
4. Identify support systems; initiate referral to psychologic counseling if indicated for coping with effects on body image and self-concept and feelings of loss, grief, or isolation (any visit).
5. Refer client to social services for assistance with occupation changes (first visit).
6. Refer client to National Psoriasis Foundation for information and support (first visit).

CLIENT AND FAMILY/CAREGIVER INTERVENTIONS

1. Client verbalizes chronicity and limitations imposed by condition.
2. Client actively uses general measures to reduce relapses or recurrences: avoids skin injury or irritation, avoids overexposure to sunlight, manages emotional stress constructively, and avoids infections.
3. Consult with appropriate agencies or individuals for assistance, information, and support.

REPRODUCTIVE SYSTEM

❋ *Mastectomy*

Mastectomy, or the surgical removal of a breast, is usually performed to treat breast malignancy. A radical mastectomy is the removal of an entire breast, including the pectoral muscles, the lymph nodes of the axilla, and the pectoral fascia; a modified radical mastectomy does not include the pectoral muscles and pectoral fascia; and a simple mastectomy is the surgical removal of an entire breast. Mastectomy may be followed by the surgical reconstruction of the breast (i.e., mammoplasty).

Home care is primarily concerned with functional maintenance of the operative side and with the psychologic consequences of such a loss.

Primary Diagnosis:
Malignant Neoplasm of the Breast—ICD code: 174.9

NURSING DIAGNOSIS | DISTURBED BODY IMAGE

▌**Related Factors:** Loss of body part; psychosocial effect on self-concept, sexuality

▌**Defining Characteristics:** Verbalization of actual change in structure of body part, missing breast, disfigurement, significance of part in regard to sexual function and desirability, negative feelings about body, change in social involvement

OUTCOMES

▌**Short Term**
Progressive improvement in body image and adaptation to changes in function and structure, as evidenced by client's expressing feelings and concerns and considering prosthetic purchase, reconstructive surgery, and sexual activity alterations (expected in 1 to 2 weeks)

▌*Long Term*

Optimal acceptance of changes in body structure, with positive self-concept and body image (expected in 1 to 2 months)

NURSING INTERVENTIONS/INSTRUCTIONS

1. Assess client's mental and emotional status and ability to adapt and cope (see Psychosocial Assessment, p. 52, for guidelines) (first visit).
2. Accept client's feelings of mutilation, grief, depression, and anxiety as result of surgery (each visit).
3. Allow time and opportunity for client to express feelings and concerns and to ask questions. Note nonverbal and verbal cues for assistance in communicating feelings (each visit).
4. Explore client's perception of effect of breast loss on self-concept, self-image, and sexuality (first and second visits).
5. Give specific and accurate information about sexual activity (third or fourth visit):
   · Fear of exposure, rejection, or pain is common.
   · Sexual activity may be resumed in 4 to 6 weeks with physician approval.
   · Initial use of breast prosthesis during sexual activity may be a transitory buffer.
   · Instruction in sensate focusing can increase awareness of other sensitive and erogenous zones.
6. Discuss availability of a proper prosthesis; include types of prostheses, emotional readiness for fitting, clothing to be worn when shopping for prosthesis, and cost. Refer to durable medical equipment supplier as indicated (first visit).
7. Initiate referral to social services or counseling if appropriate (fourth or fifth visit).

CLIENT AND FAMILY/CAREGIVER INTERVENTIONS

1. Client verbalizes feelings and concerns and asks questions if needed.
2. Client participates in personal care and grooming; client selects clothing that enhances body image without revealing prosthesis.
3. Client initiates purchase of a breast prosthesis.
4. Client considers sexual options, with gradual resumption of activity and satisfaction.

5. Client considers reconstructive breast surgery; client speaks with others who have had this surgery.

NURSING DIAGNOSIS   EXCESS FLUID VOLUME

▌*Related Factors:* Compromised regulatory mechanisms

▌*Defining Characteristics:* Lymphedema in arm on operative side; fear or refusal to exercise arm and shoulder

OUTCOMES

▌Short Term
Minimal or absence of fluid accumulation in operative arm, as evidenced by arm circumference at baseline measurements and client's compliance with postoperative mastectomy exercises (expected in 1 to 2 weeks)

▌Long Term
Adequate lymph drainage with absence of arm swelling, optimal fluid balance, and full range of motion (ROM) in arm on operative side (expected in 1 to 2 months)

NURSING INTERVENTIONS/INSTRUCTIONS

1. Assess operative site, chest wall, posture, bilateral upper arm circumference (6 cm above elbow), and complaints of arm heaviness (each visit).
2. Assess client's ability to demonstrate hospital exercise regimen for baseline; note instructions given at discharge (first visit).
3. Encourage self-care in activities of daily living (e.g., bathing, grooming, dressing, and washing and brushing hair) (first and second visits).
4. Demonstrate and establish an activity and exercise regimen as ordered (first visit).

   · Avoid strenuous activity and heavy lifting or carrying until sutures are removed and incision is healed.
   · Begin resumption of light tasks at home and work as tolerated.
   · Exercise regularly, three or four times a day; stop when pulling or pain occurs, and resume when discomfort ceases.

- Practice fist clenching, ROM, and other exercises to promote circulation and prevent limitation of movement of arm and shoulder.
- Rest affected arm above heart level; elevate arm during sleep.

CLIENT AND FAMILY/CAREGIVER INTERVENTIONS

1. Client participates in self-care, including activities that involve raising the arms over the head.
2. Client performs exercises three or four times per day, takes analgesic before exercise if needed, and stops and rests between exercises when needed.
3. Client resumes household, occupational, and recreational tasks and activities.
4. Client participates in community-sponsored programs for rehabilitation.
5. Client uses pneumatic sleeve or elastic arm stocking to relieve edema.

NURSING DIAGNOSIS DEFICIENT KNOWLEDGE

■ **Related Factors:** Lack of knowledge about disease and postoperative care

■ **Defining Characteristics:** Request for information about and instruction in postoperative care regimen and chemotherapy regimen

OUTCOMES

■ Short Term

Adequate knowledge, as evidenced by client's statements about disease, treatment expectation and progression, and measures to prevent injury or infection (expected in 1 week)

■ Long Term

Optimal knowledge, as evidenced by compliance with treatment regimens, resulting in optimal health and return to optimal functioning (expected in 1 month)

NURSING INTERVENTIONS/INSTRUCTIONS

1. Assess lifestyle, ability to adapt, learning abilities, and family participation and support (first visit).

2. Assess operative site for size, color, temperature, approximation of edges of incision, presence of drainage, and need for dressing change (each visit).

3. Instruct client to notify physician of changes in incisional area or temperature elevation (first visit).

4. Assess changes in vital signs, posture, gait, balance, and use of operative side (each visit).

5. Instruct client in administration of analgesics, including dose, frequency, side effects, and food, drug, and alcohol interactions. Differentiate between operative and phantom breast pain and numbness and pins-and-needles sensation in area, and advise client that these will eventually disappear (first visit).

6. Instruct client in measures to prevent or minimize injury or infection; to protect arm from exposure and bumping; and to have all blood pressure checks, injections, and blood withdrawals performed on unaffected arm (first visit; reinforce on second visit).

7. Instruct client to avoid any burns, cuts, nicks, scratches, or insect bites or stings of affected arm on operative side (first visit).

8. Instruct client to wear clothing over arm that is protective, loose, and nonrestrictive and to avoid carrying purse or parcels with arm on affected side (first visit).

9. Instruct client to always cleanse and apply antiseptic to all skin breaks and to notify physician if arm becomes red, hot, or swollen (first visit).

10. Discuss and provide written information about prescribed adjuvant therapy, such as chemotherapy or radiation, and inform client of protocols regarding these treatments and when to appear at clinic or agency for therapy (each visit).

11. Demonstrate and instruct client in breast self-examination (BSE) for remaining breast and to perform examination each month (third or fourth visit).

12. Instruct client to keep physician appointments and to have yearly mammogram, and ultrasound if needed, on remaining breast (fourth visit).

13. Initiate referral to support groups such as Reach for Recovery, American Cancer Society, or YWCA or to psychologic counseling if appropriate (first visit).

CLIENT AND FAMILY/CAREGIVER INTERVENTIONS

1. Client monitors wound healing and notifies physician of changes at site or of fever.
2. Client administers analgesic for pain and verbalizes pain descriptors and causes.
3. Client prevents any injury to arm on operative side and protects and supports arm as needed.
4. Client reads and interprets written information on adjuvant therapies and asks questions to clarify information and modify behaviors.
5. Client performs monthly BSE correctly and has yearly mammogram.
6. Client keeps appointments with physician and for therapies and tests.
7. Client participates in support group and/or counseling focusing on breast diseases and surgery.

✳ *Auditory/Visual Impairment*

Auditory impairment is the inability to hear adequately as a result of the aging process (presbycusis) or other physical or psychologic conditions. Visual impairment is the inability to see adequately as a result of the aging process (presbyopia) or other physical or psychologic conditions. Each type of loss imposes lifestyle changes on an individual that require the use of an aid (e.g., hearing aid or glasses) to compensate for the impairment.

Home care is primarily concerned with teaching of the use and care of sensory aids and with prevention of injury as a result of the deficit.

> Primary Diagnoses:
> Ocular Hypertension—ICD code: 365.04
> Visual Loss—ICD code: 369.9

NURSING DIAGNOSIS DISTURBED SENSORY PERCEPTION (AUDITORY, VISUAL)

■ *Related Factors:* Chronic illness; aging; neurologic disease or deficit; altered status of sense organ; psychologic stress

■ *Defining Characteristics:* Hypoxia; electrolyte imbalance; use of drugs that affect the central nervous system (stimulants or depressants, mind altering); anxiety (narrowed perceptual fields); visual and auditory distortions; change in usual response to stimuli; expressed impairment in auditory and/or visual perception

OUTCOMES

■ Short Term
Adequate sensory perception, as evidenced by client's awareness of need for lifestyle changes to compensate for auditory or visual loss (expected in 3 to 7 days)

▌*Long Term*

Optimal sensory perception, as evidenced by incorporation of lifestyle changes into activities of daily living (ADL) and other activities to achieve health and functioning within identified limitations (expected in 1 month)

NURSING INTERVENTIONS/INSTRUCTIONS

1. Assess sensory abilities, limitations in ADL imposed by sensory loss, and need for supplementary aids (see Eye, Ear, Nose, and Throat Assessment, p. 48, for guidelines) (first visit).

2. Interact with client in a well-lit, quiet room free from external distractions, and allow time to process communication and respond (each visit).

3. Use as many sensory modalities as the client is comfortable with (each visit).

4. When communicating with a hearing impaired individual, remember the following guidelines (each visit):

   · Avoid covering mouth or chewing gum when speaking.
   · Face client.
   · Speak slowly and clearly and avoid shouting; using a lower-pitched voice may help.
   · Repeat instruction or conversation if client does not respond or responds inappropriately.
   · Be sure client's hearing aid is turned on if present or that hearing aid is used.

5. When communicating with a visually impaired individual, remember the following guidelines (each visit):

   · Announce arrival and departure.
   · Use touch only if you have indicated that you will do so and if client does not object.
   · Include client in all conversation, and speak in a moderate tone.
   · Sit directly in front of client in a well-lit room.
   · Be sure client uses glasses or contact lenses are used.

6. Encourage use of assistive aids or devices, such as large-print reading material or Braille, large-numbered telephone dials, amplified telephone box, and closed-caption or narrative television (first visit).

7. Instruct client about importance of annual examination for eye or ear disorders or deficits (first visit).
8. Instruct client in administration of eyedrops, ointments, eardrops, or other prescribed treatments (first visit).
9. Support referral to community resources for assistance and information (first visit).

CLIENT AND FAMILY/CAREGIVER INTERVENTIONS

1. Family members and/or caregiver use communication skills that are meaningful for client with a particular sensory deficit.
2. Client uses supplementary and assistive aids.
3. Client consults physician about changes in perception and for yearly or more frequent examinations.
4. Client seeks out community resources that assist hearing or visually impaired individuals and families.

NURSING DIAGNOSIS RISK FOR TRAUMA

■ *Related Factors:* Poor vision or hearing; lack of safety precautions and education

■ *Defining Characteristics:* Request for information on preventing falls or other injury; reluctance to engage in activities (self-care and social)

OUTCOMES

■ *Short Term*

Absence of injury, as evidenced by compliance with safety precautions and use of assistive aids (expected in 2 days)

■ *Long Term*

Maintenance of optimal health and functioning without injury (expected in 2 weeks and ongoing)

NURSING INTERVENTIONS/INSTRUCTIONS

1. Assist client in identifying limitations and safety hazards in the environment (first visit).
2. Assess ability of client to solve problems and to resolve these threats to safety (first visit).

3. Instruct client and family to provide and maintain clear pathways, to remove throw rugs and clutter, and to maintain intact cords and electrical appliances (first visit).
4. Instruct family to provide constant, adequate, well-distributed, glare-free light in all rooms and to place night light in bathroom (first visit).
5. Instruct client to take time when adjusting to changes in light intensity, especially when climbing stairs (first visit).
6. Emphasize importance of using aids at all times (first visit).
7. Supply client with a list of available supplemental aids for telephone, reading material, doorbell, and others specific to client (first visit).
8. Instruct family and client to retain furniture placement and familiarity of environment and to provide rails or objects to hold on to when moving about (first visit).

CLIENT AND FAMILY/CAREGIVER INTERVENTIONS

1. Client identifies hazards and eliminates or modifies them.
2. Client allows time for all activities; seeks assistance when needed.
3. Client uses assistive and supplemental aids.
4. Client maintains familiar environment; obtains assistance from trained pet for hearing or vision if appropriate.

✴ *Cataract Removal and Lens Implantation*

Cataract removal is the surgical removal of a lens that has become cloudy or opaque, causing visual impairment. Cataract development may be caused by senile degeneration, congenital trauma, disease (e.g., diabetes mellitus), or drug therapy (e.g., corticosteroids). The method of removing a cataract depends on a client's particular type of cataract and particular eye, and the time for removal is determined by the extent of impairment experienced (reading, driving, or participating in activities). A cataract may be removed by intracapsular extraction, in which the entire lens is removed (including the capsule that surrounds it) by touching the lens with a cold probe that freezes the lens and then removes it from the eye. Another method is extracapsular extraction, in which the back portion of the capsule is left behind to help secure an intraocular lens implant and hold the vitreous fluid in proper position inside the eye. A third method is extracapsular extraction in which the cataract is broken into small particles by ultrasound and then suctioned out of the eye. A hard or soft lens may be implanted to replace the lens that has been removed. An alternative to the intraocular lens implant is the use of cataract glasses or contact lenses.

Home care is primarily concerned with the teaching of medication regimens (eyedrops and ointment) and measures to prevent complications of infection, glaucoma, retinal detachment, or corneal damage.

Primary Diagnosis:
Cataract—ICD code: 013.19

NURSING DIAGNOSIS: DISTURBED SENSORY PERCEPTION (VISUAL)

▌*Related Factors:* Altered status of sense organ

▌*Defining Characteristics:* Bandaged eye; reduced visual acuity in nonoperative eye; change in visual acuity until operative eye stabilizes

OUTCOMES

▌*Short Term*
Improved visual acuity in operative eye, as evidenced by client's statements that vision is improving to baseline expectation and by compliance with postoperative eye medication regimen (expected in 3 days)

▌*Long Term*
Return of visual acuity and stabilization, as evidenced by return to 20/20 or 20/30 vision (expected in 4 weeks)

NURSING INTERVENTIONS/INSTRUCTIONS

1. Announce your presence when entering the room while client's eye is covered; use normal tone of voice (each visit).
2. Advise client that another person should be present while anesthesia is metabolized and eye is covered (first visit).
3. Inform client of activities that require assistance, and determine if referral for home health aide is needed (first visit).
4. Inform client of postoperative visits to physician on first, second, and seventh postoperative days for examination of operative eye and possible suture removal (first visit).
5. Inform client of visual progression (first visit):

   · Dark glasses may be suggested to reduce glare.
   · New prescription for lens in glasses on operative eye may be secured.
   · Diplopia may result after unilateral correction.
   · Use of interim glasses will result in clear central vision only, and head must be turned to bring peripheral objects into central vision.
   · Depth perception will be affected if one eye is covered or implant is not performed.
   · Contact lenses may be used in some instances and require fewer adaptations.
   · If lens is not implanted, permanent lenses in glasses will be prescribed 4 to 12 weeks postoperatively.
   · Gradual adaptation and full adjustment occur for optimal vision.

CLIENT AND FAMILY/CAREGIVER INTERVENTIONS

1. Client participates in ADL and other activities (driving, reading, watching television) in 1 week of surgery with physician recommendation.
2. Client wears corrective lenses as prescribed.
3. Client notifies physician if vision changes or decreases.
4. Client complies with postoperative physician visits until discharged.

NURSING DIAGNOSIS: DEFICIENT KNOWLEDGE

▮**Related Factors:** Lack of exposure to information about postoperative care

▋*Defining Characteristics:* Request for information about medication regimen to prevent infection, prevent increased intraocular pressure, and reduce inflammation and about protection of eye from trauma

OUTCOMES

▋*Short Term*

Adequate knowledge, as evidenced by client's stating responsibilities to be carried out postoperatively to prevent complications (expected in 2 to 3 days)

▋*Long Term*

Optimal knowledge, as evidenced by absence of infection, glaucoma, or trauma of operative eye and by compliance with treatment regimen (expected in 4 weeks)

NURSING INTERVENTIONS/INSTRUCTIONS

1. Inspect eye after dressing is removed; note color and check for edema and presence of purulent drainage (each visit).
2. Assess for return of vision and increased acuity (each visit).
3. Assess for headache or pain and severity; instruct client to notify physician if pain is sharp and sudden and is not relieved (first visit).
4. Instruct client in eye care (cleansing from inner to outer area), handwashing, and administration of eyedrops and eye ointment (e.g., steroids, antibiotics, and mydriatics), and include dose, technique, frequency, side effects, and implications for activity (first visit).
5. Instruct client to protect eye with shield during sleep for 1 week after physician removes initial dressing and shield (first visit).
6. Instruct client to avoid lifting, stooping, straining, bending, rubbing or bumping eye, or sneezing; instruct client to use stool softener and/or cough suppressant if needed (first visit).
7. Instruct client in positioning during sleep: rest on back or on nonoperative side, avoid lying flat, and use small pillow or raise head of bed with foam rubber wedge (first visit).
8. Instruct client to ambulate carefully to avoid bumping or jostling (first visit).
9. Instruct client to use eye medications until entire amount is administered or to follow physician's instructions for length of therapy (first visit).

CLIENT AND FAMILY/CAREGIVER INTERVENTIONS

1. Client performs medical asepsis procedures before eye care and medication administration.
2. Client uses warm compress to remove discharge from operative eye.
3. Client protects eye with shield, glasses, or both.
4. Client avoids activities that will cause injury or increase intraocular pressure.
5. Client participates in ADL with assistance if needed or independently.
6. Client instills eyedrops or applies eye ointment correctly and safely, as instructed and prescribed.
7. Client rests and sleeps in optimal position without placing pressure on eye.
8. Client immediately reports to physician any sudden pain or change in vision.

PSYCHIATRIC CARE PLANS

✳ *Alcohol/Drug Abuse*

Alcohol or drug abuse is a progressive disorder that affects all body systems. It can precipitate cirrhosis of the liver, esophageal varices, coma, and death. Several theories describe the alcoholic or drug abuser as having a fixed outlook, retarded emotional development, poor impulse control, chronic low self-esteem, and low frustration tolerance and as being highly dependent. Serious family dysfunction can contribute to alcohol or drug abuse.

Home care primarily focuses on the teaching of a medication regimen and on lifestyle changes.

> Primary Diagnoses:
> Alcoholism—ICD code: 303.9
> Alcoholic Psychosis—ICD code: 291.0
> Drug Addiction—ICD code: 304.9
> Drug Psychosis—ICD code: 292.0

NURSING DIAGNOSIS DISTURBED THOUGHT PROCESSES

■ *Related Factors:* Physiologic changes; impaired judgment

■ *Defining Characteristics:* Inaccurate interpretation of environment; distractibility; egocentricity; hypervigilance or hypovigilance

OUTCOMES

■ Short Term
Adequate thought processes, as evidenced by client correctly identifying activities happening in his or her environment and by client being oriented to surroundings after prompting by health care worker (expected in 3 days)

■ Long Term
Functional thought processes, as evidenced by client verbalizing that alcohol or drugs have caused alteration in thought (expected in 2 months)

NURSING INTERVENTIONS/INSTRUCTIONS

1. Assess for memory deficits (long-term, short-term) by asking questions about the past and the present (first visit).
2. Provide the client with an unhurried, patient, reassuring approach that is both positive and empathetic (each visit).
3. Assist in helping the client put recent events in order according to time sequence. Provide support for correct answers (each visit).
4. Explore with the client his or her perception of self; reinforce reality when appropriate (each visit).
5. Plan and implement a consistent approach to the client's care (each visit).
6. Repeat instructions or information for the client; ask the client to restate information in his or her own words (each visit).
7. Use patterns of recall (each visit).
8. Limit sensory input and choices to decrease distractions and frustrations (each visit).
9. Ask the client to make realistic commitments, and hold the client accountable for fulfillment of commitments (any visit).

CLIENT AND FAMILY/CAREGIVER INTERVENTIONS

1. Family maintains calm, caring attitude during treatment; stays with client.
2. Client attempts to prevent or discourage stressful situations.
3. Client develops and uses effective coping skills that decrease anxiety.

NURSING DIAGNOSIS INEFFECTIVE COPING

▌*Related Factors:* Personal vulnerability; difficulty handling new situations; previous ineffective or inadequate coping skills; inadequate coping skills, with substitution of alcohol; anxiety; fear

▌*Defining Characteristics:* Verbalization of inability to cope or inability to ask for help; inability to meet role expectations, to meet basic needs, and to solve problems; alteration in societal participation; destructive behavior toward self or others; inappropriate use of defense mechanisms; change in usual communication patterns; verbal manipulation

OUTCOMES

▌*Short Term*

Effective coping, as evidenced by client's attending support group (such as Alcoholics Anonymous) and verbalizing relationship of alcohol or drug abuse to difficulty in present life situation (expected in 7 days)

▌*Long Term*

Effective coping, as evidenced by client's making necessary lifestyle changes (expected in 2 months)

NURSING INTERVENTIONS/INSTRUCTIONS

1. Assess for psychosomatic symptoms; sleeping, eating, and bowel problems (each visit).
2. Assess support system, how the system functions, and whether it is adequate (first visit).
3. Establish rapport, show acceptance of the person, and establish a positive relationship with him or her (each visit).
4. Reduce the number of decisions that the client must make, including the need to solve problems (first visit).
5. Allow client sufficient time to make decisions; start with decisions that have only two options (first and second visits).
6. Discuss alternative ways of coping; allow these new coping techniques to be tried in a safe, nondestructive environment (each visit).
7. Use positive rather than negative reinforcement during the testing of new coping mechanisms (each visit).
8. Allow client time to verbalize feelings of denial, anger, guilt, or grief regarding crisis situation (each visit).
9. Acknowledge the validity of client's fear and other feelings (each visit).
10. Encourage client to talk about the changes the crisis will cause (each visit).
11. Listen to and clarify the client's perception of the crisis situation (each visit).
12. Assist client in sorting out the facts concerning the crisis (any visit).
13. Assist client in seeking and accepting help, and provide referral to psychiatrist or psychologist if needed (each visit).

14. Identify defense mechanisms used and whether they are being used positively or negatively. Reinforce positive coping mechanisms that have been successfully used in the past but that are not being used now (any visit).

CLIENT AND FAMILY/CAREGIVER INTERVENTIONS

1. Client includes the family in sorting out information regarding the crisis.
2. Client discusses with the family the need to avoid judgments regarding the client's behavior.
3. Client refers family to Al-Anon or other support group.

NURSING DIAGNOSIS DEFICIENT KNOWLEDGE

▌*Related Factors:* Lack of recall; misinterpretation of information; cognitive limitation; lack of interest in learning

▌*Defining Characteristics:* Verbalization of the problem; inappropriate or exaggerated behavior (e.g., hysterical, hostile, agitated, apathetic); inaccurate follow-through of instructions; inaccurate performance on test

OUTCOMES

▌*Short Term*

Adequate knowledge, as evidenced by client's explaining needed lifestyle changes and medication regimen and by client's ability to verbalize the effects of substance abuse and its effects on therapies (expected in 5 days)

▌*Long Term*

Functional knowledge, as evidenced by client's demonstrating change in lifestyle, following through with medication regimen and rehabilitation, and verbalizing the advantages of abstaining from alcohol or drug abuse (expected in 1 month)

NURSING INTERVENTIONS/INSTRUCTIONS

1. Assess client's strengths and weaknesses through interviewing, and determine previous interests or areas of success (first visit).

2. Assess client's knowledge regarding disulfiram (Antabuse) therapy: action, side effects, and response if patient drinks alcohol while taking Antabuse (first visit).
3. Assess client's developmental level, educational level, vocabulary level, and past decisions regarding health practices (first visit).
4. Assess information client has about changes needed in lifestyle by asking specific questions (first visit).
5. Discuss what needs to be taught and who needs to be taught, including family members who may be responsible for health care (first and second visits).
6. Provide positive feedback for participation and adequate information (each visit).
7. Demonstrate techniques using several sessions; increase difficulty at each session; require return demonstration after each session (each visit).
8. Evaluate teaching plan (any visit).

CLIENT AND FAMILY/CAREGIVER INTERVENTIONS

1. Family determines progress with the client and revises schedules based on observed progress.
2. Family uses available resources for health maintenance and delivery with client's input.
3. Client institutes appropriate referrals and use of support systems through community agencies.

✳ *Depression*

Depression is an affective disorder characterized by an altered mood with symptoms of diminished interest, poor self-esteem, sadness, guilt, hopelessness, emptiness, and despondency. Views about the cause of depression include environmental, societal, genetic, and biomedical theories.

Home care is primarily concerned with the teaching of medication regimens and lifestyle changes that may be needed, providing a safe environment (commonly after hospitalization), and maintenance of daily well-being.

Primary Diagnoses:
Depression—ICD code: 311.0
Depression, Reactive (Situational)—ICD code: 300.4
Suicide—ICD code: 300.9

NURSING DIAGNOSIS HOPELESSNESS

■ *Related Factors:* Prolonged activity restriction, creating isolation; failing or deteriorating physiologic condition; long-term stress; abandonment; lost belief in transcendent values (e.g., God)

■ *Defining Characteristics:* Passivity; pessimism; decreased verbalization; decreased affect; verbal cues (despondent content); turning away from speaker; closing eyes; decreased appetite; increased sleep; lack of initiative; decreased response to stimuli

OUTCOMES

■ *Short Term*
Decreased hopelessness, as evidenced by decreased negative verbalization and increased eye contact with health care provider (expected in 3 days)

■ *Long Term*
Decreased hopelessness, as evidenced by increased involvement in care and activities (expected in 1 month)

NURSING INTERVENTIONS/INSTRUCTIONS

1. Assess for isolation (physical, emotional, and spiritual), chronic stress, and poor physical health (first visit).
2. Assess for defense mechanisms: denial, isolation, and regression (first visit).
3. Assess for nonverbal and verbal indicators of hopelessness: poor eye contact, slumped posture, flat affect, monotone speech, and retarded speech (first visit).
4. Discuss how client's life used to be and activities performed when client was happy (first visit).
5. Allow client to take as much responsibility as possible in own care (each visit).
6. Assist client in setting realistic goals in areas of life that he or she can control (first and second visits).

7. Discuss how client's life has changed and what would make life satisfying again (any visit).
8. Provide referral to appropriate groups, depending on client's condition (any visit).

CLIENT AND FAMILY/CAREGIVER INTERVENTIONS

1. Client includes family in planning, including referrals to outside agencies for help.
2. Client attempts to prevent or discourage stressful situations.
3. Client develops and uses effective coping skills that decrease depression.

NURSING DIAGNOSIS   INEFFECTIVE COPING

Related Factors: Personal vulnerability; difficulty in handling new situations; previous ineffective or inadequate coping skills; inadequate coping skills, with substitution of alcohol; anxiety; fear

Defining Characteristics: Verbalization of inability to cope or inability to ask for help; inability to meet role expectations, to meet basic needs, and to solve problems; alteration in societal participation; destructive behavior toward self or others; inappropriate use of defense mechanisms; change in usual communication patterns; verbal manipulation

OUTCOMES

Short Term
Effective coping, as evidenced by client's statement of lifestyle changes that relieve depression (expected in 5 days)

Long Term
Effective coping as evidenced by client's achievement of necessary lifestyle changes and by client's understanding of relationship between feelings and antecedent event (expected in 1 month)

NURSING INTERVENTIONS/INSTRUCTIONS

1. Assess client for psychosomatic symptoms: sleeping, eating, and bowel problems (first visit).
2. Assess client's support system and how the system functions (first visit).

3. Encourage and assist client in identifying feelings and relationship between feelings and event or stressor when event is known (each visit).
4. Establish rapport; show acceptance of the person; and establish a positive, concerned relationship with him or her (each visit).
5. Reduce the number of decisions that the client must make, including the need to solve problems (first and second visits).
6. Allow client sufficient time to make decisions; start with decisions that have only two options (first and second visits).
7. Discuss alternative ways of coping; allow these new coping techniques to be tried in a safe, nondestructive environment (any visit).
8. Use positive rather than negative reinforcement during the testing of new coping mechanisms (each visit).
9 Allow client time to verbalize feelings of denial, anger, guilt, or grief regarding crisis situation (each visit).
10. Acknowledge the validity of client's fear, hostility, and anxiety (any visit).
11. Encourage the client to talk about the changes the situation has caused (any visit).
12. Listen to and clarify the client's perception of the situation (any visit).
13. Assist the client in sorting out the facts concerning the situation (any visit).
14. Identify defense mechanisms used and determine whether they are being used positively or negatively. Reinforce positive coping mechanisms that have been successfully used in the past but that are not currently being used (any visit).
15. Avoid giving client false reassurance (each visit).
16. Assist the client in recognizing early symptoms of depression and ways to alleviate them (first visit).

CLIENT AND FAMILY/CAREGIVER INTERVENTIONS

1. Client seeks and accepts help and uses referral to day care, crisis center, psychiatrist, or psychologist, if needed.
2. Client sorts out and analyzes information from the family regarding the crisis.
3. Family avoids judgments regarding the client's behavior.

NURSING DIAGNOSIS IMPAIRED SOCIAL INTERACTION

Related Factors: Knowledge and/or skill deficit about ways to enhance mutuality; communication barriers; absence of available significant others or peers; limited physical mobility; therapeutic isolation; sociocultural dissonance; environmental barriers; altered thought processes

Defining Characteristics: Verbalized or observed discomfort in social situation; verbalized or observed inability to receive or communicate a satisfying sense of belonging, caring, interest, or shared history; observed use of unsuccessful social interaction behaviors; dysfunctional interaction with peers, family, and/or others; family report of change of style or pattern of interaction

OUTCOMES

Short Term

Adequate socialization, as evidenced by client's communicating with significant others and requesting other people to interact with him or her (expected in 1 week)

Long Term

Adequate socialization, as evidenced by client's expressing interests that are appropriate to developmental age or stage, use of eye contact while interacting, and absence of hostility in voice and behavior (expected in 1 month)

NURSING INTERVENTIONS/INSTRUCTIONS

1. Assess for limited social contacts, preoccupation with own thoughts and feelings, and number of social contacts per week (first visit).
2. Assess client for positive feelings that occur from contact with others (first visit).
3. Discuss being alone, amount of time needed, and how client feels during this time (any visit).
4. Acknowledge client's feelings of loneliness, and discuss feelings of rejection, hostility, and insecurity (any visit).
5. Identify cultural norms and discuss how isolation occurs when social norms are not followed (any visit).

6. Identify client's behaviors that are not considered socially acceptable to dominant culture; acknowledge and reinforce acceptable behaviors (any visit).
7. Discuss frequent testing of relationships and how testing may lead to social isolation (any visit).
8. Encourage verbal communication, eye contact, and involvement in community functions (any visit).

CLIENT AND FAMILY/CAREGIVER INTERVENTIONS

1. Client attempts to prevent or discourage interactions with negative individuals.
2. Client develops and uses effective coping skills that decrease isolation.

NURSING DIAGNOSIS RISK FOR SUICIDE

Related Factors: Psychiatric illness/disorder (e.g., depression); history of previous suicide attempt, physical illness, terminal illness

Defining Characteristics: Marked changes in behavior, attitude; sudden euphoric recovery from depression; verbalization of desire to die or end it all, hopelessness, helplessness, grief

OUTCOMES

Short Term
Reduced feelings of hopelessness and helplessness, as evidenced by client's verbalization of measures that can be taken to prevent suicide (expected in 1 week)

Long Term
Minimal risk for suicide, as evidenced by client's demonstration of use of appropriate resources (expected in 1 month)

NURSING INTERVENTIONS/INSTRUCTIONS

1. Assess client's psychosocial status through use of open-ended questions for expressions of depression, hopelessness, helplessness, loneliness, social isolation, history of suicide attempt, suicide plan, coping skills, problem-solving abilities, and relationships (first visit).

2. Provide client with accepting environment to promote expressions of feelings of depression, hopelessness, and helplessness (all visits).
3. Encourage client to use effective coping and decision-making skills, support groups, and community resources (all visits).
4. Inform client of activities that help reduce feelings of hopelessness, including physical activity, social interactions, and "be kind to self" activities (first visit).
5. Inform client that feelings of depression can be treated (first visit).
6. Initiate referral to counseling or psychotherapy (first visit).
7. Inform client about resources, including suicide prevention hotline (first visit).

CLIENT AND FAMILY/CAREGIVER INTERVENTIONS

1. Client uses opportunity to express feelings of depression and thoughts of suicide.
2. Client uses coping and decision-making skills to cope with problems. Client participates in regular physical activity and support groups and uses community resources.
3. Client attends counseling/psychotherapy sessions.
4. Client uses hotline or other resources when he or she needs to talk about thoughts of suicide.

NURSING DIAGNOSIS DEFICIENT KNOWLEDGE

▌*Related Factors:* Lack of exposure to information; lack of recall; misinterpretation of information; cognitive limitation; lack of interest in learning; unfamiliarity with information resources

▌*Defining Characteristics:* Verbalization of problem; inappropriate or exaggerated behavior (e.g., hysterical, hostile, agitated, or apathetic); inaccurate follow-through of instructions; inaccurate performance on test

OUTCOMES

▌*Short Term*
Adequate knowledge, as evidenced by client's ability to explain reasons for depression (expected in 3 days)

▌*Long Term*

Optimal knowledge, as evidenced by client's ability to demonstrate needed lifestyle changes, participate in treatment programs, and identify resources (expected in 1 month)

NURSING INTERVENTIONS/INSTRUCTIONS

1. Assess client's strengths and weaknesses through interviewing, and determine previous interest areas of success (first visit).
2. Assess client's developmental level, educational level, vocabulary level, age, and past discussion regarding health practices (first visit).
3. Assess extent of client's information about depression by asking open-ended questions (first visit).
4. Provide information about drug therapy, potential side effects, precautions, and benefits, and emphasize that client is not to suddenly stop taking medication (first visit).
5. Refer client to support agencies and resources (any visit).
6. Discuss progress with client, and revise schedules based on observed progress (any visit).
7. Provide written and verbal instructions (each visit).

CLIENT AND FAMILY/CAREGIVER INTERVENTIONS

1. Client administers drug therapy correctly and consistently and notes progress to report or need for change in therapy.
2. Client uses available resources for health maintenance and delivery.

�ख *Physical/Emotional Abuse*

Physical abuse is considered to be a destructive act or injury inflicted by a caregiver. Emotional abuse includes threats and acts of degradation that are damaging to a person's self-worth.

Home care is primarily concerned with the teaching aspects of symptoms of abuse and with adequate prevention, evaluation, and reporting of abuse.

Primary Diagnoses:
Physical Abuse, Adult—ICD code: 995.81
Emotional Abuse, Adult—ICD code: 995.82

NURSING DIAGNOSIS · RISK FOR TRAUMA

■ *Related Factors:* Interactive conditions between individual and environment that pose a risk to the defensive and adaptive resources of the individual

■ *Defining Characteristics:* Internal environment: weakness; poor vision; balancing difficulties; lack of safety or drug education; lack of proper precautions; cognitive or emotional difficulties. External environment: people or caregiver

OUTCOMES

■ Short Term
Absence of trauma, as evidenced by client's statement that trauma has not occurred (expected in 1 week)

■ Long Term
Absence of trauma, as evidenced by absence of falls, injuries, or death from abuse (expected in 2 months)

NURSING INTERVENTIONS/INSTRUCTIONS

1. Assess client, situation, and environment for potentially abusive situation (first visit).
2. Identify and remove actual dangers from the client's environment (see Defining Characteristics) (each visit).

CLIENT AND FAMILY/CAREGIVER INTERVENTIONS

1. Client increases awareness of the possibility of abuse by family and caregivers.
2. Family provides for respite care of client to relieve caregiver.

NURSING DIAGNOSIS · INTERRUPTED FAMILY PROCESSES

■ *Related Factors:* Situational transition or crisis; developmental transition or crisis

■ **Defining Characteristics:** Family system unable to meet physical, emotional, and spiritual needs of its members; inability to
express or accept wide range of feelings; inability to express or
accept feelings of members; family unable to meet security needs
of its members; family members unable to relate to each other for
mutual growth and maturation; family uninvolved in community
activities; inability to accept or receive help appropriately; rigidity
in function and roles; family not demonstrating respect for indi-
viduality and autonomy of its members; family unable to adapt to
change or deal constructively with traumatic experience; family
failure to accomplish current or past developmental tasks;
unhealthy family decision-making process; failure to send and
receive clear messages; inappropriate boundary maintenance; inappropriate or poorly communicated family rules, rituals, symbols;
unexamined family myths; inappropriate level and direction of
energy

OUTCOMES

■ **Short Term**
Family allows for individual differences of its members (expected
in 1 week)

■ **Long Term**
Family allows for all individuals to be involved in the decision-
making process; all family members state that basic needs (physical, emotional, and spiritual) are being met in the family (expected
in 3 months)

NURSING INTERVENTIONS/INSTRUCTIONS

1. Assess decision-making or problem-solving techniques used in
   the family (who influences the decisions in the family, who
   makes the final decision, and all persons involved in the
   process) (first visit).
2. Assess the developmental stage of the family and of each member (Are there developmental lags in any one of the members?)
   (first visit).
3. Assess for coalitions in the family (who takes whose side during arguments), triangulating, and scapegoating (first visit).
4. Assess the realistic view of the crisis (first visit).
5. Assess the availability of support systems outside the family
   (any visit).

6. Identify ineffective coping mechanisms used; acknowledge and encourage positive coping mechanisms (each visit).
7. Discuss ambivalence, hostility, guilt, and anxiety and how these emotions affect the family; discuss verbalizing these feelings and emotions (each visit).
8. Assist the family in identifying the major stressors in the family (each visit).
9. Allow client and family to verbalize about situational or maturational crises that are occurring in the family; determine whether family crises are occurring at the same time as individual crises (each visit).
10. Discuss the concept of tolerance and how nonjudgmental attitudes lead to feelings of security in the family (first visit).
11. Identify the family's need for further professional help, and refer the family to appropriate agencies (any visit).

CLIENT AND FAMILY/CAREGIVER INTERVENTIONS

1. Family is involved in decision making related to the client.
2. Family members avoid severe stressors in the family and develop more appropriate coping mechanisms.
3. Family members use resources when indicated.

NURSING DIAGNOSIS IMPAIRED HOME MAINTENANCE

Related Factors: Disease or injury of family member; insufficient family organization or planning; insufficient finances; unfamiliarity with neighborhood resources; impaired cognitive or emotional functioning; lack of knowledge; lack of role modeling; inadequate support systems

Defining Characteristics: Household members express difficulty in maintaining their home in a comfortable fashion; household members request assistance with home maintenance; household members describe outstanding debts or financial crises; disorderly surroundings; unwashed or unavailable cooking equipment, clothes, or linens; accumulation of dirt, food wastes, or hygienic wastes; offensive odors; inappropriate household temperature; overtaxed family members (e.g., exhausted, anxious); lack of necessary equipment or aids; presence of vermin or rodents; repeated hygienic disorders, infestations, or infections

OUTCOMES

▌*Short Term*

Absence of dirt, food wastes, or hygienic waste; absence of offensive odors; washed or available cooking equipment, clothing, and linens; absence of hygienic disorders, infestations, and infections; absence of vermin (expected in 1 week)

▌*Long Term*

Household members state ease in maintaining home in comfortable fashion (expected in 3 months)

NURSING INTERVENTIONS/INSTRUCTIONS

1. Assess mental status, including orientation, affect, and level of consciousness (first visit).
2. Assess mobility (ambulation and equipment needed) (first visit).
3. Assess self-care abilities (hygiene, dressing, and eating) (first visit).
4. Assess housekeeping skills (first visit).
5. Assess ability to organize housekeeping activities (first visit).
6. Provide referral for outside help or preparation of meals if needed (any visit).
7. Discuss making an organizational plan to be followed daily; include all family members (first visit).
8. Discuss rotation of household chores (first visit).
9. Discuss preparation of meals for 2 days or for the entire week (any visit).

CLIENT AND FAMILY/CAREGIVER INTERVENTIONS

1. Family reorganizes family chores.
2. Client uses family and persons in the community who may help with home maintenance.

NURSING DIAGNOSIS DEFICIENT KNOWLEDGE

▌*Related Factors:* Lack of exposure to information; lack of recall; misinterpretation of information; cognitive limitation; lack of interest in learning; unfamiliarity with information resources

Defining Characteristics: Verbalization of the problem; inappropriate or exaggerated behavior (e.g., hysterical, hostile, agitated, or apathetic); inaccurate follow-through of instructions; inaccurate performance on test

OUTCOMES

Short Term
Adequate knowledge, as evidenced by client's ability to verbalize definition of signs and symptoms of abusive behavior (expected in 3 days)

Long Term
Optimal knowledge, as evidenced by client's ability to report abuse (expected in 2 weeks)

NURSING INTERVENTIONS/INSTRUCTIONS

1. Assess strengths and weaknesses of relationship between caregiver and client (first visit).
2. Assess information known about abuse; ask specific questions (first visit).
3. Discuss what needs to be taught (first visit).
4. Discuss abuse, symptoms, and prevention (any visit).

CLIENT AND FAMILY/CAREGIVER INTERVENTIONS

1. Caregiver uses available resources for prevention of abuse; uses client's input.
2. Client institutes appropriate use of support systems and referrals to community agencies.

SPECIAL CARE PLANS

❊ Chemotherapy and External Radiation Therapy

Chemotherapy and radiation therapy are treatment modalities that are used to cure, control, or palliate cancer. Radiation therapy may be administered alone or in combination with surgery or chemotherapy. Chemotherapy protocols include alkylating agents, antimetabolites, antitumor antibiotics, plant alkaloids, nitrosoureas, corticosteroids, hormones, and unclassified miscellaneous and investigational drugs. These agents are given in combination for prescribed periods and frequency, depending on the malignancy being treated. They may be administered by oral, intramuscular, intravenous, intrathecal, intraarterial, intracavity, subcutaneous, topical, intraperitoneal, or perfusion routes, depending on tumor site.

Home care is primarily concerned with administration of chemotherapy, teaching of the physical and emotional effects and resulting care and needs during administration of chemotherapy and/or radiation therapy, and assessment and treatment of side effects.

Primary Diagnosis:
Cancer (Location of Malignancy)—ICD code relates to location

NURSING DIAGNOSIS INEFFECTIVE COPING

■ **Related Factors:** Multiple life changes; inadequate coping methods

■ **Defining Characteristics:** Verbalization of inability to cope or ask for help; inability to solve problems; chronic worry and anxiety; inappropriate use of defense mechanisms

OUTCOMES

▌Short Term

Improved coping, as evidenced by client's statement of understanding of need for adaptations in lifestyle and positive coping strategies (expected in 1 week)

▌Long Term

Optimal coping, as evidenced by client's participation in and adaptation to altered lifestyle and by client's compliance with medical regimen to maintain optimal health and functioning (expected in 1 to 2 months)

NURSING INTERVENTIONS/INSTRUCTIONS

1. Assess client for developmental level and dependency needs, mental status, behavioral and emotional changes, use of defense mechanisms and their effectiveness, and ability to solve problems (first visit).
2. Establish a trusting relationship and facilitate an open discussion to explore options and develop skills in coping and problem solving (each visit).
3. Help client identify coping skills that work, and encourage positive feeling about success of any adaptation or changes (each visit).
4. Include client in all planning and formulation of realistic goals; assist if requested to do so (each visit).
5. Provide an accepting, nonjudgmental attitude and environment when teaching and discussing needs and changes to be made in lifestyle (each visit).
6. Encourage expressions of fears, concerns, and questions regarding therapy and effects (each visit).
7. Initiate referral to support group, social services, and counseling (any visit).

CLIENT AND FAMILY/CAREGIVER INTERVENTIONS

1. Client develops coping strategies for long-term treatment and possible outcome.
2. Client shares feelings, fears, and concerns with caregiver and family.
3. Client plans and participates in own care and health promotion.
4. Client sets goals and strategies for coping with lifestyle changes.

5. Client participates in support group with those who have similar conditions.
6. Client uses social services, counseling, and clergy as needed.

NURSING DIAGNOSIS	IMBALANCED NUTRITION: LESS THAN BODY REQUIREMENTS

▌**Related Factors:** Inability to ingest and absorb nutrients because of biologic factors (chemotherapy and/or radiation therapy)

▌**Defining Characteristics:** Anorexia; lack of interest in food; weakness; fatigue; weight loss; inadequate nutritional intake; stomatitis; vomiting; altered taste perception; mucositis of bowel

OUTCOMES

▌**Short Term**

Adequate nutrition, as evidenced by intake of prescribed dietary regimen and stabilization of weight without anorexia, nausea, and vomiting (expected in 1 to 2 weeks)

▌**Long Term**

Adequate nutritional status, as evidenced by intake of required nutrients for optimal health and functioning during and after therapy (expected in 1 month and ongoing)

NURSING INTERVENTIONS/INSTRUCTIONS

1. Assess client's nutritional status, including food preferences, cultural and religious restrictions, caloric requirements, and effect of different medications on food intake (first visit).
2. Calculate ideal weight for size, sex, frame, and height; instruct client in measuring weight weekly (first visit).
3. Assess client for diarrhea, nausea, vomiting, anorexia, weight loss, fatigue, malaise, and reactions to meals (each visit).
4. Instruct client to schedule rest periods after meals and to get 6 to 8 hours of sleep per night (first visit).
5. Inform client of measures to facilitate eating, including the following: eliminating odors; providing a relaxed atmosphere and quiet environment; eating smaller, more frequent, attractively prepared meals; and taking antiemetic medications 30 minutes before meals (first visit).

6. Inform client of newer antiemetic medications and their success in controlling nausea and vomiting, and instruct in administration (first visit).
7. Instruct client to maintain a food diary for 1 week that includes types and amounts of foods consumed and methods of preparation (first and second visits).
8. Instruct and include client in food selections for a high-protein, high-carbohydrate, high-calorie diet and to avoid hot, spicy foods; incorporate assessment data and food diary into menu planning (first and second visits).
9. Provide information for calorie and vitamin supplements (first visit).
10. Suggest oral hygiene before each meal (first visit).
11. If client's appetite is poor, suggest eating more frequent meals in smaller amounts and increasing amounts slowly as tolerated (first visit).
12. Initiate referral to nutritionist if needed (any visit).
13. Refer home health aide (HHA) to assist with feeding and meal preparation as needed.

CLIENT AND FAMILY/CAREGIVER INTERVENTIONS

1. Client maintains or gains weight as determined.
2. Client participates in planning and ingestion of well-balanced diet with restrictions as determined.
3. Client promotes pleasant environment, preferred food preparation, and dietary pattern that enhances intake.
4. Client weighs weekly using same scale, at same time of day, wearing same amount of clothing and records in a log.
5. Client maintains a 7-day food diary listing types and amounts of all foods eaten.
6. Client eats a high-protein, high-carbohydrate, high-calorie diet; to assist with meal preparation, client secures a cookbook for individuals with cancer.
7. Client uses high-calorie supplements as needed.
8. Client takes daily vitamins.
9. Client administers antiemetic medications 30 minutes before meals as needed.

NURSING DIAGNOSIS | DIARRHEA

■*Related Factors:* Inflammation or irritation of bowel; malabsorption of bowel (chemotherapy and/or radiation therapy)

■*Defining Characteristics:* Abdominal pain; cramping; increased frequency of bowel eliminations; loose, liquid stools; urgency; mucus in stool; increased frequency of bowel sounds; mucositis

OUTCOMES

■Short Term
Return of baseline bowel pattern, as evidenced by decrease in the frequency of bowel eliminations and by stool characteristics in baseline parameters (expected in 1 week)

■Long Term
Minimal or absence of diarrheal bowel eliminations, as evidenced by soft formed stools eliminated according to baseline pattern (expected in 2 weeks)

NURSING INTERVENTIONS/INSTRUCTIONS

1. Assess client's bowel elimination patterns and stool characteristics (see Gastrointestinal System Assessment, p. 22, for guidelines) (first visit).
2. Instruct client to maintain a record of bowel movements, including number and when they occur and characteristics such as color; amount; consistency; odor; and presence of mucus, blood, or pus (first visit).
3. Monitor medication administration, and instruct client in intake and output, about antidiarrheals and anticholinergics, and to monitor intake and output ratio with increased fluid intake (each visit).
4. Instruct client to notify physician if diarrhea becomes more severe or frequent, if bleeding is noted, or if fatigue or weakness is noted (first visit).

CLIENT AND FAMILY/CAREGIVER INTERVENTIONS

1. Client administers antidiarrheal correctly as needed.

2. Client reports diarrhea that is not controlled or reveals blood, pus, or mucus.
3. Client adjusts diet and avoids foods irritating to bowel.
4. Client monitors fluid intake and output and increases fluid intake up to 3000 ml/day as needed.

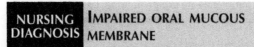

| NURSING DIAGNOSIS | IMPAIRED ORAL MUCOUS MEMBRANE |

▌*Related Factors:* Medication (chemotherapeutic agents)

▌*Defining Characteristics:* Stomatitis; oral lesions or ulcers; oral pain or discomfort

OUTCOMES

▌Short Term
Minimal changes in oral mucous membrane, as evidenced by decreased inflammation and oral pain and by intact mucous membrane (expected in 4 to 7 days)

▌Long Term
Oral mucous membrane maintained intact, as evidenced by absence of stomatitis and associated signs and symptoms (expected in 1 to 2 weeks and ongoing during therapy)

NURSING INTERVENTIONS/INSTRUCTIONS

1. Assess oral cavity for redness, pain, ulcerations, dysphagia, and dryness (each visit).
2. Instruct client to provide mouth care after meals, to rinse mouth with an alkaline mouthwash or viscous lidocaine every 2 hours or as needed, and to avoid commercial mouthwashes or alcohol (first visit).
3. Instruct client to avoid mouth breathing, smoking, and eating hot and spicy or irritating foods (first visit).
4. Instruct client to avoid using a hard toothbrush and to remove dentures except for meals (first visit).
5. Instruct client to apply petroleum jelly or cocoa butter to lips and artificial saliva preparation to oral cavity; instruct client to use topical anesthetic and fungal antibiotic medication if prescribed (first visit).

6. Instruct client to consume cool beverages, popsicles, and ice cream to soothe oral cavity (first visit).

CLIENT AND FAMILY/CAREGIVER INTERVENTIONS

1. Client assesses oral cavity for stomatitis and reports condition that deteriorates despite treatments.
2. Client performs oral care using soft brush, unwaxed floss, soft-tipped applicator, and mouthwash consisting of acceptable solution.
3. Client applies topical preparations for dryness.
4. Client avoids commercial products for mouth care and irritants to oral cavity, such as hot, spicy foods; alcohol; and tobacco. Client ingests cool fluids and bland, smooth foods.

NURSING DIAGNOSIS IMPAIRED SKIN INTEGRITY

▌*Related Factors:* Internal factor of medication (chemotherapy); external factor of radiation

▌*Defining Characteristics:* Disruption of skin surfaces; dryness; pruritus; blistering, allergic rashes; hyperpigmentation; irritation and excoriation of perianal area from diarrhea

OUTCOMES

▌*Short Term*
Skin intact, as evidenced by absence of irritation, dryness, rash, or breaks (expected in 1 week)

▌*Long Term*
Skin integrity maintained, as evidenced by absence of skin disruption and by skin protection to achieve optimal condition during treatments (expected to be ongoing during treatments)

NURSING INTERVENTIONS/INSTRUCTIONS

1. Assess for skin condition at irradiation site, itching, irritation at perianal area; assess skin for dryness, pruritus, rashes; and review skin care protocol for clients receiving chemotherapy and/or radiation therapy (each visit).
2. Instruct client to cleanse skin with mild soap and warm water and pat dry and to avoid using soap, lotions, or deodorants or

washing or removing marks of any kind placed on skin at ir-radiation site (first visit).

3. Instruct client to avoid any massage, scratching, adhesive tape, pressure, or sun exposure to skin; to wear soft, loose clothing; and to use a sun screen for a year following treatment (first and second visits).

4. Instruct client to expose irradiation site to the air and to apply only prescribed preparations to skin twice a day, such as a water-soluble lubricant for dryness, cornstarch to absorb moisture, and hydrocortisone cream to reduce inflammation (first visit).

5. Instruct client to cleanse and dry perianal area after each bowel elimination and to apply a water-soluble lubricant or karaya gel to area (first visit).

6. Instruct client to assess skin for breakdown and to report any open areas to physician (first visit).

CLIENT AND FAMILY/CAREGIVER INTERVENTIONS

1. Client performs measures to protect skin integrity during chemotherapy and/or radiation therapy.

2. Client provides safe cleansing and protection to skin.

3. Client avoids exposure of skin to harmful pressure, rubbing, or irritants.

4. Client applies ointments to prevent or treat dryness, itching, or irritation of skin.

5. Client preserves markings placed on skin by radiography personnel.

6. Client reports skin breakdown to physician.

NURSING DIAGNOSIS INEFFECTIVE PROTECTION

Related Factors: Abnormal blood profile (chemotherapy and/or radiation)

Defining Characteristics: Leukopenia, thrombocytopenia, anemia from bone marrow depression; proneness to bleeding, infection, fatigue, weakness

OUTCOMES

▌Short Term
Control of bleeding or infection tendency, as evidenced by absence of bleeding or infection at any site (expected in 1 week)

▌Long Term
Absence of bleeding or infectious process, with blood profile in acceptable parameters during therapy (expected for duration of therapy)

NURSING INTERVENTIONS/INSTRUCTIONS

1. Assess client for bleeding, including petechiae, ecchymoses, oozing or frank bleeding from any orifice or skin site, or blood in stool or urine; assess joints for pain and swelling; assess for increased weakness and fatigue (each visit).
2. Assess client for fever; chills; decreased breath sounds; dyspnea with or without exertion; cough; chest pain; cloudy, foul-smelling urine; and frequency, burning, and urgency in urinary elimination (each visit).
3. Assess, as available, levels of white blood cells, red blood cells, hematocrit, hemoglobin, and platelets and urine or sputum culture results, and compare with levels at which bleeding or infection is probable (any visit).
4. Instruct client to avoid any trauma to skin and to take measures to prevent falls or other injury in the home environment (first visit).
5. Instruct client to avoid exposure to others with infections or illnesses that might be transmitted (first visit).
6. Instruct client in handwashing technique, to wear mask if needed, to avoid eating uncooked foods such as raw vegetables as indicated, and to avoid sharing utensils or articles such as linens or clothing (first visit).
7. Instruct client to avoid using a safety razor, hard tooth brushing, hard nose blowing, or straining at defecation (first visit).
8. Inform client of importance of having laboratory tests performed as scheduled to determine bone marrow function and possible effects (first visit).
9. Instruct client to report any persistent symptoms to physician (each visit).

CLIENT AND FAMILY/CAREGIVER INTERVENTIONS

1. Client takes and records temperature, respirations, and pulse rate as needed.
2. Client adapts activities of daily living (ADL) and other activities to physical tolerance and rests when feeling fatigued.
3. Client assesses daily for bleeding or infectious process and reports any findings to physician.
4. Client avoids trauma to skin or mucous membranes resulting from straining or using harsh implements.
5. Client administers stool softeners and vitamin K as prescribed; avoids aspirin or aspirin products.
6. Client avoids exposure to persons with infections, crowded places, and use of or exposure to contaminated articles.
7. Client provides protective isolation measures based on laboratory results.
8. Client reports for all appointments for laboratory tests and physician follow-up.
9. Client secures and transports blood, urine, and sputum specimens to laboratory.

NURSING DIAGNOSIS DISTURBED BODY IMAGE

Related Factors: Biophysical effect of chemotherapy and/or radiation

Defining Characteristics: Alopecia; negative feeling about body; physical changes caused by therapy or surgery

OUTCOMES

Short Term
Improved body image, as evidenced by client's statement of reason for change and measures to take to disguise the change (expected in 2 to 3 days)

Long Term
Enhanced body image, as evidenced by client's verbalization of more positive feelings about appearance and the temporary state of the changes caused by chemotherapy and/or radiation (expected in 2 to 4 weeks and ongoing for duration of therapy)

NURSING INTERVENTIONS/INSTRUCTIONS

1. Before therapy, inform client of potential for hair loss, and instruct client to prepare with purchase of a wig or to use a scarf, turban, or large hat (first visit).
2. Allow client to express, in an accepting and nonjudgmental environment, feelings about hair loss, weight loss, nail changes, skin discoloration, and surgical scarring (each visit).
3. Instruct client to use a mild shampoo and to avoid use of curlers, dryers, hair spray, or hot iron and harsh brushing of hair (first visit).
4. Inform client that hair will grow back after treatment regimen but may be coarser and a slightly different color (first visit).
5. Inform client of clothing with high necks, loose fit, long sleeves, or leg covering (slacks) to select to cover exposed surgical areas or prostheses (first visit).

CLIENT AND FAMILY/CAREGIVER INTERVENTIONS

1. Client secures wig, hairpiece, scarf, or other clothing to deal with concerns such as hair loss, thinness, skin discoloration, scarring, or prosthesis.
2. Client uses makeup to cover discoloration of skin.
3. Client expresses feelings about appearance and coping skills to maintain lifestyle and improved body image.
4. Client avoids actions that injure hair, skin, or nails.

NURSING DIAGNOSIS | DEFICIENT KNOWLEDGE

▌*Related Factors:* Lack of information about therapy

▌*Defining Characteristics:* Request for information about chemotherapy and/or radiation therapy and effects and about health maintenance needs

OUTCOMES

▌*Short Term*
Adequate knowledge, as evidenced by client's statement of therapy regimen and of its temporary effect on health status (expected in 2 to 3 days)

▌*Long Term*

Adequate knowledge, as evidenced by client's compliance with medical protocol and actions to maintain optimal health and functioning during therapy (expected for duration of therapy)

NURSING INTERVENTIONS/INSTRUCTIONS

1. Assess client's lifestyle, ability to adapt, and learning ability and interest; family participation and support; and availability of community agencies that offer information and support (first visit).
2. Assess client's knowledge of reason for therapy and what effects can be expected (first visit).
3. Instruct client in administration of each chemotherapeutic drug, including what action the drug has on the malignant cells, route of administration, dose, frequency, and combination protocols, with length of time given, side effects, and treatments given to prevent or control them; provide client with a written protocol and check-off sheet to take to physician for administration of chemotherapy (first and second visits).
4. Instruct client in radiation site, effect of radiation, frequency of treatment, length of therapy, and protection of irradiated area (first visit).
5. Inform client that fatigue and other effects of therapy begin during the first week and gradually disappear 2 to 4 weeks after therapy ends (first visit).
6. Inform client of medications administered to counteract toxic effects of therapy and those given to treat complications of therapy (first visit).
7. Assist client in planning for fluid, nutritional, activity, rest, and sleep requirements and in modifying them according to effects of therapy (each visit).
8. Instruct client to notify physician of any severe side effects and to keep all follow-up appointments for medications, treatments, and laboratory tests (first visit).
9. Initiate referral to American Cancer Society, community agencies, and social and economic services to assist with transportation, meals, homemaking, shopping, economic problems, medical equipment and supplies, information, and psychologic support (any visit).

CLIENT AND FAMILY/CAREGIVER INTERVENTIONS

1. Client meets fluid, dietary, exercise, and sleep requirements based on assessment and abilities.
2. Client verbalizes chemotherapy and/or radiation protocol and measures to take to promote desired effect.
3. Client maintains positive attitude regarding effect and result of treatment.
4. Client administers medications as instructed to treat side effects of therapy.
5. Client reports uncontrolled side effects to physician.
6. Client keeps all appointments during therapy.
7. Client contacts American Cancer Society or other agencies as appropriate for needs.

❋ *Hospice Care*

Hospice care is a concept of holistic care that provides compassion, concern, support, and skilled care for the terminally ill client. It includes physical, psychologic, social, and spiritual care by a medically supervised interdisciplinary team of professionals and volunteers. Hospice care in the home is based on client and family need and may be part time, intermittent, scheduled on a regular basis, or provided on a 24-hour on-call basis. Support for grieving before and after the death of the client is included in the care plan for client and family.

Home care is primarily concerned with the control of symptoms and promotion of comfort through palliative care.

Primary Diagnosis:
Diagnosis of terminal illness and appropriate ICD code

NURSING DIAGNOSIS CHRONIC PAIN

❚ *Related Factors:* Chronic physical disability; progressive invasion of malignant tumor

■ *Defining Characteristics:* Altered ability to continue previous activities; long-term pain that becomes progressively more severe; tumor metastasis and pressure as mass becomes larger

OUTCOMES

■ *Short Term*
Pain decreased, as evidenced by client's statement that severity has been reduced with appropriate analgesic therapy (expected in 1 week)

■ *Long Term*
Pain absent or controlled with continuous or intermittent analgesic therapy administered orally or parenterally and based on need (expected for duration of terminal state)

NURSING INTERVENTIONS/INSTRUCTIONS

1. Assess status of pain and client's ability to tolerate pain (each visit).
2. Intravenously administer analgesic of choice that will achieve pain control, or instruct client in self-administration with a pump device, orally, and/or transdermally (first and second visits).
3. Provide a quiet, restful environment, and reduce stimuli to a minimum (first visit).
4. Instruct client to place self in position of comfort and to change positions gently and carefully to prevent additional pain (first visit).
5. Instruct client in guided imagery or relaxation techniques and provide music if these actions are appropriate (any visit).

CLIENT AND FAMILY/CAREGIVER INTERVENTIONS

1. Client or caregiver administers analgesic therapy as needed to relieve or control pain.
2. Caregiver maintains quiet, well-ventilated, temperature-controlled, restful environment.
3. Client avoids any stressful or anxiety-provoking situations.
4. Caregiver provides music or other desirable diversions as appropriate.

NURSING DIAGNOSIS: RISK FOR POWERLESSNESS

▮ *Related Factors:* Illness-related regimen

▮ *Defining Characteristics:* Expressions of uncertainty about fluctuating energy levels; resentment; anger; guilt; passivity; depression regarding physical deterioration; dependence on others; verbal expressions of having no control

OUTCOMES

▮ Short Term
Improved perception of control over current situation, as evidenced by client's expressions of increased input into care (expected in 1 week)

▮ Long Term
Optimal perception of ability to affect care outcome, as evidenced by client's participation in planning care

NURSING INTERVENTIONS/INSTRUCTIONS

1. Assess client's mental and emotional status; expressions of degree of control over situation; behavioral changes indicating resentment, anger, guilt, passivity, frustration; and use of defense mechanisms and coping and problem-solving skills (first visit).
2. Provide an accepting environment to promote expressions of frustrations and concerns (all visits).
3. Encourage client to participate in administering and planning care. Provide choices in areas of client's control (all visits).
4. Initiate referral to social services, support groups, counseling, or psychotherapy as indicated (any visit).
5. Inform client about the American Cancer Society as a resource for support (first visit).

CLIENT AND FAMILY/CAREGIVER INTERVENTIONS

1. Client expresses feelings about ability to control the situation.
2. Client participates in the planning and administration of care.
3. Client makes choices in areas of control.
4. Family/caregiver allows and encourages participation of client.
5. Client uses social services, support groups, and counseling as appropriate.

NURSING DIAGNOSIS COMPROMISED FAMILY COPING

▐ *Related Factors:* Situational crisis of dying family member

▐ *Defining Characteristics:* Significant persons preoccupied with personal reactions of fear, grief, guilt, and anxiety regarding client's condition

OUTCOMES

▐ Short Term
Improved coping, as evidenced by client's and family's acknowledgment of terminal state of illness and ability to grieve and support palliative treatment of family member (expected in 1 week)

▐ Long Term
Optimal coping abilities and support of family members to facilitate client's comfort and care (expected during hospice experience)

NURSING INTERVENTIONS/INSTRUCTIONS

1. Assess family interactions, ability to cope, strengths and inner resources, ability to support family member who is terminally ill, and presence of or need for an advance directive in compliance with the Patient Self-Determination Act (each visit).
2. Inform family that care and concern extend to all family members according to their needs (first visit).
3. Provide accurate information to family about treatment and goal of hospice care and about what can and cannot be changed; allow for questions and clarifications (each visit).
4. Provide client with written information about right to know what treatment is planned and his or her right to decide in advance what treatment is wanted or not wanted under special or serious conditions, to control medical treatment decisions. Inform client of right to execute advance directives through a living will or a durable power of attorney for health care according to state laws (first visit).
5. Encourage family to discuss strengths and options for use of coping skills that are helpful (each visit).
6. Include family members in as much care of client as they feel ready and able to perform; allow family to plan client's needs around family routines if possible (each visit).

7. Allow for family members to grieve in an accepting and nonjudgmental environment; assist family to identify grieving behaviors (each visit).
8. Inform family of government and community agencies and referral to interdisciplinary caregivers as needed and as available for hospice care (any visit).
9. Encourage family to accept social services, counseling from clergy, and psychotherapy as needed (first visit).

CLIENT AND FAMILY/CAREGIVER INTERVENTIONS

1. Client completes an advance directive stating choice for health care or names someone to make these choices if unable to make decisions about medical treatment.
2. Family members support and perform care if possible.
3. Family members verbalize concerns and feelings about client's condition during terminal stage of illness.
4. Family members cope with the imminent loss of a loved one.
5. Family members participate in planning and assisting with care.
6. Family members seek assistance from other professionals as needed.
7. Family members progress through grieving process.
8. Family prepares for death of family member.
9. Family maintains an open, honest approach and communication among family members and client.

NURSING DIAGNOSIS **FATIGUE**

▌**Related Factors:** Overwhelming psychologic or emotional demands; state of physical discomfort

▌**Defining Characteristics:** Weakness; inability to maintain and perform usual routines and ADL

OUTCOMES

▌**Short Term**
Minimal fatigue, as evidenced by client's obtaining needed assistance in personal care (expected in 1 to 2 weeks)

▌*Long Term*

Optimal level of energy maintained and fatigue level minimized during terminal phase of illness (expected during length of hospice care)

NURSING INTERVENTIONS/INSTRUCTIONS

1. Provide assistance or complete care, including bathing, grooming, personal hygiene, toileting or urinary and bowel elimination care, feeding and drinking as appropriate, and gown changing (each visit).
2. Provide position changes, skin care, and aids to prevent pressure on susceptible areas (each visit).
3. Provide clean linens, massage with lotion, glycerin to lips, and mouth care with rinses or glycerin swabs (each visit).
4. Perform range-of-motion exercises for all joints, and maintain body alignment without compromising comfort (each visit).
5. Provide necessary assistance and care for all body processes as needed, support all body parts, and provide for every physical need without causing additional fatigue to client (each visit).
6. Anticipate needs of client and family, and pace activities according to energy level of client and family; instruct about energy conservation (each visit).
7. Use touch to exhibit caring (each visit).
8. Provide all interventions on a continuous basis (each visit).

CLIENT AND FAMILY/CAREGIVER INTERVENTIONS

1. Client accepts total physical care and support of all failing systems on a continuous basis.
2. Family promotes quality of life with comfort and support to client.
3. Family conserves client's energy and preserves client's emotional and physical status.
4. Family and caregiver comply with legal and ethical issues regarding terminal care (e.g., withholding basic needs and non-resuscitation).

✳ *Neoplasms (Malignant)*

Malignant neoplasms, or cancer, is a term used to identify disease processes characterized by unregulated cell changes that are capable of metastasis or spread to other organs of the body. Cancer is classified according to the type of tissue involved: lymphomas originate in the lymphatic or infection-preventing system organs; leukemias originate in the blood-forming organs; sarcomas originate in connective tissue, bone, or muscle; and carcinomas originate in the epithelial cells of organs. Metastasis occurs via the vascular system or the lymphatic system or by implantation from the primary site of the tumor. In addition to the classification of cancer by anatomic site or tissue of origin, the cells are graded by appearance and differentiation, from grade I through grade IV, and the extent of the disease is described by staging, from stage 0 through stage IV. Typing, grading, and staging are used as a basis to determine treatment modalities, whose goal may be cure, control, or palliation of the disease. At least 200 diseases are included in this group, and this care plan for clients with malignant conditions is presented to assist with the problems common to all or most of these clients who receive care in the home. Because treatment for this condition consists of surgical intervention, chemotherapy, and/or radiation therapy, the Postoperative and Chemotherapy and External Radiation Therapy care plans should be used in conjunction with this one for a comprehensive approach to care of the client with cancer.

Home care is primarily concerned with the teaching and caring aspects of the client's physical and emotional needs and with implementation of the medical protocol to preserve and maintain optimal physical health and function.

Primary Diagnosis:
Diagnosis and ICD code relate to type and location
of malignancy

NURSING DIAGNOSIS **ANXIETY**

▌ *Related Factors:* Threat of death; threat to or change in health status

▌*Defining Characteristics:* Apprehension; uncertain outcome; increased tension and helplessness; fearfulness; poor prognosis; possible early death; changes in lifestyle and temperament; powerlessness; depression; withdrawal

OUTCOMES

▌*Short Term*

Decreased anxiety, as evidenced by client's statement of reduced fear, worry, and apprehension regarding change in health status and possible poor prognosis (expected in 1 to 3 weeks)

▌*Long Term*

Management or control of anxiety level, as evidenced by client's adaptation to change in lifestyle and by compliance with and acceptance of treatment regimen to achieve desired goal of medical protocol (expected in 1 to 2 months and ongoing)

NURSING INTERVENTIONS/INSTRUCTIONS

1. Assess client's mental and emotional status regarding life-threatening illness (see Psychosocial Assessment, p. 52, for guidelines) (first visit).
2. In an accepting environment, encourage expressions of fears and concerns and questions regarding therapy and its effects (each visit).
3. Assist client in identifying needed changes in lifestyle and methods to make necessary changes (first visit; reinforce each visit).
4. Inform client of all activities, treatments, tests, and effects to expect; reinforce information about the disease and client condition given by the physician (each visit).
5. Allow client to direct own care and make own choices when possible regarding treatment regimen and plan of care (each visit).
6. Initiate referral to counseling, support group, and agencies that may assist with social services and economic and health care needs (first visit).
7. Instruct client in relaxation exercises, music therapy, or imagery, or introduce other techniques to reduce anxiety (first and second visits).

CLIENT AND FAMILY/CAREGIVER INTERVENTIONS

1. Client develops coping methods for long-term treatment and possible outcome.
2. Client maintains manageable level of anxiety.
3. Client seeks information that will reduce anxiety.
4. Client expresses fears and concerns about necessary changes in lifestyle.
5. Client contacts and consults with available support services.

NURSING DIAGNOSIS ANTICIPATORY GRIEVING

■ *Related Factors:* Perceived potential loss of physiopsychosocial well-being

■ *Defining Characteristics:* Expression of distress at potential loss; anger; guilt; denial of potential loss; sorrow; choked feelings; changes in sleep, eating, and activity patterns

OUTCOMES

■ *Short Term*
Progress in grieving, as evidenced by attitude and behavior changes manifested by stage in process (expected in days)

■ *Long Term*
Grief process resolving, as evidenced by client's resumption of lifestyle with or without changes as needed and by integration of grieving stage into lifestyle and activities (expected in 2 to 3 months and ongoing)

NURSING INTERVENTIONS/INSTRUCTIONS

1. Assess degree and stage of grief (each visit).
2. Inform client of stages of grieving process and that behavior is acceptable for specific stage, that progress goes back and forth, and that acceptance will be final stage (first visit).
3. Allow expression of feelings and perception of effects of therapy, potential loss, and death in a nonjudgmental environment (each visit).
4. Initiate referral for social service, psychologic, and spiritual counseling as appropriate (any visit).

CLIENT AND FAMILY/CAREGIVER INTERVENTIONS

1. Client progresses through grief process to acceptance.
2. Client seeks counseling as needed.
3. Client verbalizes stages and behaviors during grief process.

NURSING DIAGNOSIS DEFICIENT KNOWLEDGE

Related Factors: Lack of information about disease

Defining Characteristics: Request for information, at understandable level, about cancer, treatment modalities, and limitations imposed by the disease

OUTCOMES

Short Term
Adequate knowledge, as evidenced by client's statement of disease process and type of cancer, diagnostic and classification methods, proposed treatment, and expected results (expected in 1 week)

Long Term
Optimal knowledge, as evidenced by client's understanding of and compliance with treatment protocol to achieve optimal physical and functional status in identified therapeutic goal (expected in 2 to 3 months and ongoing, depending on disease progression)

NURSING INTERVENTIONS/INSTRUCTIONS

1. Assess client's lifestyle, ability to adapt, learning ability and interest, family participation and support, and need for reinforcement of information given by physician (first visit).
2. Inform client of disease process, possible causes, reasons for signs and symptoms, and changes in body appearance and function (first visit).
3. Inform client of importance of maintaining all follow-up care and appointments with physician, for laboratory testing, and for scheduled chemotherapy and/or radiation therapy during treatment protocol (first visit; reinforce on second visit).
4. Provide client with accurate information about the benefits of proven therapies and fallacies of unproven methods of cancer treatment, which might include chemicals or drugs, dietary

supplements, and occult or mechanical devices or techniques (first visit).

5. Outline treatment protocol, length of therapy, expected discomforts and results, and side effects in honest, understandable terms (each visit).

6. Inform client of any limitations or restrictions to follow during therapy, including performing ADL within energy tolerance, avoiding sun exposure and alcohol intake, and arranging for leaving work or loss of work during therapy.

7. Inform client of common problem of fear associated with the disease and methods of coping with and reducing it after diagnosis and during the initial phases of treatment (first visit).

8. Inform client of and refer to hospice care if appropriate, and explain the availability of this care in the future if appropriate (any visit).

9. Refer client to American Cancer Society for information, support groups, and equipment or supplies as needed (any visit).

10. In a realistic manner, inform client of importance of a hopeful attitude about the disease and the progress that has been made in curing the disease (any visit).

CLIENT AND FAMILY/CAREGIVER INTERVENTIONS

1. Client verbalizes information about the disease and important factors that contribute to its effect on the body.

2. Client verbalizes needed changes in lifestyle to accommodate treatment regimen.

3. Client establishes and maintains hope.

4. Client adapts to presence of cancer and complies with scheduled follow-up appointments.

5. Client avoids unproven therapies and methods of controlling disease.

6. Client contacts and uses community agencies for information and support.

7. Client participates in goal setting and decision making regarding care.

✳ *Postoperative Care Following Inpatient or Outpatient Surgery*

Postoperative care involves the physical and emotional care of a client following surgery and discharge from the hospital or care of a client after surgery performed in an outpatient surgical unit and discharge to home on the day of surgery. Outpatient surgery usually involves minor procedures that are performed with administration of local anesthetics and/or short-acting inhalation anesthetics.

Home care is primarily concerned with the teaching of safety management and preservation of health and function following outpatient surgery and with maintenance and reinforcement of the hospital discharge teaching for follow-up care at home.

Primary Diagnoses:
Diagnosis and ICD code will usually relate to
condition for which the surgery is performed
Nonhealing Surgical Wound—ICD code: 998.83
Wound Infection, Postoperative—ICD code: 998.59

NURSING DIAGNOSIS RISK FOR INFECTION

▌*Related Factors:* Inadequate primary defenses; invasive procedure

▌*Defining Characteristics:* Surgical wound (broken skin) with redness, swelling, pain, and drainage; respiratory changes (stasis of secretions) with decreased breath sounds and shortness of breath; urinary changes (stasis of body fluids) with cloudy, foul-smelling urine with or without indwelling catheter

OUTCOMES

▌Short Term
Reduced risk of infectious process following surgery, as evidenced by client's compliance with postoperative measures to prevent bacterial contamination (expected in 1 to 2 weeks)

▌*Long Term*

Absence of infectious process, as evidenced by wound healing without complication and by absence of postoperative complications, with return of optimal health and functional status (expected in 1 to 2 months)

NURSING INTERVENTIONS/INSTRUCTIONS

1. Assess and instruct client to assess wound site(s) for edge approximation and healing; drainage device for characteristics and amount of wound drainage; changes in color, temperature, or drainage; presence of swelling at surgical site; and increased pain (each visit).
2. Assess urine for characteristic changes and catheter for patency if one is in place; assess for respiratory changes in rate, depth, and ease and for changes in sputum to yellow or other color (each visit).
3. Instruct client in handwashing technique and to perform before direct care, before meals, and after using bathroom (first visit).
4. Instruct client in continued use of incentive spirometry and coughing and deep breathing exercises, and assist client in planning daily schedule for times and frequency (first visit).
5. Instruct client in wound care and dressing change using sterile technique; how to care for and dress wound drains and device; how to remove dressing and apply smaller dressing; and to report pain, redness, or swelling at site. Allow for return demonstration (first visit; reinforce on second visit).
6. Instruct client in need to void every 2 hours and to report any change in color or odor; teach client how to care for catheter and prevent entry of bacteria into the bladder (first visit).
7. Instruct client to monitor temperature and to note chilling or elevation to higher than 1.00° F and to report to physician (first visit).
8. Instruct client in administration of antibiotic therapy to prevent or treat infection, whether oral or topical (ointment, drops), including route, dose, time, frequency, side effects, and drug and food interactions, and instruct client to complete entire prescription (first visit).
9. Instruct client to avoid exposure to people with upper respiratory infections or who are ill (first visit).

CLIENT AND FAMILY/CAREGIVER INTERVENTIONS

1. Client administers antibiotic therapy correctly and as prescribed.
2. Client provides care to surgical site as needed, using aseptic technique.
3. Client monitors temperature and condition of site(s).
4. Client assesses respiratory and urinary function and reports signs and symptoms of infection.
5. Client uses handwashing technique when appropriate.
6. Client avoids exposure to persons with infections or touching wound site.

NURSING DIAGNOSIS **BATHING/HYGIENE, DRESSING/GROOMING, TOILETING SELF-CARE DEFICIT**

■*Related Factors:* Pain; discomfort with movement; intolerance to activity

■*Defining Characteristics:* Decreased strength and endurance; inability to perform or complete ADL independently; reluctance to attempt movement and activity; fear of injury to incision

OUTCOMES

■*Short Term*
Improvement in self-care performance, as evidenced by client's progressive participation in ADL and increased activity within prescribed limitations (expected in 1 to 2 weeks)

■*Long Term*
Independence in ADL, as evidenced by client's meeting requirements for self-care within limitations or restrictions for optimal postoperative health and function and return to work (expected in 2 months, depending on surgical procedure)

NURSING INTERVENTIONS/INSTRUCTIONS

1. Assess client's ability to perform ADL; fatigue level; pain on movement or during activity; and need for special procedures or treatments before, during, or after ADL (see Functional Assessment, p. 55, for guidelines) (each visit).

2. Instruct client to assist with ADL as needed without compromising client independence or progressive self-care (first visit).
3. Allow client to develop own plan of progressive care and goals to achieve during convalescence and to revise plan as needed (each visit).
4. Instruct client to accept assistance when needed until weakness and fatigue diminish (first visit).
5. Instruct client to avoid strenuous activity or activities (first visit).
6. Instruct client in use of energy-saving devices and techniques for ADL (first visit).
7. Instruct client in administration of analgesics for pain based on assessment before activities (first visit).
8. Instruct client to rest after activity, pace activities, and set limits if needed (first visit).
9. Refer HHA to assist with ADL as needed (first visit).

CLIENT AND FAMILY/CAREGIVER INTERVENTIONS

1. Client schedules rest and activity based on individual needs and condition.
2. Client participates in ADL in set limits, with goals for daily or weekly progress toward independence.
3. Client assists with any activity requiring support; asks for assistance when needed until independence is achieved.
4. Client uses energy-saving devices or aids in ADL.
5. Client administers analgesics when needed, based on assessment, to allow for optimal activity and ADL performance.

NURSING DIAGNOSIS DEFICIENT KNOWLEDGE

Related Factors: Lack of information about follow-up postoperative care

Defining Characteristics: Request for information about postoperative activity restrictions, nutrition and fluid needs, bowel and urinary elimination, and prevention of complications

OUTCOMES

Short Term
Adequate knowledge, as evidenced by client's statement of postoperative medical regimen requirements and performance of

postoperative procedures and treatments (expected in 1 to 2 weeks)

▌*Long Term*

Optimal knowledge, as evidenced by client's compliance with postoperative care regimen to achieve return to optimal health and functioning (expected in 4 to 6 weeks)

NURSING INTERVENTIONS/INSTRUCTIONS

1. Assess client's lifestyle, ability to adapt, learning ability and interest, and family participation and support (first visit).
2. Assess client's knowledge of surgical procedures, reason for surgical intervention for correction of problem, and where procedure was performed (hospital or outpatient unit); provide information needed or reinforce information already received if necessary (first visit).
3. Instruct client in medication administration as ordered, including times, dose, frequency, side effects, and food and drug interactions (first and second visits).
4. Inform client of bowel and bladder elimination changes and causes and about use of stool softener, fluid intake, and exercising to assist in return to normal pattern (first visit).
5. Inform client of importance of compliance with activity and exercise regimen proposed, and instruct client to avoid activities that place stress on operative area (e.g., changing position, lifting, pushing, pulling, stooping) and to avoid heavy lifting, carrying, or straining (first visit).
6. Instruct client in incision care and in protecting the incision during bathing with a plastic cover taped to skin on the sides in shape of a picture frame (first visit).
7. Instruct client in appropriate amount of daily fluid intake, up to 3 L/day, and inclusion of protein and vitamin C in dietary planning; offer food lists and sample menus and assist client in coordinating them with food and fluid preferences (first and second visits).
8. Inform client of time to resume work schedule and activities to avoid (any visit).
9. Instruct client to report incisional pain, increased drainage, elevated temperature, or any discomfort or changes in other body areas (first visit).
10. Instruct client to comply with follow-up schedule to see physician as advised after surgery or hospital discharge (first visit).

CLIENT AND FAMILY/CAREGIVER INTERVENTIONS

1. Client administers all medications accurately; uses check-off sheet as a reminder and to avoid errors.
2. Client establishes and maintains bowel and urinary elimination patterns.
3. Client reports adverse effects of medications, treatments, and surgical intervention if appropriate.
4. Client participates in approved activities and avoids those that place stress on incisional area.
5. Client provides and ingests fluids and nutrients to facilitate health.
6. Client maintains a written daily plan for compliance with post-operative requirements.
7. Client returns to work or seeks occupational rehabilitation or retraining if appropriate.

✸ *Appendixes* ✸

✳ *Documentation/Insurance Payment Guidelines*

BASIC CONSIDERATIONS

1. The Outcome and Assessment Information Set (OASIS) data of Medicare and Medicaid clients should be accurately documented at the designated points of care (Start of Care [SOC], recertification, transfer, resumption of care, discharge, death), which maintains required timelines. (OASIS data are identified in the Assessment section of this book.) Accuracy of the data gathered is crucial because these data help determine reimbursement under the Prospective Payment System (PPS). An accurate primary diagnosis and its International Classification of Diseases (ICD) code are included in these data.

2. Homebound status must be documented at least weekly, with specific notations of physical, mental, or emotional limitations or restrictions that require a considerable and taxing effort to leave home except for church, therapy, physician, or laboratory appointments (usually determined by payor); examples of limitations or restrictions include bed- or wheelchair-bound status; severe pain, shortness of breath with slight exertion, indwelling catheter, poor balance, or unsteady gait as a result of surgery or illness; and fractures or other disabilities that prevent ambulation without assistance or use of aids; draining wounds or dressing change; partial or complete paralysis; mental confusion; and extreme anxiety or paranoia.

3. Documentation of home care includes the criteria needed to meet state and federal certification and licensure requirements.

4. Documentation of the plan of care and the client's progress toward goals supports reimbursement requirements of Medicare, Medicaid, and third-party payors.

5. Documentation allows for continuity of planned care by providing a method of communication among all of the disciplines involved in the provision of care.

6. Documentation and maintenance of an accurate record is essential because the record is considered to be a legal document that ensures that professional standards have been followed in the delivery of home care.
7. Documentation and maintenance of an accurate record provides data for research and audits for payor and accreditation surveys.
8. Documentation must be factual, objective, succinct, descriptive, and relevant.
9. Teaching of clients and family members must be clearly recorded.

GENERAL DOCUMENTATION REQUIREMENTS FOR ALL CARE PLANS

1. Date and signature of nurse preparing the care plan
2. Assessment data and client status in major areas affected
3. Changes in client's health status
4. Client and family response and adaptation to illness
5. Plan of care with inclusion of all accepted components (i.e., primary diagnosis, ICD code, client goals, expected outcome dates, frequency and duration of care, physician signature)
6. Nursing skills provided, including all assessments and teaching
7. Client progress toward goals
8. Need for further assessment, instruction, or referral
9. Plan for and time of next visit
10. Readiness and plan for discharge from home visits
11. Dates and signatures of all professional and nonprofessional personnel performing care, and evaluation when and where appropriate
12. Copy of the plan available for client and family

ESSENTIAL DOCUMENTATION COMPONENTS

1. OASIS data, health history, and physical assessment with emphasis on system(s) related to the client's medical diagnosis (listing all relevant diagnoses and designating the principal or primary diagnosis and all related ICD codes).
2. Dates of onset or exacerbation for diagnoses, including the primary diagnosis (establishes reasonable and necessary requirement). The primary diagnosis reflects the predominant reason skilled services are required.

3. Identified nursing diagnoses, based on analysis of assessment data, with dates for each problem on the care plan.

4. Client-focused, measurable, realistic goals or outcomes (short- and long-term in collaboration with the client) and achievement dates documented at least weekly, with the nursing interventions to achieve the specific outcomes and personnel responsible for the activities.

5. Specific skilled-nursing interventions implemented to achieve client goals and client response to these actions.

6. Evaluation of goal fulfillment at designated time intervals based on changes in client condition and any modification of the care plan resulting from the assessment.

7. Time frames in which care will be provided (frequency and duration), depending on client need.

8. All care (specific and general) that relates to the medical diagnoses and physician orders; physician signature should appear on the document according to agency and payor requirements. Payor approvals, when required, are documented for each visit.

9. Unstable state or technology dependence that requires skilled nursing care and client response to changes in treatments or care.

10. Treatments, exercise, and other rehabilitation regimens to restore function lost because of illness or disability; any obstacles (e.g., mental capabilities, language barrier) that need to be overcome to achieve optimal health.

11. All teaching to client and family to develop ability to perform care and procedures, including disease-related information, assessments, strategies, demonstrations, and record keeping; note poor comprehension by and lack of capability of client and need to reteach.

12. Referrals to professional therapists, social services, and community resources. Ongoing documentation of communication between all disciplines.

13. Supervisory visits (frequency depending on payor requirements) noting evaluation of licensed vocational nurse, home health aide (HHA), client and family response to care, and need for care plan revision or restatement of existing plan.

14. Discharge plan and instructions, physician orders, summary to physician, case closing date; discharge must be considered if the client does not progress toward goals after a reasonable

time or if he or she no longer meets criteria for service eligibility.

UNACCEPTABLE WORD USAGE AND STATEMENTS

1. Use of *chronic* instead of *an acute exacerbation*
2. Use of *monitor* instead of *assess* or *evaluate* if condition has stabilized
3. Use of *discussed* instead of *instructed*
4. Use of *check* instead of *assess*
5. Use of words such as *stabilized* instead of *responding to treatment*
6. Use of *provide emotional support* instead of *making a referral*
7. Use of *prevent* if instruction has already been given
8. Use of *improvement* instead of specific assessment data
9. Use of a subjective general statement (e.g., *general weakness*) instead of an objective statement (e.g., *ambulates only 10 feet without fatigue, dizziness, dyspnea*)
10. Statements of *lack of progress when progress should be seen* instead of *inability to participate in therapy because of mental or physical disabilities*
11. Statements of repetitive teaching, except if client has limited intelligence or increased anxiety; *limitations must be reflected in documentation*
12. Statements about trips that client takes that imply non–homebound status (Medicare clients must be discharged when no longer homebound)
13. Statements of medications reviewed
14. Statements of maintenance care
15. Statements of *unstable* states instead of noting *specific interventions* and *changes in client condition and treatment*

PAYOR REIMBURSEMENT GUIDELINES*

1. Usually all clients who are older than 65 years of age, who have been disabled for 2 years or more, or who have end-stage renal disease are eligible to receive Medicare benefits for health care. These clients may also have supplemental private

*Requirements and benefits for government and private insurance plans change periodically, and guidelines should be compared and validated as to what is and what is not covered at a given time.

health insurance (Medi-Gap) that covers expenses not paid for by Medicare or may belong to a health maintenance organization (HMO) that accepts Medicare benefits without additional private coverage; these plans vary and benefits are policy specific. Medicare-eligible individuals who belong to an HMO do not receive benefits from both Medicare and the HMO.

2. The PPS is a standardized reimbursement system for home care provided for Medicare-eligible clients. PPS reimbursement rate is adjusted based on case mix to reflect the severity of the client's condition. The adjustment is based on certain clinical, functional, and service items of the OASIS assessment called *Home Health Resource Groups* (HHRGs). The reimbursement covers a 60-day period called an *episode*.

3. Medicaid is a government assistance plan that differs from state to state. Coverage is reserved for a segment of the population whose economic status complies with the payment standards set by government regulations (usually 50% federally and 50% state funded).

4. Civilian Health and Medical Program of the Uniformed Services (CHAMPUS) insurance benefits and coverage are reserved for government employees who are eligible to receive these payments via past or present employment or service to the government.

5. Private health insurance can be individually owned and paid for or part of a group policy sponsored and paid for completely or in part by the client's employer. The coverage also can include varied options for deductibles, prescription drugs, vision and dental health, HMOs, preferred provider organizations (PPOs), and others.

6. Private long-term facility care insurance can include home care benefits following a hospitalization or long-term facility stay or private home care exclusively as a single policy or as a rider to a long-term nursing home policy.

7. Private combination health care insurance plans may cover long-term facility care, alternate or assistive facility care, and home care that includes case management planning.

8. Major areas of coverage usually include assessment, teaching, and performing complex hands-on care and procedures, with hours or number of visits allowed depending on acuity and type of skilled care needed; skilled care and lack of someone to perform personal care is needed before an HHA is assigned and will be paid.

9. Medicare, Medicaid, and some third-party payors require documentation of homebound status and skilled care need with specific detailed functional limitations, dates of onset, and appropriate descriptive adjectives included in the medical diagnoses; a medical plan of care; and medical orders for home care.

10. The frequency of paid visits depends on the diagnosis, acuteness of the illness, homebound status, client or caregiver ability to learn, presence of a caregiver to teach, stability of client's condition, multiple medical diagnoses, and finally insurance criteria. Parameters may or may not be given as a basis for the acceptable number of visits. Care usually begins with a higher frequency of visits, tapers down if possible, and schedules for two or three times per week. Daily visits may be allowed for a limited period; however, documentation must justify the need, and an end date is required if the daily visits extend beyond 21 days.

11. Private home care insurance usually provides a designated amount of money available for daily care for a specified number of years based on the amount selected by the client. Criteria for payment commonly includes medical necessity and need for care in at least two or three of the five activities of daily living (ADL).

12. Written approvals for all visits are required by most payors other than Medicare and must be obtained before the visit is made.

13. Nursing history, assessments, OASIS data, and care plan documentation that include all of the specific requirements identified in the Essential Documentation Components must be present.

EXAMPLES OF ACTIVITIES USUALLY COVERED

1. New diagnosis of diabetes requiring instruction for insulin administration, glucose monitoring, foot care, dietary regimen

2. New intestinal or urinary diversion surgical care

3. Unstable hypertension or other cardiac conditions requiring medication, dietary changes

4. Intramuscular (IM), intravenous (IV) injections or infusion therapy

5. Renal or peritoneal dialysis

6. Nasogastric, gastrostomy feedings and care

7. Tracheostomy care and tube change, assisted ventilation

8. Wound care and dressing changes
9. Foley catheter changes, disimpaction
10. Medication regimen related to disease, one medication per visit
11. Disease pathology and signs and symptoms
12. Any assessment and teaching function that is reasonable and necessary

EXAMPLES OF ACTIVITIES NOT USUALLY COVERED (UNLESS NOT ABLE TO BE PERFORMED BY CLIENT OR CAREGIVER)

1. Vital signs, intake and output
2. Stable client who continues to be monitored
3. Repetition and reinforcement of instruction (medications, treatments)
4. Any preventive care, especially if previously taught (pressure ulcers)
5. Emotional support
6. Positioning in bed, active or passive range-of-motion exercises
7. Medication injections if not medically necessary
8. Procedures performed by person not considered to be skilled
9. Venipunctures, except when another skilled service is required

EXAMPLES OF PROBLEM AREAS FOR COVERAGE

1. Frequent physician contacts with no new orders
2. Chronic diagnosis with no change in treatment plan by physician and no evidence of exacerbation
3. Too few or too many visits
4. Procedures not corresponding with diagnoses
5. Rehabilitative claims of more than 3 months unless properly documented
6. Repeated instruction
7. Custodial care
8. Not homebound (varies with different payors)
9. Unskilled or intermittent care with no skilled need
10. Daily visits for more than 3 weeks unless estimated time of healing and necessity of teaching are documented
11. Duplication of services

✳ *Indications for Referrals to Therapy/Social Services*

The following lists examples of indications necessitating referrals to therapy or social services. This list is not all-inclusive; other indications may also apply.

PHYSICAL THERAPY (LOWER EXTREMITY)

Abnormality of gait
Ambulation difficulty
Amputation (lower extremity)
Amyotrophic lateral sclerosis
Ankylosis
Arthritis
Back pain
Burns
Contractures
Coordination disorder
Disuse/atrophy of muscles
Fracture (lower extremities)
Hip replacement
Knee replacement
Lumbar stenosis
Muscle weakness
Paralysis
Parkinson's disease
Rotator cuff syndrome
Spinal cord disorder
Weakness, general

OCCUPATIONAL THERAPY (UPPER EXTREMITY)

ADL decline
Amputation (upper extremity)
Ankylosis
Arthritis
Burns
Cerebrovascular accidents
Contractures
Disuse/atrophy of muscles

Fracture (upper extremity)
Muscle weakness
Paralysis
Parkinson's disease
Reduced energy
Spinal cord disorder
Weakness, general

SPEECH/LANGUAGE PATHOLOGY

Aphasia
Cognitive deficits
Communication disorder
Developmental delays
Dysarthria
Dyslexia
Dysphagia
Dysphasia
Hearing loss
Language delay
Language disorder
Mental/behavioral problems
Reading disorder
Speech disturbance
Vocal cord paralysis

MEDICAL SOCIAL WORKER

Cognitive therapy
Community resource needs
Crisis intervention
Dementia management
Depression/anxiety/fear
Emotional/mental problems
Environmental issues
Family conflict
Grief and loss
Long-term planning
Memory loss
Pain/discomfort
Safety issues
Short-term therapy
Stress management
Substance abuse
Suicidal behaviors

✳ *Laboratory Values**

Test	Value Range	SI Range
BLOOD		
Acid phosphatase	0.13-0.63 U/L at 37° C	2.2-10.5 U/L at 37° C
Albumin	3.5-5 g/dl	35-50 g/L
Aldolase	3-8.2 U/dl at 37° C	22-59 mU/L at 37° C
Alkaline phosphatase	30-120 IU/L at 37° C	30-120 U/L at 37° C
Ammonia	80-110 µg/dl	47-65 µmol/L
Amylase	16-120 Somogyi units/dl	30-220 U/L
Arterial blood gases		
pH	7.35-7.45	7.35-7.45
P_{CO_2}	35-45 mm Hg	
P_{O_2}	80-100 mm Hg	
Bilirubin		
Total	0.3-1.0 mg/dl	5.1-17 µmol/L
Direct	0.1-0.3 mg/dl	1.7-5.1 µmol/L
Indirect	0.2-0.8 mg/dl	3.4-12 µmol/L
Calcium		
Total	7.6-10.4 mg/dl	1.9-2.6 mmol/L
Ionized	4.5-5.6 mg/dl	1.05-1.3 mmol/L
Chloride	98-106 mEq/L	98-106 mmol/L
Cholesterol	<200 mg/dl	<5.2 mmol/L
(age, diet related)		
Complete blood count		
Hematocrit (male)	42%-52%	0.42-0.52
Hematocrit (female)	37%-47%	0.37-0.47
Hemoglobin (male)	14-18.0 g/dl	8.7-11.2 mmol/L
Hemoglobin (female)	12.0-16.0 g/dl	7.4-9.9 mmol/L
Red cell count (male)	$4.7\text{-}6.1 \times 10^6/\mu l$	$4.7\text{-}6.1 \times 10^{12}/L$
Red cell count (female)	$4.2\text{-}5.4 \times 10^6/\mu l$	$4.2\text{-}5.4 \times 10^{12}/L$
White cell count	$5000\text{-}70,000/mm^3$	$5\text{-}10 \times 10^9/L$
Creatine kinase		
Male	55-170 U/L at 37° C	55-170 U/L at 37° C
Female	30-135 U/L at 37° C	30-135 U/L at 37° C
Creatinine	0.6-1.2 mg/dl	53-106 µmol/L

*Modified from Pagana KD, Pagana TJ: *Mosby's diagnostic and laboratory test reference*, ed 5, St Louis, 2001, Mosby.

Test	Value Range	SI Range
Erythrocyte sedimentation rate (male)	<15 mm/hr	
Erythrocyte sedimentation rate (female)	<20 mm/hr	
Folate	5-25 ng/ml	11-57 nmol/L
Glucose	70-105 mg/dl (fasting)	3.9-5.8 mmol/L
Immunoglobulins		
IgG	565-1765 mg/dl	
IgA	85-385 mg/dl	
IgM	55-375 mg/dl	
IgD	minimal	
IgE	minimal	
Iron	60-160 µg/dl (total)	11-29 µmol/L
Lactate dehydrogenase	100-190 U/L at 37° C	100-190 U/L at 37° C
Lipase	0-160 U/L	0-160 U/L
Magnesium	1.3-2.1 mEq/L	0.65-105 mmol/L
Partial thromboplastin time (activated)	30-40 sec	
Phosphorus	3-4.5 mg/dl	0.97-1.45 mmol/L
Platelet count	150,000-450,000/mm^3	150-400 × 10^9/L
Potassium	3.5-5.0 mEq/L	3.5-5.0 mmol/L
Proteins		
Total	6.4-8.3 g/dl	64-83 g/L
Albumin	3.5-5 g/dl	35-50 g/L
Globulin	2.3-3.4 g/dl	
Prothrombin time	11-12.5 sec	
Reticulocyte count	0.5%-2% of total red blood cells	
Sodium	136-145 mEq/L	136-145 mmol/L
Thyroid tests		
Thyroxine (total)	5-11 µg/dl	64-142 nmol/L
Thyroxine (free)	0.8-2.8 ng/dl	10-36 pmol/L
Triiodothyronine	75-220 ng/dl	1.21-3.4 nmol/L
Transferases		
Aspartate aminotransferase	0-35 U/L	0-0.58 µKat/L
Alanine aminotransferase	4-36 U/L at 37° C	4-36 U/L
γ-Glutamyl	8-38 U/L at 37° C	8-38 U/L
Triglycerides	40-160 mg/dl	0.4-1.81 mmol/L
Urea nitrogen	10-20 mg/dl	3.6-7.1 mmol/L
Uric acid (male)	4.0-8.5 mg/dl	0.24-0.51 mmol/L

Test	Value Range	SI Range
Uric acid (female)	2.7-7.3 mg/dl	0.16-0.43 mmol/L
URINE		
Creatinine clearance (male)	107-130 ml/min	1.78-2.32 ml/sec
Creatinine clearance (female)	87-107 ml/min	1.45-1.78 ml/sec
Glucose	Negative (random) 130 mg/24 hr	Negative 0.72 mmol/24 hr
Ketones	Negative	Negative
Osmolality	850 mOsm/kg water (fluid restriction)	>850 mmol/kg
Specific gravity	1.005-1.030	1.010-1.025
Uric acid	250-750 mg/24 hr	1.48-4.43 mmol/24 hr
Vanillylmandelic acid	<6.8 mg/24 hr	<35 µmol/24 hr
FECES		
Bile	Negative (random)	Negative
Fat	2-6 g/24 hr (total)	7-21 mmol/24 hr
Occult blood	Negative	Negative

THERAPEUTIC DRUG LEVELS

	Therapeutic Level	Toxic Level
Digoxin	0.8-2 ng/ml	>2.4 ng/ml
Gentamicin	5-10 µg/ml	>12 µg/ml
Lithium	0.8-1.2 mEq/L	>2.0 mEq/L
Phenytoin	10-20 µg/ml	>30 µg/ml
Salicylate	100-250 µg/ml	>300 µg/ml
Theophylline	10-20 µg/ml	>20 µg/ml

❋ *Medication Administration and Teaching Guidelines*

Medication administration to clients in the home by the caregiver or self-administration is the focus of these guidelines. Major responsibilities of the home care nurse are teaching the client and/or family to perform these procedures correctly and assessing the effects. Some of the more complex administration methods and routes require adequate or more extensive instruction and practice time to ensure safe compliance with a medication regimen. Medications administered in the home are prescribed by the physician or other prescriber and include those given orally, sublingually, topically, intramuscularly, subcutaneously, intrathecally, intravenously, by inhalation, and by feeding tube and are scheduled for regular administration or in response to requests when needed. The following information provides helpful tips, as well as actual procedures and teaching performed by the nurse for the client and/or family to ensure safe administration and effective results from drug therapy.

TIPS FOR TEACHING SAFE ADMINISTRATION

1. Assess for age, weight, and drug allergies.
2. Teach about compatibility with foods and other medications.
3. Note medications taken, both prescribed and over the counter.
4. Assess past dependency or risk for present dependency on drugs.
5. Instruct regarding use of alcohol, caffeine-containing beverages, herbal products, and tobacco.
6. Provide information about each drug and special recommendations for administration.
7. Determine daily routines and best times for medication administration.
8. Assess ability to swallow medications and use of alternative forms or routes.
9. Assess client's cognitive and intellectual capacity, developmental level, readiness to learn, past learning experiences, and understanding of drug administration.
10. Give thorough instructions that include the drug name, reason for use, dose, frequency, route, form, length of time, measurement device to use, expected effects, and adverse side effects to report and what actions to take.
11. Encourage return demonstrations until client shows competency with the procedure (usually more appropriate for injections).
12. Provide a written procedure and time schedule for administration of medications, check sheet, and compartmental medication boxes as indicated.
13. Inform client that if drug is forgotten, to wait until next dosage time unless dose can be taken in 1 hour after scheduled time (depends on frequency of dosage).
14. Note expiration dates and store in a cool, dry, locked cabinet with lid tightly fixed on the original container and labeled with the written instructions; refrigerate if medicine is to be kept at a lower temperature.

15. Instruct client to discard all expired medications.
16. Ensure that devices used in medication administration are accompanied by inserts with instructions for use or pamphlet with manufacturer's directions for use, care, and type of administration set to use.

ORAL MEDICATIONS

1. Check medication label for the name, amount, and time before, during, and after administration to ensure accuracy; compare with drug container or checklist.
2. Administer according to special instructions such as before or after meals, at bedtime, number of times per day, with or without food, use of a straw, under the tongue, or in the cheek.
3. Select device to give the medication based on form and ability to swallow and prepare medications:
   - Measuring spoon, calibrated cup for liquid form, paper medicine cup
   - Pill crusher to crush tablets and water, juice, or soft food for mixing
4. Place tablet toward the back of the mouth and offer a glass of water to swallow.
5. Note side effects and instruct client to stop the medication and report to the physician immediately.

TOPICAL MEDICATIONS (TRANSCUTANEOUS, SUPPOSITORY, OINTMENT)

Gloves and sterile technique are used to perform all topical procedures when exposure to body fluid or breaks in skin are anticipated or present.

1. Check medication label for the name, amount, and time.
2. Expose area to be treated, position client and provide privacy if needed, and remove dressings.
3. Uncap ointment and squeeze small amount and discard, apply to affected area with a sponge or applicator.
4. Cleanse skin and apply patch to administer via transcutaneous route for prescribed time.
5. Insert correct dosage suppository, removed from wrapper, into the rectum past the internal sphincter with a cotton-protected finger that has been moistened with water; hold buttocks together for approximately 5 minutes to prevent expulsion if needed.

EYE, EAR, AND NOSE MEDICATIONS

▋*Eye Administration*

1. Cleanse around eyes with a warm, damp cloth to remove any secretions; leave in place if crusted material is present until soft enough to be wiped away; draw medication up into the eyedropper.
2. Position client in a supine position with head slightly tilted backward and to the side of the eye to receive the medication.
3. Ask the client to look up; gently pull the lower lid downward and place the correct number of drops into the lower lid using the other hand; avoid allowing the tip of the dropper to touch any part of the eye or skin.
4. Ask client to close eyes tightly and open again to disperse the fluid; wipe any excess medication from around the eye with tissue.
5. For eye ointment, follow same procedure and squeeze the ointment across the inner aspect of the lower lid from the canthus to the outer aspect of the eye.

▋*Ear Administration*

1. Warm bottle of medication in a pan of water and check to assess warmth to avoid cold or hot drops; draw up medication into the ear dropper.
2. Cleanse outside of ears to remove any drainage with a tissue or cotton-tipped applicator; avoid touching the external ear canal.
3. Place client on side to expose ear to receive medication and then on the other side to receive the medication.
4. Pull the outer ear upward and backward to straighten canal; place correct number of drops in each ear toward the side of the canal; avoid allowing tip of dropper to touch ears.
5. Maintain position of the head for a minute following the drops in each ear and wipe away excess from the outer ear if needed.
6. Place a cotton ball in each ear to prevent medication from leaking; change with each administration of drops to ears.

▋*Nose Administration*

1. Cleanse around nose and remove any accumulated secretion from the nares with a warm, damp cloth; leave in place if crusted secretions are present until soft enough to be wiped away; draw up medication into the nose dropper.

2. Place client in a supine position and gently tilt head backward to rest on a small pillow or over side of the bed.
3. Place the correct number of drops into each side of the nose and retain head in tilted position for a minute; avoid allowing tip of dropper to touch nose.
4. Wipe excess from nose and allow client to resume normal position.

INHALATION MEDICATIONS

▌*Handheld Small-volume Nebulizer (SVN) Administration*

1. Prepare nebulizer by attaching tubing and plugging into electric outlet with machine OFF.
2. Assemble nebulizer chamber by attaching mouthpiece to the piece that is connected to the cap of the chamber containing prescribed medication dose (measured and poured or pre-measured unit dose and poured).
3. Place cap on chamber by turning clockwise and attach the tubing from the nebulizer (compressor) to the chamber.
4. Ensure that all connections are tight, turn machine to ON, and note mist coming from the mouthpiece.
5. Place the mouthpiece into the client's mouth with lips around it and inform client to breathe through mouth.
6. Allow client to breathe slowly and deeply; to turn machine OFF to rest if fatigued; and to continue when able, until all solution is gone.
7. Turn machine OFF, disassemble chamber and cleanse with mild detergent, rinse with warm water, and air dry on paper towel.

▌*Handheld Metered-dose Inhaler (MDI) Administration*

1. Insert metal canister tightly into the holder and shake well to mix medication with the propellant.
2. Remove cap; ask client to exhale fully, place the inhaler in an upright position, and hold mouthpiece up to mouth or in the mouth resting on lower teeth with lips around it.
3. Ask client to press on top of canister with finger and inhale slowly and deeply, then hold breath for 5 to 10 seconds or as long as possible.
4. Instruct client to release finger and remove from mouth, wait for 30 seconds, and repeat the procedure for a second dose.
5. Repeat the procedure if a second medication is to follow by inhalation.

6. Perform at frequency prescribed, remove canister, rinse holder daily, and allow to dry on paper towel.
7. Instruct client to rinse mouth following inhalation of corticosteroid medication.

ENTERAL TUBE MEDICATIONS

Indwelling tubes include nasogastric and gastrostomy types. They are placed in position for short- or long-term feedings when the oral route is not possible. Medications administered via these small-bore feeding tubes are in liquid form or are crushed tablet(s) mixed in a small amount of liquid (10 ml) and administered by the gravity method as follows:

1. Unclamp tube and check for placement in stomach and amount of residual, and discontinue or delay any feeding for 15 minutes before medication administration.
2. Place the prescribed dose in the barrel of a syringe, unclamp the tube end, and connect the barrel to the tubing.
3. Hold barrel 6 inches above insertion site and allow the liquid to flow into the tube by gravity; when the syringe barrel is almost empty, add 30 ml of water and allow to flow and clear the tubing to ensure that all the medication has reached the stomach.
4. Check patency of tubing for clogging if crushed or viscous medications are administered.

INTRAMUSCULAR AND SUBCUTANEOUS MEDICATIONS

Medication Preparation

1. Open proper-sized packaged syringe and needle; assemble if needed.
2. Cleanse top of vial with alcohol swab or remove top of ampule.
3. Remove cap from needle, draw in amount of air equal to amount of medication needed, place needle into top of vial, inject air into the vial, and withdraw the amount of medication needed; or place needle into the ampule and withdraw amount of medication needed.
4. Remove the needle from the vial or ampule, remove any air bubbles, and replace the cap loosely for easy removal when ready to administer the injection.

Medication Administration

1. Place client in sitting or lying position with proposed site exposed.

2. Don gloves and cleanse the site with an alcohol swab in a circular motion from center outward and allow to air dry.
3. Remove cap from needle, hold the skin firmly at the appropriate site, and insert the needle at a 90-degree angle (IM) or 45-degree angle with bevel of point facing upward (SC).
4. Pull the plunger to check for blood; remove and change needle if blood appears or inject contents of syringe if blood does not appear.
5. Quickly and smoothly withdraw syringe and gently swab area with a tissue; apply an adhesive strip.
6. Dispose of syringe and needle, without recapping or breaking needle, in a waterproof, puncture-proof, unbreakable container (covered coffee can or hard plastic container) for proper disposal of hazardous materials.

SYRINGE PUMP SUBCUTANEOUS MEDICATIONS

A syringe pump contains a battery-powered motor that pushes fluid through the syringe in measured amounts and intervals for infusion of medication. It is usually used for insulin administration when multiple injections are necessary to receive insulin therapy. Gloves and sterile technique are used to perform syringe pump procedures.

1. Fill syringe, with the infusion tubing attached, with the prescribed type and amount of insulin (usually a 24-hour supply of fast-acting insulin) and place in the pump correctly; close the cover while leaving the tubing clamped and exposed on the outside of the pump.
2. Attach needle to the tubing, unclamp, and prime; insert into the prepared abdominal site subcutaneously at a 30- to 60-degree angle, secure in place on the abdomen with a transparent dressing over the needle and tubing to prevent dislodgment, and allow for site assessment.
3. Set the program pump for continuous dose injections or manually for dose intervals with amounts (as before meals) that are balanced with activities and dietary regimens.
4. Place pump in carrying case and attach to belt or place in pocket.
5. Perform pump alarm checks, alternate the injection sites, change tubing and needle every 48 hours, and change batteries as needed.
6. Instruct client to perform blood glucose and urine testing and report altered levels that indicate need for modifi-

cation of insulin dosage or dietary regimen. (See Diabetes Mellitus).

MEDIFUSE SYRINGE PUMP INTRAVENOUS MEDICATIONS

A Medifuse syringe is a portable, disposable, nonelectric mechanical system for a continuous delivery of medications. It is an infusion device that contains a mechanism that applies the force needed to push the medication through a syringe that holds 10 to 35 ml. Small, predictable amounts of 0.25 ml or less in a set infusion time and rate can be delivered. The infusion device system contains the infusion holder, the syringe to hold the medication, the administration set-up (tubing), and a belt. It is used to deliver analgesic, antibiotic, or chemotherapeutic agents intravenously at a preset volume, time, and rate. Gloves and sterile technique are used to perform any Medifuse procedures.

1. Prepare the syringe containing the appropriate amount and dose of medication (can be prepared by a pharmacist), connect to the administration set, expel air, and cover end of tubing.
2. Position the syringe in the holder in the infuser device and set the time and rate ordered (set is color-coded for time).
3. Attach to access site and start infusion; flow will cease when correct amount of medication has been administered without allowing a backflow of blood.
4. Carry device in a case attached to a belt and hang over shoulder or place in a pocket.
5. Remove when completed, provide site care, and dispose of syringe.

HOMEPUMP INTRAVENOUS MEDICATIONS

A Homepump is a single-use, disposable, small (3 inches in height), lightweight (2 oz if empty) infusion pump available in various sizes to administer antibiotics and chemotherapy medications intravenously in home care. It is an infusion pump that controls the flow rate by the pressure of an elastometric membrane and microbore cannula. It is a one-piece closed system that can deliver 50 to 200 ml of antibiotics per hour in single doses and 2 to 5 ml of chemotherapeutic agents per hour. It consists of a pump device with a port cap, a container, tubing and a clamp, a filter, an adapter, a cap, and a carrying pouch. Gloves and sterile technique are used when performing Homepump procedures.

1. Select the proper-sized pump, close the clamp, and place the proper dose of medication at room temperature through the top port with a syringe into the multilayer membrane.
2. Remove the cap of the pump set-up at the distal end to release air from the line, then reclamp and attach the Luer-Lok adapter to the IV access site.
3. Unclamp pump set-up and begin the infusion.
4. Place in a carrying bag or pocket to permit mobility.
5. At conclusion of medication administration, disconnect the pump and set-up and dispose of the entire device because it cannot be reused.
6. Provide site care and apply dressing.

VERIFUSE INFUSION PUMP FOR INTRAVENOUS MEDICATIONS OR FLUIDS

A Verifuse infusion pump is capable of multiple therapy delivery of medications by continuous, intermittent, or continuous with bolus methods and has tapering capabilities for delivery of total parenteral nutrition (TPN). It is a single-channel peristaltic pump that can be powered by battery or AC electric power. It includes the small, lightweight pump device, remote bolus control, programing software, administration set-up with filter and multiple injection ports, a universal spike, a TPN kit, a battery pack, an AC power adapter, and a carrying case.

1. Have the client's protocol or prescription parameters entered into the computer to convert the data into a bar code by the software.
2. Print bar is printed onto a label for the medication container or entered by the nurse (bar code simplifies programing of an infusion and prevents client tampering, improper programing, and prolonged instruction).
3. Spike administration set tubing into the solution container, clamp and thread through the pump, unclamp and prime the tubing, reclamp, and attach to the IV access.
4. Scan bar code, press VERIFY, and check for the correct protocol on the pump's display screen.
5. Unclamp tubing, press START, and initiate infusion to deliver as little as 0.1 ml/hr or a total of 0.1 ml with a maximal rate of 300 ml/hr, with the capability to deliver a total of 6000 ml.
6. Place carrying case in pocket or in reach during infusion.

7. Press STOP to discontinue intermittent or bolus infusion, disconnect from IV site, remove set-up for proper disposal.
8. Attach Homebase to the side of the pump for remote programming of the pump or to check infusion status by telephone via a built-in modem to a computer for viewing by the pharmacist (allows for Homebase to receive a new protocol and send pump status for evaluation and client compliance, which can reduce home visits to monitor IV therapy).

PATIENT-CONTROLLED ANALGESIA

Patient-controlled analgesia is a method of self-administering drugs that uses a programmable infusion pump for IV and SC routes to allow for intermittent doses at preset time intervals. The analgesic can be administered by initial bolus and then continuous infusion. Time between doses is known as the *lockout interval* and should be the length of time needed for the onset of drug action. Infusion of medication is initiated by pushing a button when pain is experienced.

EPIDURAL OR INTRATHECAL MEDICATIONS

Medication administration via epidural or intrathecal routes is usually reserved for terminal care. A catheter is inserted into the epidural or intrathecal space for intermittent or continuous infusion of analgesic to provide consistent drug levels and a long-lasting effect by the direct action on receptors in the spinal cord.

INFUSION PUMPS FOR INTRAVENOUS MEDICATIONS OR FLUIDS

A variety of ambulatory, small, portable microcomputer-controlled peristaltic infusion pumps are available to deliver prescribed amounts of medications, fluids, or TPN via central venous lines (e.g., right atrial catheter, port catheter). The infusion pump controller is used when a sustained slow flow rate is desired. Another available infusion pump delivers fluids at a high flow rate. Both of these stationary types of pumps have safety alarms that go off when air gets in the line, the line becomes occluded, or the infusion has been completed. In general, ambulatory and stationary pumps are selected according to the type of infusion fluid, amount and rate of infusion, and route of administration.

They are selected for use depending on their capability of delivering continuous (with or without bolus) and intermittent infusion of analgesic, antibiotic, and chemotherapeutic agents; TPN; and hydration fluids. Depending on the model, they can deliver 1 to 400 ml/hr for 1 minute to 100 hours and deliver two independent programs with one device for bolus, intermittent, or continuous infusion. The ambulatory devices operate via internal or external battery power. The device and solution container(s) can be placed in a carrying case and hung over the shoulder or kept in the open for viewing.

HEPARIN-LOCK INTRAVENOUS MEDICATIONS

A catheter is inserted into a vein and maintained over time to eliminate the need for multiple peripheral venipunctures to administer IV medication in the home. The primary care involves maintaining and monitoring tube for patency and insertion site for infection and ensuring safe medication administration. Gloves and sterile technique are used when performing heparin-lock procedures.

▌*Site Assessment and Protection*

1. Note redness, edema, pain, and drainage at the site daily.
2. Change sterile dressing over the heparin lock, tape in place with capped end exposed, cleanse around the insertion site with antiseptic, cover the tube and area with plastic when bathing to protect from wetness.
3. Change catheter periodically according to policy or if problem develops.

▌*Patency and Use of Heparin Lock*

1. Prepare heparin and medication in separate syringes as outlined in IM and SC injections.
2. Flush catheter with a specified amount of heparin solution at prescribed frequency and after all medication administration.
3. Cleanse heparin-lock hub or cap with antiseptic, insert needle of syringe with the medication into the hub or cap center, and inject the contents slowly over 3 to 4 minutes or as indicated.
4. Remove the needle from the heparin lock and inject the prepared heparin into the hub or cap to ensure patency of the device, withdraw the needle and cover the catheter end for protection from trauma and dislodgment.

CENTRAL VENOUS CATHETER INTRAVENOUS MEDICATIONS

An indwelling catheter is inserted through an SC tunnel into a central vein near the heart and is maintained for long-term continuous or frequent-intermittent IV administration of fluids, nutrients, and medications. Tissue growth to the cuff around the portion in the SC tissue provides anchoring of the catheter in place. Catheters commonly used include the Hickman, Broviac, and Groshong.

▌*Site Assessment and Protection*

1. Note redness, edema, pain, and drainage at the site through a transparent dressing daily or during dressing changes; assess for temperature elevation.
2. Cover the site with plastic when bathing to protect from wetness.
3. Cover site with a shirt or clothing; avoid handling the tube end.
4. Report any signs of infection, damage, or occlusion to the catheter and clamp if a Hickman or Broviac is in place.

▌*Patency and Care of Central Catheter*

1. Prepare syringe with a specified amount of heparin solution (Broviac) or 5 ml saline (Groshong) as outlined in IM and SC injections to flush catheter (prescribed frequency is daily and after all medication administrations for Broviac, weekly and after all medication administrations for Groshong).
2. Use gloves and sterile technique for care of a central line.
3. Cleanse injection cap of catheter with antiseptic, insert needle of syringe with the flushing solution into the cap center, and inject the contents slowly.
4. Remove the needle from the cap (Groshong) and while the injection of the last 0.2 ml of the prepared heparin is injected (Broviac) to ensure patency of the device.
5. To replace an injection cap (frequency determined by policy), clamp the tube in the area between the end of the tube and the skin (Broviac), on the area prepared for clamping found on some catheters, or not at all on the Groshong; cleanse around the tip below the cap with an antiseptic swab, remove the old cap, attach the new cap, and remove the clamp if used.

6. To change a transparent dressing (frequency determined by policy or if soiled or insecure), gently peel off dressing, assess skin and site, cleanse around insertion site with a circular motion from center outward using hydrogen peroxide swabs and then again using antiseptic, and allow to air dry; loop the tube at the insertion site with the cap below the area to be covered by the dressing, place the window frame type of dressing on the skin, gently pressing from top to bottom while eliminating any air bubbles, and secure cap area in place with tape for easy access but covered with clothing.

7. To change a gauze dressing, follow the same procedure as for a transparent dressing through cleansing of the site, applying antiseptic ointment around the insertion site, positioning gauze dressing over the site, looping catheter over the gauze and covering with another gauze dressing, securing the edges with tape, and leaving the cap area exposed for easy access but covered with clothing.

▮ *Medication Preparation and Administration*

1. Prepare medication in syringe as outlined in IM and SC injections.

2. Cleanse cap with antiseptic, insert needle of syringe with the medication into the cap center, and inject the contents slowly over 3 to 4 minutes or as indicated.

3. Remove the needle of the empty syringe from the cap and insert the needle of the prepared heparin or saline into cap and inject to ensure patency of the catheter, withdraw the needle, and cover the catheter end with clothing for protection from trauma and dislodgment.

✳ *NANDA-approved Nursing Diagnoses 2001-2002*

Activity intolerance
Activity intolerance, risk for
Adjustment, impaired

Airway clearance, ineffective
Allergy response, latex
Allergy response, risk for latex
Anxiety
Anxiety, death
Aspiration, risk for
Attachment, risk for impaired parent/infant/child
Autonomic dysreflexia
Autonomic dysreflexia, risk for
Body image, disturbed
Body temperature, risk for imbalanced
Bowel incontinence
Breastfeeding, effective
Breastfeeding, ineffective
Breastfeeding, interrupted
Breathing pattern, ineffective
Cardiac output, decreased
Caregiver role strain
Caregiver role strain, risk for
Communication, impaired verbal
Conflict, decisional
Conflict, parental role
Confusion, acute
Confusion, chronic
Constipation
Constipation, perceived
Constipation, risk for
Coping, compromised family
Coping, defensive
Coping, disabled family
Coping, ineffective
Coping, ineffective community
Coping, readiness for enhanced community
Coping, readiness for enhanced family
Denial, ineffective
Dentition, impaired
Development, risk for delayed
Diarrhea
Disuse syndrome, risk for
Diversional activity, deficient
Energy field, disturbed
Environmental interpretation syndrome, impaired

Failure to thrive, adult
Falls, risk for
Family processes, dysfunctional: alcoholism
Family processes, interrupted
Fatigue
Fear
Fluid volume, deficient
Fluid volume, excess
Fluid volume, risk for deficient
Fluid volume, risk for imbalanced
Gas exchange, impaired
Grieving, anticipatory
Grieving, dysfunctional
Growth and development, delayed
Growth, risk for disproportionate
Health maintenance, ineffective
Health-seeking behaviors
Home maintenance, impaired
Hopelessness
Hyperthermia
Hypothermia
Identity, disturbed personal
Incontinence, functional urinary
Incontinence, reflex urinary
Incontinence, stress urinary
Incontinence, total urinary
Incontinence, urge urinary
Incontinence, risk for urge urinary
Infant behavior, disorganized
Infant behavior, risk for disorganized
Infant behavior, readiness for enhanced organized
Infant feeding pattern, ineffective
Infection, risk for
Injury, risk for
Injury, risk for perioperative-positioning
Intracranial adaptive capacity, decreased
Knowledge, deficient
Loneliness, risk for
Memory, impaired
Mobility, impaired bed

Mobility, impaired physical
Mobility, impaired wheelchair
Nausea
Neglect, unilateral
Noncompliance
Nutrition, imbalanced: less than body requirements
Nutrition, imbalanced: more than body requirements
Nutrition, risk for imbalanced: more than body requirements
Oral mucous membrane, impaired
Pain, acute
Pain, chronic
Parenting, impaired
Parenting, risk for impaired
Peripheral neurovascular dysfunction, risk for
Poisoning, risk for
Posttrauma syndrome
Posttrauma syndrome, risk for
Powerlessness
Powerlessness, risk for
Protection, ineffective
Rape-trauma syndrome
Rape-trauma syndrome: compound reaction
Rape-trauma syndrome: silent reaction
Relocation stress syndrome
Relocation stress syndrome, risk for
Role performance, ineffective
Self-care deficit, bathing/hygiene
Self-care deficit, dressing/grooming
Self-care deficit, feeding
Self-care deficit, toileting
Self-esteem, chronic low
Self-esteem, situational low
Self-esteem, risk for situational low
Self-mutilation
Self-mutilation, risk for
Sensory perception, disturbed
Sexual dysfunction
Sexuality patterns, ineffective
Skin integrity, impaired
Skin integrity, risk for impaired

Sleep deprivation
Sleep pattern, disturbed
Social interaction, impaired
Social isolation
Sorrow, chronic
Spiritual distress
Spiritual distress, risk for
Spiritual well-being, readiness for enhanced
Suffocation, risk for
Suicide, risk for
Surgical recovery, delayed
Swallowing, impaired
Therapeutic regimen management, effective
Therapeutic regimen management, ineffective
Therapeutic regimen management, ineffective community
Therapeutic regimen management, ineffective family
Thermoregulation, ineffective
Thought processes, disturbed
Tissue integrity, impaired
Tissue perfusion, ineffective
Transfer ability, impaired
Trauma, risk for
Urinary elimination, impaired
Urinary retention
Ventilation, impaired spontaneous
Ventilatory weaning response, dysfunctional
Violence, risk for other-directed
Violence, risk for self-directed
Walking, impaired
Wandering

Modified from North American Nursing Diagnosis Association: *Nursing diagnoses: definitions and classifications 2001-2002*, Philadelphia, 2001, NANDA.

✳ Resources for Home Care and Selected National Agencies

Administration on Aging
U.S. Department of Health and Human Services
330 Independence Avenue, SW
Washington, DC 20201
www.aoa.gov

Alcoholics Anonymous
475 Riverside Drive
11th Floor
New York, NY 10115
www.alcoholics-anonymous.org

Alzheimer's Association
919 North Michigan Avenue
Suite 1100
Chicago, IL 60611-1676
www.alz.org

American Cancer Society
1599 Clifton Road, NE
Atlanta, GA 30329
www.cancer.org

American Chronic Pain Association
PO Box 850
Rocklin, CA 95677-0850
www.theacpa.org

American Council of the Blind
1155 15th Street, NW, Suite 1004
Washington, DC 20005
www.acb.org

American Diabetes Association
1701 North Beauregard Street
Alexandria, VA 22311
www.diabetes.org

American Geriatrics Society
The Empire State Building
350 Fifth Avenue, Suite 801
New York, NY 10118
www.americangeriatrics.org

American Heart Association
7272 Greenville Avenue
Dallas, TX 75231-4596
www.cpr-ecc.org

American Lung Association
1740 Broadway
New York, NY 10019
www.lungusa.org

American Parkinson Disease Association, Inc.
1250 Hylan Boulevard, Suite 4B
Staten Island, NY 10305-1946
www.apdaparkinson.com

Arthritis Foundation
1330 West Peachtree Street
Atlanta, GA 30309
www.arthritis.org

Centers for Disease Control and Prevention
1600 Clifton Road
Atlanta, GA 30333
www.cdc.gov

Centers for Medicare & Medicaid Services (CMS; formerly
HCFA)
7500 Security Boulevard
Baltimore, MD 21244-1850
www.hcfa.gov
http://cms.hhs.gov

Infusion Nurses Society
220 Norwood Park South
Norwood, MA 02062
www.ins1.org

Joint Commission on Accreditation of Healthcare Organizations
One Renaissance Boulevard
Oakbrook Terrace, IL 60181
www.jcaho.org

MedicAlert Foundation
2323 Colorado Avenue
Turlock, CA 95382
www.medicalert.org

Medic ID's International
PO Box 571687
Tarzana, CA 91357
www.medicid.com

National Association of the Deaf
814 Thayer Avenue
Silver Spring, MD 20910-4500
www.nad.org

National Association for Home Care
228 Seventh Street, SE
Washington, DC 20003
www.nahc.org

National Hospice and Palliative Care Organization
1700 Diagonal Road, Suite 625
Alexandria, VA 22314
www.nhpco.org

National Kidney Foundation
30 East 33rd Street, Suite 1100
New York, NY 10016
www.kidney.org

National Mental Health Association
1021 Prince Street
Alexandria, VA 22314-2971
www.nmha.org

National Multiple Sclerosis Society
733 Third Avenue
New York, NY 10017
www.nmss.org

Occupational Safety & Health Administration
U.S. Department of Labor
200 Constitution Avenue, NW
Washington, DC 20210
www.osha.gov

United Ostomy Association, Inc.
19772 MacArthur Boulevard, Suite 200
Irvine, CA 92612-2405
www.uoa.org

U.S. Department of Health & Human Services
200 Independence Avenue, SW
Washington, DC 20201
www.dhhs.gov

Wound, Ostomy and Continence Nurses Society (WOCN)
National Office
4700 W. Lake Avenue
Glenview, IL 60025
www.wocn.org

�֍ *Self-Determination Guidelines (Advance Directives)**

The Patient Self-Determination Act requires Medicare- and Medicaid-certified hospitals, long-term care facilities, hospice care, home care agencies, HMOs, and other health care providers and organizations to give clients information about their rights to make their own health care decisions, including the right to accept or refuse medical treatment. It also includes the provision for providers to educate their staffs on issues related to advance directives. The advance directive is a written statement completed in advance of a serious illness about how one wants medical decisions to be made. The act was incorporated into the Omnibus

---

*Modified from Health Care Financing Administration, U.S. Department of Health and Human Services: *Advanced directives*, HCFA Publication No. 02175, Washington, DC, 1995, DHHS.

Budget Reconciliation Act of 1990 (OBRA 1990) and took effect on December 1, 1991. This does not preclude the need for advance directives for those receiving care from any agency or institution not certified by Medicare and Medicaid.

PROVISIONS OF THE LAW

1. Provide all adult individuals with written information about their rights under state law to make health decisions, including the right to execute advance directives. State laws are developed, and federal law does not override any law that would allow a health provider to object, based on conscience, to implementing an advance directive.
2. Inform clients and residents about the facility or agency policy on implementing advance directives. At the time of admission, written information must be provided to an inpatient entering a hospital, a resident of a nursing facility, an outpatient of a home health provider, an enrollee of a prepaid health plan, and a recipient of hospice care.
3. Document in the medical record whether an advance directive has been executed.
4. Do not discriminate against an individual based on the existence of an advance directive.
5. Provide staff and community education on advance directives.

DEFINITION OF ADVANCE DIRECTIVE

An *advance directive* is a written statement completed in advance of a serious illness, or in the presence of a chronic illness, about how an individual wants medical decisions to be made. It allows clients to state choices for health care or to name someone to make those choices if unable to make decisions about medical treatment now or in the future. It allows the individual to control medical treatment decisions and to say "yes" to treatment that is wanted or "no" to treatment that is not wanted. Advance directives are not required and may be canceled at any time.

TYPES OF ADVANCE DIRECTIVES

1. *Living Will.* A written form approved by a state that specifies the kind of medical care wanted or not wanted if the client becomes unable to make the decisions. A living will can be initiated by using a form developed by the state, completing and signing a preprinted form available in the community, developing

one's own form, or writing a statement of treatment preference. Advice can be solicited from an attorney or physician to ensure that one's wishes are understood and followed.

2. *Durable Power of Attorney for Health Care.* A signed, dated, and witnessed paper naming another person, such as a spouse, an adult child, or a close friend, as the client's agent or proxy to make medical decisions if the client should become unable to make them. It may include instructions about any treatment the client wishes to avoid. Some states have specific laws allowing for health care power of attorney and provide printed forms.

APPLICATION TO HEALTH CARE IN THE HOME

The most important directive applicable to the client who has a serious chronic illness and who is at home is probably the decision to call 911 emergency services in cases of heart or respiratory arrest and if cardiopulmonary resuscitation (CPR) should be administered. Unless a directive is available to the respondents, CPR would be administered regardless of the consequences of such an action. The client would be well advised to clearly indicate his or her directive in this regard.

Other home care should be provided totally or in part according to the client's directive if possible, or care can be provided by a hospice or a long-term care facility.

GENERAL REMARKS

Some state laws make it better to have one or the other type of directive, and it may be possible to have both or to combine the two types (in a document that describes treatment choices in specific situations and names someone to make decisions for the client when necessary). Either of these can be changed or canceled at any time. Some states allow a change by oral statement.

An advance directive should be signed and dated, and copies should be given to the physician and other health care providers as needed. A copy should be given to the client's attorney if a durable power of attorney exists, to the physician to become a part of the permanent record, and to an agent or proxy, and a copy should be put in a safe place with easy access if needed. A card 'that states the existence of an advance directive, where it is located, and the name of the agent or proxy should be placed in the client's purse or wallet if appropriate.

❋ *Standard (Universal) Precautions and Guidelines for Control of Body Substances*

Standard (universal) precautions is a method to prevent or minimize exposure to blood and potentially infectious materials. Blood of infected individuals can contain pathogenic microorganisms (e.g., human immunodeficiency virus, hepatitis B or C virus) called *blood-borne pathogens* that can be transmitted to others by the blood and other body fluids. All body fluids are to be considered potentially infectious. The standards require that every health worker or caregiver must take protective measures when in contact with any client, whether known or suspected to be infected. The standards also require that health care facilities provide supplies and equipment and offer hepatitis B vaccine to employees, free of charge. The goal is to practice controls that decrease the possibility of exposure by changing the way a task or procedure is performed. These include hand protection, personal protective clothing, handling of equipment and supplies, and other techniques to prevent transmission to a home health nurse or caregiver. The selection of protective safeguards to use or teach to the caregiver depends on specific situations. The following guidelines are outlined for home implementation.

HAND PROTECTION

- Wash hands with soap and water, rinse, and dry before and after client contact for care or treatments; wash hands even if gloves are worn; and wash bare hands immediately following exposure to blood or body secretions or excretions (count to 10 for thorough wash).
- Wear gloves if possibility of touching blood, body fluids, secretions, or excretions on any item or article or specimen exposed to these fluids exists.
- Change gloves if soiled or torn before client contact.

- Wear gloves if rash, cuts, or open areas are present on hands, or avoid any contact with body fluids or contaminants.
- Wear gloves if collecting blood, urine, feces, or other specimens for dipstick or laboratory examination.
- Wear gloves to administer parenteral medications or fluids; take precautions to prevent accidental needlesticks to hands.

PROTECTIVE WEAR

- Wear disposable plastic apron or gown during direct or close contact if soiling of clothing is likely or if spattering of body fluids is possible.
- Anticipate splashing of blood or body fluids and protect face with shield or goggles.

EQUIPMENT AND SUPPLIES

- Gloves should not be washed, disinfected, and reused. Discard used gloves, dressings, cleansing articles, and other disposable supplies in a waterproof, leak-proof bag for proper disposal.
- Use safety protection needles whenever possible. Dispose of used lancets; syringes with needle attached and not recapped; and cut, bent, and other sharp articles in a hard container (coffee can with lid) and label for future disposal of hazardous material.
- Dispose of catheters and bags, IV tubing and bags, and medication vials in labeled biohazard container for disposal.
- Dispose of suction canister fluid by tightly closing and discarding, without emptying contents, in a biohazard container.
- Wash soiled linens, clothing, bathing articles, dishes, and eating utensils in hot water and detergent, rinse, and dry well for reuse.
- Label specimen of blood or body fluids for special precautions, place in a container that prevents leakage and breakage in transport, and label again before transport to laboratory.

DISINFECTION

- Wash article in warm, soapy water and rinse inside and outside with hot running water to prepare for further disinfection.
- Moist heat: boil in water in a covered container for 10 minutes after water has boiled for 1 hour.
- Dry heat: place cloth-wrapped article on a flat pan and bake in an oven at 350 degrees for 1 hour.
- Prepare commercial solution according to instructions and submerge article for 10 minutes, rinse well, and air dry on paper towel.

· Spilled liquids: Cleanse liquids such as vomitus, blood, or others containing blood by putting on gloves; wiping with paper towels; preparing and pouring a solution of bleach and water (1:10) onto the area; wiping clean with paper towels; and finally, placing used towels in a waterproof, leak-proof bag with gloves and other used articles for disposal.

BAG TECHNIQUE

· Barriers: Use barrier before placing nursing bag and equipment on furniture in the home. Barriers are never reused.
· Handwashing: Hands must be washed before removing supplies from clean section of the bag.
· Supplies/equipment: Clean supplies are kept separate from soiled equipment. Equipment is cleansed with disinfectant after each client use.

BIBLIOGRAPHY

Alzheimer's Association: *Steps to ensuring safety: preventing wandering and getting lost*, Chicago, 1999, Alzheimer's Disease & Related Disorders Association, Inc.

American Diabetes Association: Standards of medical care for patients with diabetes mellitus, *Diabetes Care*, 24:S33, 2001.

American Heart Association Scientific Publishing: *Basic life support for healthcare providers*, Dallas, 2001, American Heart Association.

Apter J: 8 tips to avoid top HHA ICD-9 coding mistakes, *Home Health Line* 26(33), 2001. Available at: http://www.homehealthline.com

Bickley LS, Hoekelmen RA: *Bates' guide to physical examination and history taking*, ed 7, Philadelphia, 1999, Lippincott.

Church V: Staying on guard for DVT & PE, *Nursing2000* 30(2):34, 2000.

Eliopoulos C: *Gerontological nursing*, ed 5, Philadelphia, 2001, Lippincott Williams & Wilkins.

Garvey C: Pulmonary rehabilitation for the elderly client, *Medscape Nursing*, 1(2), 2001. Available at: http://www.medscape.com

Glajehen M: Chronic pain: treatment barriers and strategies for clinical practice, *J Am Board Fam Practice*, 14:178, 2001.

Health Care Financing Administration: *Advanced directives*, Washington, DC, 1996, U.S. Department of Health and Human Services. Available at: http://www.hcfa.gov/pubforms/advdir.htm.

Health Care Financing Administration: *OASIS implementation manual: general OASIS instructions*, Washington, DC, 1998, Department of Health and Human Services.

Makleburst J: Wound care: preventing pressure ulcers in home care patients, *Home Healthcare Nurse*, 17:229, 1999.

Makleburst J: Wound care: treating pressure ulcers in the home, *Home Healthcare Nurse*, 17:307, 1999.

Marrelli TM: *Handbook of home health standards and documentation guidelines for reimbursement*, ed 4, St Louis, 2001, Mosby.

Monahan FD, Neighbors M: *Medical-surgical nursing foundations for clinical practice*, ed 2, Philadelphia, 1998, WB Saunders.

Monks KM: *Pocket guide to home health care*, Philadelphia, 2000, WB Saunders.

Neabel B: Family assessment tools: a review of literature from 1978-1997, *Heart and Lung* 29(3), 2000.

North American Nursing Diagnosis Association: *Nursing diagnoses: definitions and classifications 2001-2002*, Philadelphia, 2001, NANDA.

Occupational Safety and Health Administration: *Regulations: bloodborne pathogens*, Washington, DC, 2001, OSHA.

Pagana KD: *Mosby's diagnostic and laboratory test reference*, ed 5, St Louis, 2001, Mosby.

Skidmore-Roth L: *Mosby's 2001 nursing drug reference*, St Louis, 2001, Mosby.

Sparks M: Assessment and management of Alzheimer's disease, *Medscape Nursing* 1(2), 2001. Available at: http://www.medscape.com

St Anthony, Medicode: *2002 Expert ICD-9-CM for home health services, nursing facilities, and hospices*, Salt Lake City, 2001, Ingenix.

INDEX

Printed and bound by CPI Group (UK) Ltd, Croydon, CR0 4YY

08/06/2025

01896874-0001